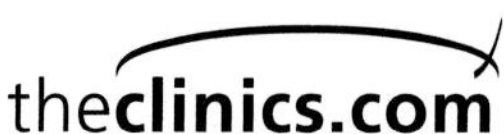

BURTON P. DRAYER, MD, Consulting Editor

# NEUROIMAGING CLINICS of North America

## Ophthalmologic Neuroimaging

MAHMOOD F. MAFEE, MD
Guest Editor

February 2005 • Volume 15 • Number 1

SAUNDERS

An Imprint of Elsevier, Inc.
PHILADELPHIA LONDON TORONTO MONTREAL SYDNEY TOKYO

**W.B. SAUNDERS COMPANY**
*A Division of Elsevier Inc.*

1600 John F. Kennedy Boulevard • Suite 1800 • Philadelphia, Pennsylvania 19103-2899

http://www.theclinics.com

**NEUROIMAGING CLINICS OF NORTH AMERICA** **Volume 15, Number 1**
**February 2005** **ISSN 1052-5149**
Editor: Barton Dudlick **ISBN 1-4160-2732-7**



*Neuroimaging Clinics of North America* (ISSN 1052-5149) is published quarterly by Elsevier Inc. Corporate and editorial offices: 1600 John F. Kennedy Boulevard, Suite 1800, Pennsylvania, PA 19103-2899. Accounting and circulation offices: 6277 Sea Harbor Drive, Orlando, FL 32887-4800. Periodicals postage paid at Orlando, FL 32862, and additional mailing offices. Subscription prices are USD 190 per year for US individuals, USD 290 per year for US institutions, USD 95 per year for US students and residents, USD 214 per year for Canadian individuals, USD 352 per year for Canadian institutions, USD 255 per year for international individuals, USD 352 per year for international institutions and USD 128 per year for Canadian and foreign students/residents. To receive student/resident rate, orders must be accompanied by name of affiliated institution, date of term and the *signature* of program/residency coordinator on institution letterhead. Orders will be billed at individual rate until proof of status is received. Foreign air speed delivery is included in all *Clinics* subscription prices. All prices are subject to change without notice. POSTMASTER: Send address changes to *Neuroimaging Clinics of North America*, W.B. Saunders Company, Periodicals Fulfillment, Orlando, FL 32887-4800. **Customer Service: 800-654-2452 (US). From outside of the US, call (+1) 407-345-4000. E-mail: hhspcs@harcourt.com.**

*Reprints.* For copies of 100 or more, of articles in this publication, please contact the Commercial Reprints Department, Elsevier Inc., 360 Park Avenue South, New York, New York 10010-1710. Tel.: (+1) 212-633-3813; Fax: (+1) 212-462-1935; E-mail: reprints@elsevier.com.

*Neuroimaging Clinics of North America* is covered by *Excerpta Medica/EMBASE,* the RSNA Index of Imaging Literature, Index Medicus, MEDLINE/MEDLARS, SciSearch, Research Alert, and Neuroscience Citation Index.

Printed in the United States of America.

## GOAL STATEMENT

The goal of *Neuroimaging Clinics of North America* is to keep practicing radiologists and radiology residents up to date with current clinical practice in radiology by providing timely articles reviewing the state of the art in patient care.

## ACCREDITATION

The *Neuroimaging Clinics of North America* is planned and implemented in accordance with the Essential Areas and Policies of the Accreditation Council for Continuing Medical Education (ACCME) through the joint sponsorship of the University of Virginia School of Medicine and Elsevier. The University of Virginia School of Medicine is accredited by the ACCME to provide continuing medical education for physicians.

The University of Virginia School of Medicine designates this educational activity for a maximum of 60 category 1 credits per year, 15 category 1 credits per issue, toward the AMA Physician's Recognition Award. Each physician should claim only those credits that he/she actually spent in the activity.

The American Medical Association has determined that physicians not licensed in the US who participate in this CME activity are eligible for AMA PRA category 1 credit.

Category 1 credit can be earned by reading the text material, taking the CME examination online at ***http://www.theclinics.com/home/cme***, and completing the evaluation. Each test question must be answered correctly; you will have the opportunity to retake any questions answered incorrectly. Following successful completion of the test and the evaluation, you may print your certificate.

## FACULTY DISCLOSURE

As a provider accredited by the Accreditation Council for Continuing Medical Education (ACCME), the Office of Continuing Medical Education of the University of Virginia School of Medicine must ensure balance, independence, objectivity, and scientific rigor in all its individually sponsored or jointly sponsored educational activities. All authors/editors participating in a sponsored activity are expected to disclose to the readers any significant financial interest or other relationship (1) with the manufacturer(s) of any commercial product(s) and/or provider(s) of commercial services discussed in an educational presentation and (2) with any commercial supporters of the activity (significant financial interest or other relationship can include such things as grants or research support, employee, consultant, stock holder, member of speakers bureau, etc.) The intent of this disclosure is not to prevent authors/editors with a significant financial or other relationship from writing an article, but rather to provide readers with information on which they can make their own judgments. It remains for the readers to determine whether the author's/editor's interest or relationships may influence the article with regard to exposition or conclusion.

***The authors/editors listed below have identified no professional or financial affiliations related to their publication:***
Sameer A. Ansari, MD, PhD; Marsha A. Apushkin, MD; Michael A. Apushkin, MD; Larissa T. Bilaniuk, MD, FACR; Mark F. Conneely, MD; Barton Dudlick, Acquisitions Editor; Deepak P. Edward, MD; Geetanjali Kapoor, MD; Rashmi Kapur, MD; Lawrence Kaufman, MD, PhD; Reema Lamba, BSE; Vito LaRocca, MD, MPH; Mahmood F. Mafee, MD, FACR; John Pak, MD, PhD; Mark Pisaneschi, MD; Mark Rapoport, BS; Nelson R. Sabates, MD; Jay Shah, BS; Michael J. Shaprio, MD; Marc Shields, MD; and, Thasarat S. Vajaranant, MD.

***Disclosure of discussion of non-FDA approved uses for pharmaceutical products and/or medical devices.***
The University of Virginia School of Medicine, as an ACCME provider, requires that all authors/editors identify and disclose any "off label" uses for pharmaceutical products and/or for medical devices. The University of Virginia School of Medicine recommends that each reader fully review all the available data on new products or procedures prior to instituting them with patients.

***The authors who provided disclosures will not be discussing off-label uses.***

***The authors listed below have not provided disclosure or off-label information:***
Paul Caruso, MD; Gleb Gorelick, MD; Afshin Karimi, MD, PhD, JD; and, Alfred L. Weber, MD.

## TO ENROLL

To enroll in the Neuroimaging Clinics of North America Continuing Medical Education program, call customer service at 1-800-654-2452 or sign up online at ***http://www.theclinics.com/home/cme***. The CME program is available to subscribers for an additional annual fee of USD 156.

## FORTHCOMING ISSUES

May 2005

**Stroke I**
Michael Lev, MD, *Guest Editor*

August 2005

**Stroke II**
Michael Lev, MD, *Guest Editor*

## RECENT ISSUES

November 2004

**Head and Neck MR Imaging**
Suresh K. Mukherji, MD, *Guest Editor*

August 2004

**Epilepsy**
John S. Duncan, MA, DM, FRCP, *Guest Editor*

May 2004

**Genetics and Neuroimaging**
Tina Young Poussaint, MD, *Guest Editor*

# CONSULTING EDITOR

**BURTON P. DRAYER, MD,** Dr. Charles M. and Marilyn Professor and Chairman, Department of Radiology, Mount Sinai Medical Center, New York, New York

# GUEST EDITOR

**MAHMOOD F. MAFEE, MD, FACR,** Medical Director, MRI Center; Professor, Department of Radiology, University of Illinois at Chicago Medical Center; and Chief, Section of Head and Neck Radiology, Department of Radiology, University of Illinois at Chicago, Chicago, Illinois

# CONTRIBUTORS

**SAMEER A. ANSARI, MD, PhD,** Resident, Department of Radiology, University of Illinois Hospital at Chicago, University of Illinois College of Medicine, Chicago, Illinois

**MARSHA A. APUSHKIN, MD,** Fellow, Hereditary Retinal Diseases, Department of Ophthalmology and Visual Science, University of Illinois at Chicago, Chicago, Illinois

**MICHAEL A. APUSHKIN, MD,** Fellow, Cross-Sectional Imaging, Department of Radiology, University of Illinois at Chicago, Chicago, Illinois

**LARISSA T. BILANIUK, MD, FACR,** Professor, Radiology, University of Pennsylvania School of Medicine; and Staff Neuroradiologist, Department of Radiology, Children's Hospital of Philadelphia, Philadelphia, Pennsylvania

**PAUL CARUSO, MD,** Assistant Radiologist, Radiology, Massachusetts Eye and Ear Infirmary; and Instructor, Radiology, Harvard Medical School, Boston, Massachusetts

**MARK F. CONNEELY, MD,** MR Imaging Fellow, Department of Radiology, University of Illinois at Chicago Medical Center, Chicago, Illinois

**DEEPAK P. EDWARD, MD,** Director, Glaucoma Service and Ophthalmic Pathology Service; and Associate Professor, Department of Ophthalmology and Visual Sciences, University of Illinois at Chicago, Chicago, Illinois

**GLEB GORELICK, MD,** Resident, Department of Radiology, University of Illinois at Chicago, Chicago, Illinois

**GEETANJALI KAPOOR, MD,** Diagnostic Radiology Resident, Department of Radiology, John H. Stroger, Jr. Hospital of Cook County, Chicago, Illinois

**RASHMI KAPUR, MD,** Pre-Residency Fellow, Department of Ophthalmology and Visual Sciences, University of Illinois at Chicago, Chicago, Illinois

**AFSHIN KARIMI, MD, PhD, JD,** Resident, Department of Radiology, University of Illinois Hospital at Chicago, University of Illinois College of Medicine, Chicago, Illinois

**LAWRENCE M. KAUFMAN, MD, PhD,** Clinical Associate Professor, Department of Ophthalmology and Visual Sciences, University of Illinois at Chicago, Chicago, Illinois

**REEMA LAMBA, BSE,** Medical Student, Department of Radiology, University of Illinois at Chicago, Chicago, Illinois

**VITO LaROCCA, MD, MPH,** Fellow, Department of Ophthalmology and Visual Sciences, University of Illinois at Chicago, Chicago, Illinois

**MAHMOOD F. MAFEE, MD, FACR,** Medical Director, MRI Center; Professor, Department of Radiology, University of Illinois at Chicago Medical Center; and Chief, Section of Head and Neck Radiology, Department of Radiology, University of Illinois at Chicago, Chicago, Illinois

**JOHN PAK, MD, PhD,** Fellow, Division of Oculoplastic and Reconstructive Surgery, Department of Ophthalmology, University of Illinois Eye and Ear Infirmary, Chicago, Illinois

**MARK PISANESCHI, MD,** Division Chairman, Outpatient Imaging, Department of Radiology, John H. Stroger, Jr. Hospital of Cook County; and Assistant Professor, Department of Clinical Radiology, University of Illinois Hospital, Chicago, Illinois

**MARK RAPOPORT, BS,** Medical Student, Department of Radiology, University of Illinois Hospital at Chicago, University of Illinois College of Medicine, Chicago, Illinois

**NELSON R. SABATES, MD,** Associate Professor and Vice-Chairman, Department of Ophthalmology, University of Missouri at Kansas City School of Medicine; and Eye Foundation of Kansas City–Truman Medical Centers, Kansas City, Missouri

**JAY SHAH, BS,** Medical Student, Department of Radiology, University of Illinois Hospital at Chicago, University of Illinois College of Medicine, Chicago, Illinois

**MICHAEL J. SHAPIRO, MD,** Associate Professor, Ophthalmology, Department of Ophthalmology and Visual Science, University of Illinois at Chicago, Chicago, Illinois

**MARC SHIELDS, MD,** Clinical Assistant Professor, Department of Ophthalmology, University of Virginia, Charlottesville, Virginia

**THASARAT S. VAJARANANT, MD,** Resident, Department of Ophthalmology and Visual Sciences, University of Illinois at Chicago, Chicago, Illinois

**ALFRED L. WEBER, MD,** Chief, Radiology (Emeritus), Massachusetts Eye and Ear Infirmary; Professor, Radiology, Harvard Medical School, Boston, Massachusetts; Clinical Professor, Radiology, University of Missouri at Kansas City Medical School, Kansas City, Missouri; Consultant, Head and Neck and Neuroradiology, King Faisal Hospital and Research Center; and Consultant, Ophthalmologic Radiology, King Khaled Eye Hospital, Riyadh, Saudi Arabia

# CONTENTS

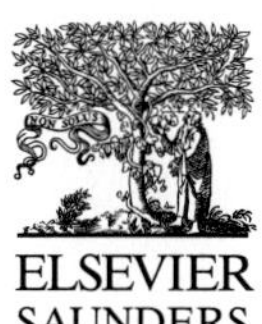
ELSEVIER
SAUNDERS

Neuroimag Clin N Am 15 (2005) xi

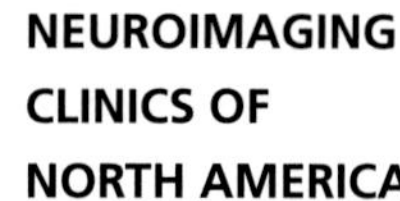


# Preface

# Ophthalmologic Neuroimaging

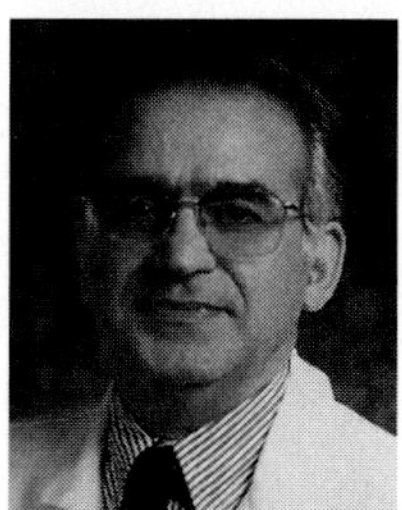

Mahmood F. Mafee, MD
*Guest Editor*

Imaging of the eye, orbit, and visual system is important not only to the neuroradiologist and head and neck radiologist but equally to the general radiologist, as well as ophthalmologist, neuro-ophthalmologist, neurologist, neurosurgeon, and otolaryngologist–head and neck surgeon. The evolution of advanced technologies in ophthalmologic diagnostic imaging has had great impact on the practice of radiology. With this in mind, we have condensed into this issue of the *Neuroimaging Clinics of North America* the essentials of radiologic imaging of ophthalmologic disorders. Although certainly not all of the aspects of the pathologic entities have been included, a comprehensive overview of the present state-of-the-art can be found herein.

The contributing authors have submitted practical and concise articles discussing a variety of important pathologic entities of the eye, orbit, and visual system. We have tried to make this issue unique by demonstrating the role of high-field (1.5- and 3-T) MR imaging in the evaluation of the eye, orbit, and visual system anatomy and pathology. This issue provides radiologists and clinicians with an opportunity to enhance their knowledge and appreciate the complex spectrum of pathology affecting the eye, orbit, and visual system. It is hoped that the exchange of thoughts and experience of the authors will provide readers with knowledge that enhance their service to their patients.

I am greatly indebted to the authors of this issue, who have generously and graciously contributed their knowledge and time; to Barton Dudlick, Editor, and the editorial and production staff of Elsevier for their patience and valuable guidance; and to Aura Smith for her diligence and forbearance in manuscript organization and typing.

## Dedication

I dedicate this issue to my father, who valued greatly intellectual pursuits; to my mother, my teachers, and my brothers and sisters for their valuable guidance; and to my beloved wife, Mahvash, and our wonderful children, Rana, Alireza, and Mariam for their patience, encouragement, and continued support.

Mahmood F. Mafee, MD
*Department of Radiology*
*University of Illinois at Chicago Medical Center*
*1740 West Taylor Street*
*MC 931*
*Chicago, IL 60612-7233, USA*
*E-mail address:* mfmafee@uic.edu

1052-5149/05/$ – see front matter 
doi:10.1016/j.nic.2005.04.001

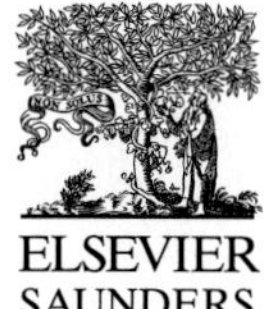
ELSEVIER
SAUNDERS

Neuroimag Clin N Am 15 (2005) 1 – 21

NEUROIMAGING CLINICS OF NORTH AMERICA

# Orbital and Ocular Imaging Using 3- and 1.5-T MR Imaging Systems

Mahmood F. Mafee, MD[a,*], Mark Rapoport, BS[b], Afshin Karimi, MD, PhD, JD[b], Sameer A. Ansari, MD, PhD[b], Jay Shah, BS[c]

[a]*Department of Radiology, University of Illinois at Chicago Medical Center, 1740 West Taylor Street, MC 931, Chicago, IL 60612, USA*

[b]*Department of Radiology, University of Illinois Hospital at Chicago, University of Illinois College of Medicine, 1801 West Taylor Street, MC 711, Chicago, IL 60612, USA*

[c]*Department of Radiology, University of Illinois at Chicago, 1801 West Taylor Street, MC 711, Chicago, IL 60612, USA*

CT scanning and MR imaging of the eye and orbit have significantly enhanced the diagnosis of ocular and orbital lesions [1–21]. The anatomy and pathologic findings of the bony orbit, surrounding structures of the eye, and optic pathways can now be visualized with exquisite detail, so that the diagnosis of pathologic conditions can be made with much more certainty than in the past [1–21]. The evolution of advanced technologies has greatly influenced and aided in the differentiation of orbital and ocular lesions. Ophthalmologic diagnostic evaluation, in particular, has significantly improved with the use of imaging modalities such as ultrasound and MR imaging. The increasing availability of clinical high-field MR imaging at 3 Tesla (3-T) scanners holds the promise of making 3-T MR imaging scanners more available for routine clinical use. The purpose of this article is to describe the application of the 3-T MR imaging scanner in orbital and ocular pathologic findings and, in particular, whether the 3-T MR imaging scanner improves the imaging evaluation of orbital and ocular lesions. In keeping with the purpose of this issue, we review the MR imaging characteristics of selected patients (Table 1) who presented with various orbital and ocular disorders and underwent scanning on a 3-T MR imaging scanner. Some of these patients also underwent scanning on a 1.5-T MR imaging unit. An attempt is made to emphasize the diagnostic patterns of common orbital and ocular lesions on 3-T MR imaging sequences.

## General considerations

Most orbital and some ocular lesions can be evaluated by CT [1,16–18]. MR imaging offers more information than CT in the differentiation of various pathologic conditions involving the eye and orbit [17]. The success of MR imaging depends on the cooperation of the patient, the use of appropriate sedation in pediatric populations, and the use of appropriate MR pulse sequences. Our sedation and MR imaging (1.5-T unit) protocols have been described in detail elsewhere [16–18,20]. Although individual examinations should always be tailored to the problems of each patient, there are general recommendations for orbital and ocular lesions. These include acquisition of T1- and T2-weighted (T1W and T2W) spin echo (SE) or fast SE (FSE) pulse sequences. The FSE T2W pulse sequences may be obtained with or without fat suppression. Precontrast and postcontrast axial T1W MR imaging sequences with and without fat suppression are obtained whenever intravenous

* Corresponding author.
*E-mail address:* mfmafee@uic.edu (M.F. Mafee).

1052-5149/05/$ – see front matter 
doi:10.1016/j.nic.2005.02.010

Table 1
Orbital and ocular lesions in our study

| Condition | No. of patients who have condition |
|---|---|
| Optic nerve sheath meningioma | 7 |
| Optic nerve glioma | 3 |
| Optic nerve neuritis | 4 |
| Optic nerve lymphoma | 1 |
| Orbital rhabdomyosarcoma | 2 |
| Orbital lymphangioma | 2 |
| Orbital cavernous hemangioma | 5 |
| Orbital and dural AVM (ophthalmic artery aneurysm) | 3 |
| Orbital lymphoma | 1 |
| Orbital pseudotumor | 2 |
| Thyroid ophthalmopathy | 3 |
| Orbital langerhans cell histiocytosis | 1 |
| Uveal melanoma | 5 |
| Optic nerve melanocytoma | 1 |
| Choroidal osteoma | 1 |
| Retinoblastoma | 5 |
| Ocular cysticercosis | 1 |
| PHPV | 1 |
| **Total** | **48** |

gadolinium (Gd)–diethylenetriamine penta-acetic acid (DTPA)–based contrast is used. We obtain at least one axial view after a contrast without fat suppression T1W MR pulse sequence because we have noticed that the magnetic susceptibility effect, dental filling, and dental brace artifacts are exaggerated on T1W fat suppression pulse sequences. Postcontrast coronal and oblique sagittal views (along the optic nerve) are routinely obtained for orbital and ocular lesions.

## Material and methods

Forty-eight patients who had various orbital and ocular pathologic findings (see Table 1) underwent MR imaging using our 3-T unit. A number of these patients also had MR imaging studies performed on a 1.5-T scanner. The 3-T studies were performed on a clinical 3-T unit (General Electric Medical Systems, Milwaukee, Wisconsin), using a head coil (quadrature or eight channels). Most studies were performed with eight-channel coils, which we found increased the signal-to-noise ratio (SNR) and gave us superior performance in terms of image quality and general clinical use compared with a quadrature head coil. The 1.5-T MR imaging studies were performed on a Signa 1.5-T unit (General Electric Medical Systems). Our protocol for orbital MR imaging at 3-T and recommendations consist of pulse sequences that are summarized as follows:

- Head coil (eight-channel coils)
- Sagittal T1W inversion recovery (IR) of the head if the quadrature head coil is used (repetition time [TR] = 2600 ms, echo time [TE] = 15 ms, time after inversion pulse [TI] = 100 ms, 512 × 192 matrix, 5-mm section thickness, 1.5-mm skip [gap], 20–24-cm field of view [FOV], and number of excitations [NEX] = 2) or sagittal T1W SE of the head if using eight-channel coils (TR = 500 ms, TE = 14 ms, 256 × 192 matrix, 5-mm section thickness 1.5-mm skip [gap], 20–24-cm FOV, NEX = 2, and 15–25-cm bandwidth).
- Precontrast T1W axial view (TR = 450–500 ms, TE = 12–20 ms, 256 × 192 matrix, 3-mm section thickness, 0.5-mm skip [gap], 14–16-cm FOV, NEX = 3, and 15–25-cm bandwidth)
- Precontrast fat suppression T1W axial view (TR = 500–600 ms, TE = 12–20 ms, 256–352 × 192 matrix, 3-mm section thickness, 0.5-mm skip [gap], 14–16-cm FOV, NEX = 3, and 15–25-cm bandwidth)
- Axial T2W view (TR = 4000–6000 ms, TE = 80–104 ms, 512 × 384 matrix, 3–4-mm section thickness, 0.5-mm skip [gap], 14–16-cm FOV, and NEX = 4)
- Postcontrast T1W axial view (TR = 500 ms, TE = 14–20 ms, 256 × 192 matrix, 3-mm section thickness, 0.5-mm skip [gap], 14–16-cm FOV, NEX = 2–4, and 15–25-cm bandwidth)
- Postcontrast T1W fat suppression (TR = 500 ms, TE = 20 ms, 256 × 192 matrix, 3-mm section thickness, 0.5-mm skip [gap], 16–18-cm FOV, NEX = 2–4, and 31.2-cm bandwidth)
- Postcontrast T1W oblique sagittal view (TR = 500–550 ms, TE = 12–20 ms, 256 × 192 or 352 × 192 matrix, 3-mm section thickness, 0.5-mm skip [gap], 14–16-cm FOV, NEX = 3, and 25-cm bandwidth)
- Postcontrast coronal and sagittal T1W pulse sequences with fast suppression are often obtained instead of regular T1W pulse sequences.

## Results

Fig. 1 shows normal ocular and orbital anatomy obtained at 3-T using thin sections (3 mm) with high (512 × 256 to 512 × 288) matrices. Optic nerve me-

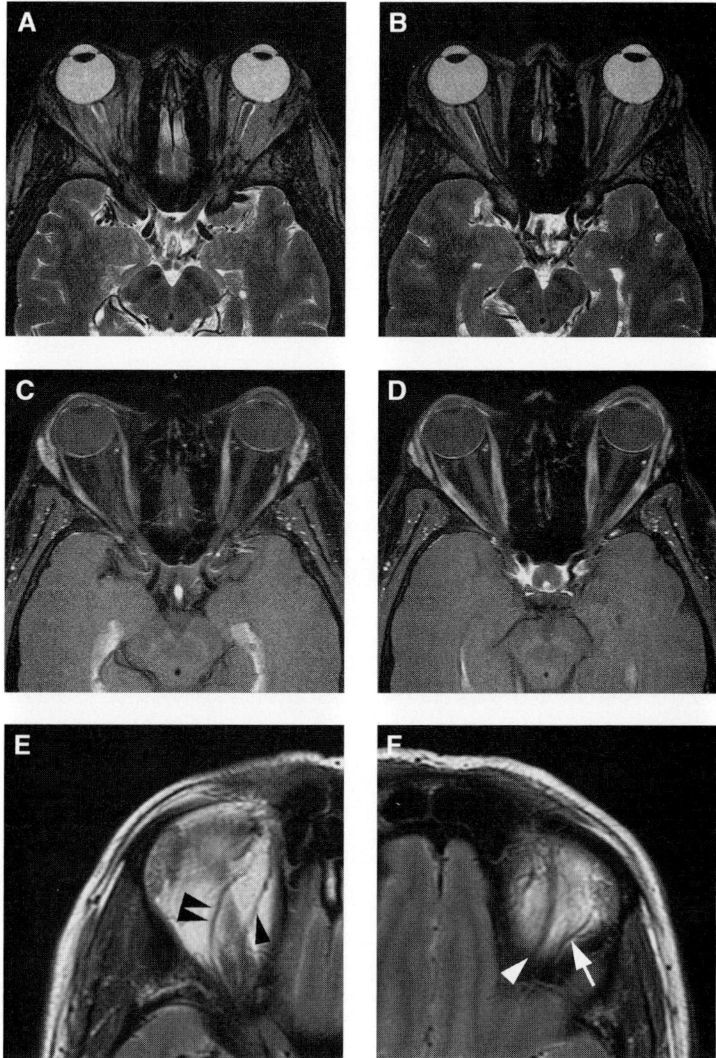


Fig. 1. 3-T MR imaging of normal ocular and orbital anatomy. (*A*, *B*) FSE scan (TR/TE: 5600/108 ms, 1.5-mm section thickness, 0.5-mm gap, 512 × 288 matrix, NEX = 4, 160-mm × 160-mm FOV). (*C*, *D*) Enhanced SE T1W scan with fat suppression (TR/TE: 500/22 ms, 3-mm section thickness, 0.5-mm gap, 512 × 256 matrix, NEX = 2, 160-mm × 160-mm FOV). These images were obtained using a quadrature head coil. (*E*) Axial T2W scan (TR/TE: 2566/88 ms, 3-mm section thickness, 0.5-mm gap, 320 × 224 matrix, NEX = 4) using an eight-channel coil shows superior orbital vein (*double black arrowheads*) and nasociliary nerve (*single black arrowhead*). (*F*) Axial T2W scan (same parameters as in *E*) shows the lacrimal nerve (*single arrow*) and frontal nerve (*arrowhead*).

ningiomas (Figs. 2–5), optic nerve gliomas (Fig. 6), optic nerve lymphoma (Fig. 7), optic neuritis (Fig. 8), orbital lymphoma (Fig. 9), cavernous hemangioma (Fig. 10), lymphangioma (venolymphatic malformation) (Fig. 11), orbital pseudotumor (Fig. 12), and thyroid myositis (Fig. 13) were delineated with exquisite detail. Malignant uveal melanoma (Fig. 14), uveal effusion (Fig. 15), retinoblastomas (Figs. 16 and 17), persistent hyperplastic primary vitreous (PHPV) (Fig. 18), and a case of ocular cysticercosis (Fig. 19) were depicted on 3-T MR imaging scans with details similar to the best of 1.5-T images.

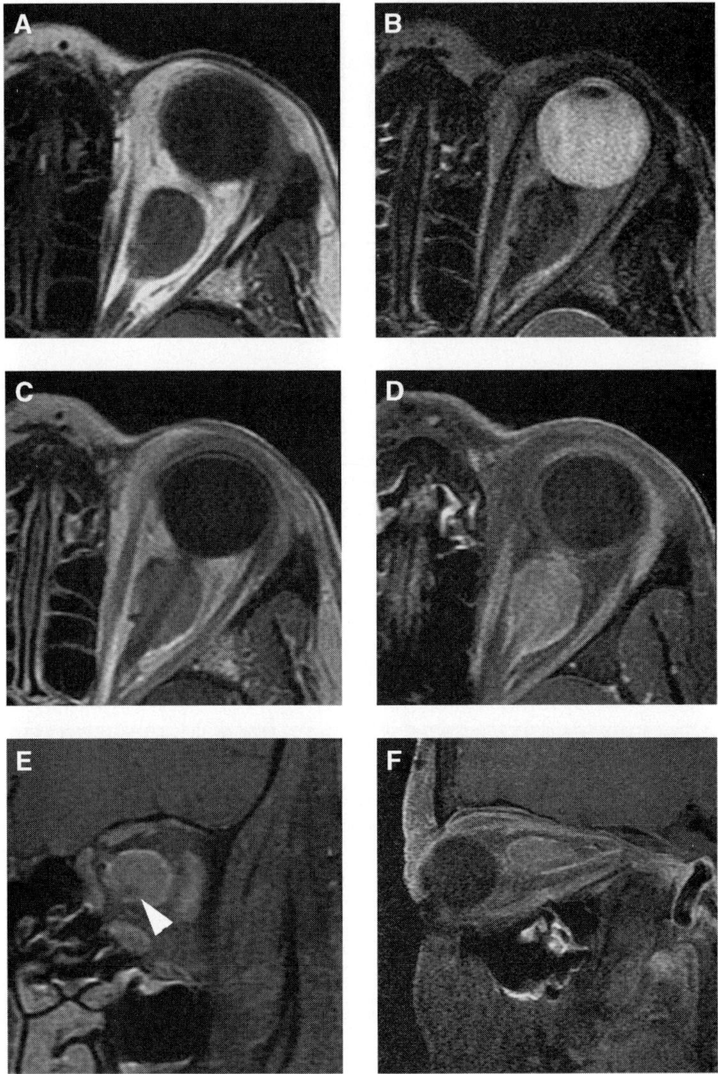


Fig. 2. Optic nerve sheath meningioma (3-T MR imaging using a head coil). (*A*) Unenhanced T1W scan (TR/TE: 550/12 ms, 2.5-mm section thickness, 352 × 192 matrix, NEX = 2). (*B*) FSE scan (TR/TE: 6016/104 ms, 1.5-mm section thickness, 0.5-mm gap, 384 × 256 matrix, NEX = 4) (*C*) Enhanced T1W scan (TR/TE: 550/12 ms, 2.5-mm section thickness, 0.3-mm gap, 352 × 192 matrix, NEX = 2). (*D*) Enhanced fat suppression T1W scan (TR/TE: 466/12 ms, 3-mm section thickness, 352 × 192 matrix, NEX = 2). (*E*) Coronal enhanced fat suppression T1W scan (TR/TE: 750/12 ms, 3-mm section thickness, 0.5-mm gap, 320 × 192 matrix, NEX = 2). (*F*) Sagittal enhanced fat suppression T1W scan (TR/TE: 466/12 ms, 3-mm section thickness, 0.3-mm gap, 320 × 192 matrix, NEX = 2). Note that the optic nerve (*arrowhead* in *E*) is surrounded by the optic nerve sheath meningioma.

Retinoblastoma appeared hyperintense on diffusion-weighted (DW) imaging (see Fig. 17C), and a case of melanocytoma of the optic disc was not detected by 3-T scanning. The same melanocytoma could not be detected by 1.5-T scanners, even when using the surface coil. The increased magnetic susceptibility effect artifacts of the 3-T scans, particularly along the planum sphenoidale, proved to be a major limiting factor in evaluating lesions involving the intracanalicular and intracranial segments of the optic nerves

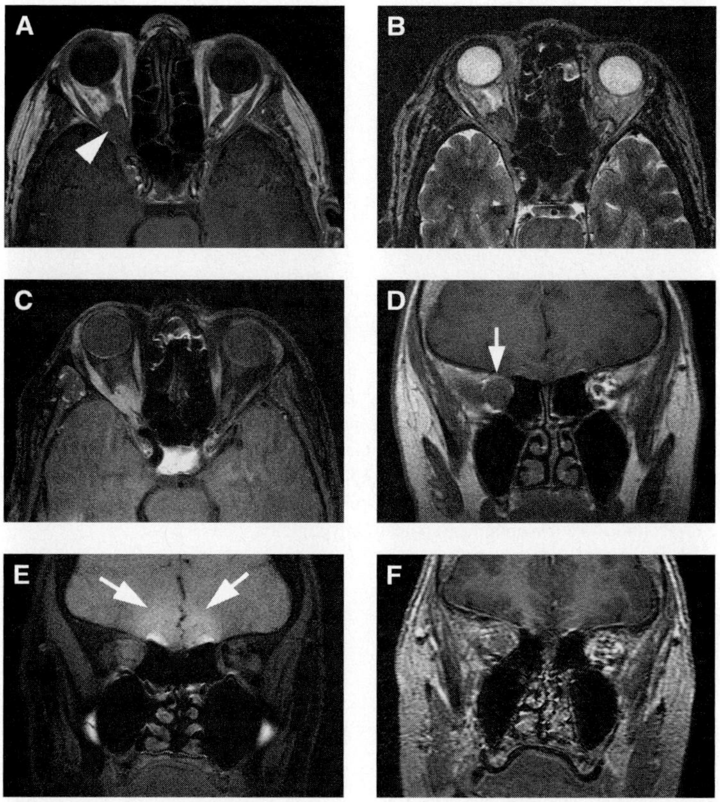


Fig. 3. Optic nerve sheath meningioma. (3-T MR imaging using a quadrature head coil). (*A*) Unenhanced axial T1W scan (3-mm section thickness, 0.4-mm gap, TR/ TE: 600/9 ms, 512 × 224 matrix, 160-mm × 160-mm FOV, NEX = 2). (*B*) axial FSE T2W scan (TR/TE: 5800/108 ms, 0.2-mm section thickness, 512 × 288 matrix, 160-mm × 160-mm FOV, NEX = 4). (*C*) Fat suppression enhanced axial T1W scan (TR/TE: 900/22 ms, 3-mm section thickness, 0.5-mm gap, 512 × 240 matrix, 160-mm × 160-mm FOV, NEX = 2). (*D*) unenhanced coronal T1W scan (TR/TE: 900/ 9 ms, 3-mm section thickness, 1-mm gap, 512 × 224 matrix, 160-mm × 160-mm FOV, NEX = 2). (*E*) Enhanced fat suppression coronal T1W scan (TR/TE: 556/22 ms, 4-mm section thickness, 0.8-mm gap, 512 × 224 matrix, 160-mm × 160-mm FOV, NEX = 2). (*F*) Enhanced coronal three-dimensional spoiled gradient echo sequence (TR/TE: 13.8/2.6 ms, 1.5-mm section thickness, 512 × 192 matrix, 220-mm × 220-mm FOV). Note the orbital apical meningioma (*arrowhead* in *A*; *arrow* in *D*) and magnetic susceptibility artifact (*arrows* in *E*).

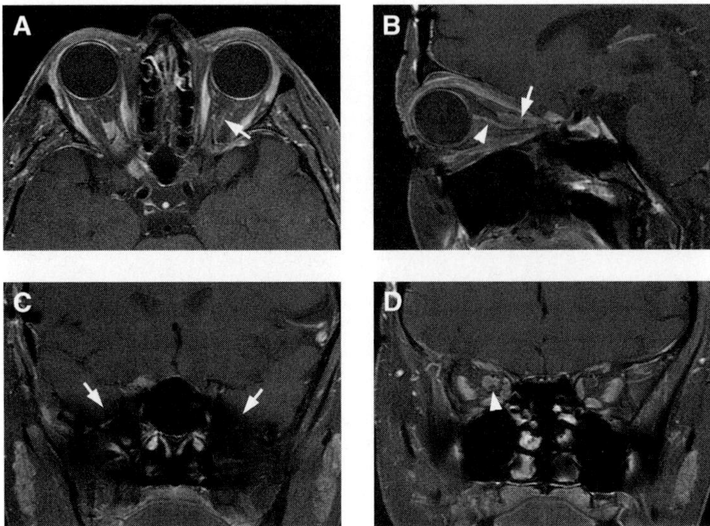


Fig. 4. Optic nerve sheath meningioma (3-T MR imaging using an eight-channel head coil). (*A*) Enhanced fat suppression axial T1W scan shows a right optic nerve sheath meningioma and normal left optic nerve (*arrow*). (*B*) Enhanced fat suppression sagittal scan shows a right optic nerve meningioma (*arrow* and *arrowhead*). (*C*) Enhanced fat suppression coronal scan shows meningioma involving the intracranial segment of the right optic nerve. Note the significant magnetic susceptibility effect artifacts (*arrows*) distorting the anatomy of the skull base. (*D*) Enhanced fat suppression coronal scan. Note the constricted right optic nerve (*arrowhead*) surrounded by the optic nerve sheath meningioma.

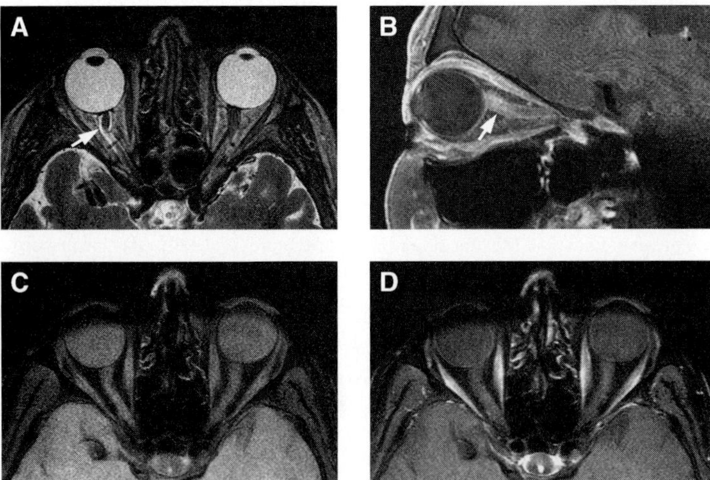


Fig. 5. Optic nerve sheath presumed meningioma (3-T MR imaging using an eight-channel head coil). Axial T2W (*A*), enhanced fat suppression sagittal T1W (*B*), unenhanced fat suppression axial T1W (*C*), and enhanced fat suppression axial T1W (*D*) scans. Note the enhancement of the meningioma (*arrow* in *B*). The meningioma is less defined in the axial section (*D*). This optic nerve sheath meningioma, which was clinically suspected for 3 years, could not be depicted on several MR imaging scans performed at 1.5-T and on one performed at 3-T using a quadrature head coil. Note effacement of CSF along the left optic nerve compared to the normal side (*arrow* in *A*).

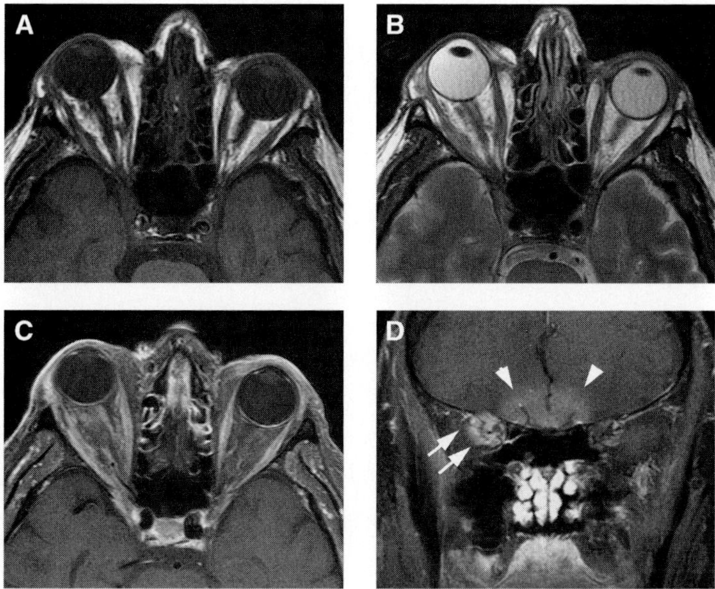


Fig. 11. Venolymphatic malformation (3-T MR imaging using an eight-channel head coil). Axial T1W (*A*), T2W (*B*), enhanced fat suppression axial T1W (*C*), and coronal (*D*) scans show enhancement of the venous component of the venolymphatic malformation (*arrows* in *D*). Note the marked magnetic susceptibility effect artifacts (*arrowheads*).

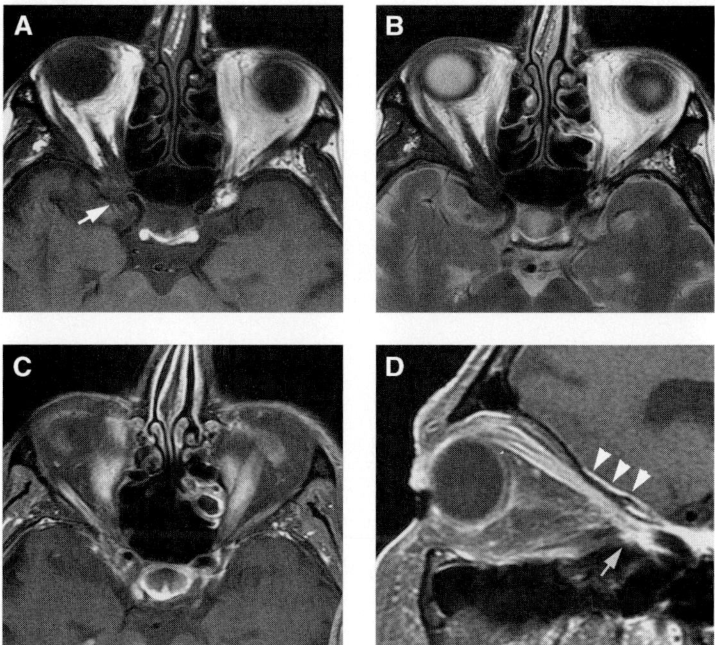


Fig. 12. Orbital pseudotumor (3-T MR imaging using an eight-channel head coil). Axial T1W (*A*), T2W (*B*), enhanced fat suppression axial T1W (*C*) and sagittal T1W (*D*) scans show an infiltrative process involving the right orbital apex (*arrows*). Note the abnormal dural enhancement (*arrowheads*). Patients responded well to a short course of steroid therapy.

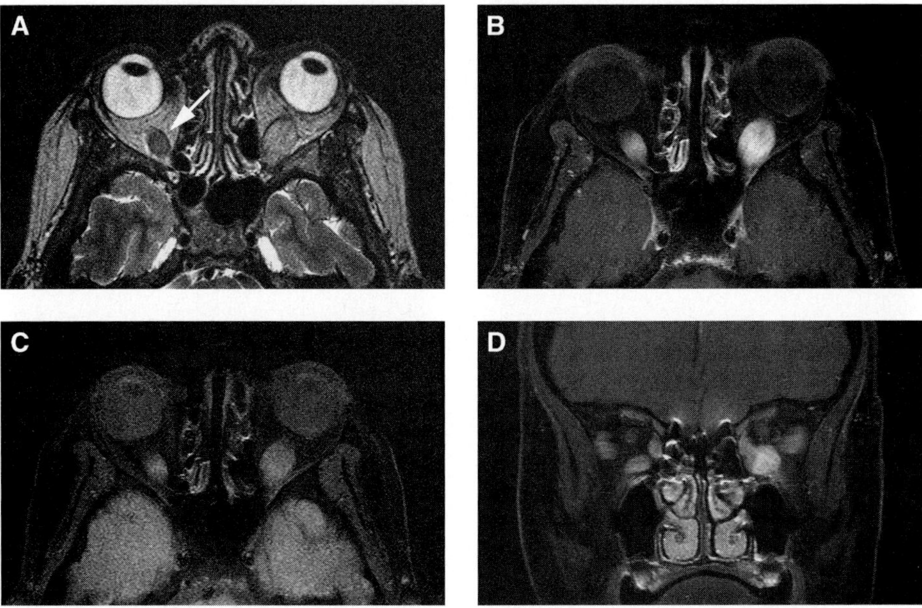


Fig. 13. Thyroid orbitopathy (3-T MR imaging using a quadrature head coil). Axial FSE T2W (*A*), enhanced fat suppression T1W (*B*), unenhanced fat suppression T1W (*C*), and enhanced fat suppression T1W coronal (*D*) scans. Note the increased size of the left inferior rectus muscle along with edema (*A*) and increased contrast enhancement (*B*, *D*).

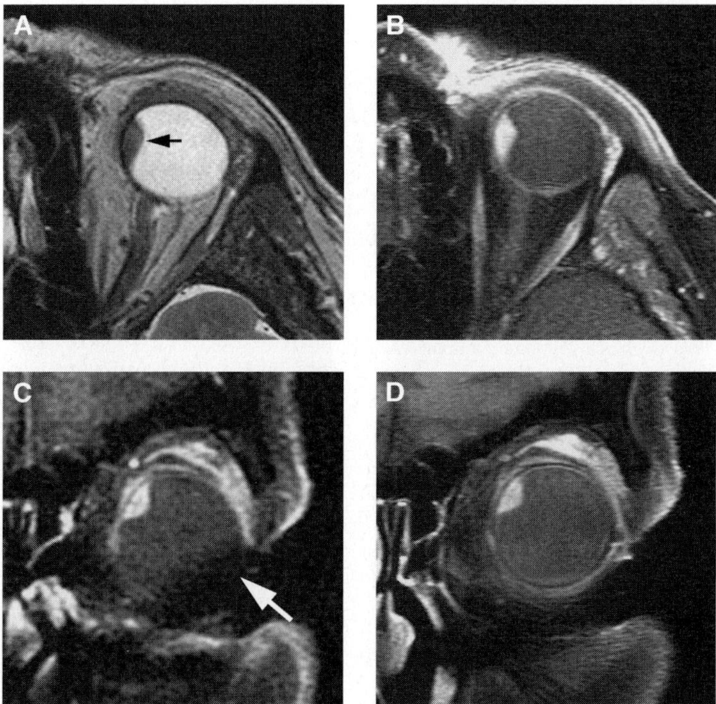


Fig. 14. Malignant uveal melanoma (3-T MR imaging using an eight-channel head coil). (*A*) Axial T2W scan (TR/ TE: 5500/ 103 ms, 1.5-mm section thickness. (*B*) Axial enhanced fat suppression T1W scan (TR/TE: 400/19 ms, 3-mm section thickness, 0.5-mm gap, 14-cm × 14-cm FOV, NEX = 4). (*C*) Coronal enhanced fat suppression T1W scan (TR/TE: 450/18 ms, 3-mm section thickness, 0.5-mm gap, 256 × 192 matrix, 14-cm × 14-cm FOV, NEX = 2). (*D*) Coronal enhanced fat suppression T1W scan (TR/TE: 600/20 ms, 3-mm section thickness, 0.5-mm gap, 512 × 192 matrix, 14-cm × 14-cm FOV, NEX = 4). A malignant uveal melanoma is shown (*black arrow* in *A*). Note the increased artifact in *C* (*white arrow*).

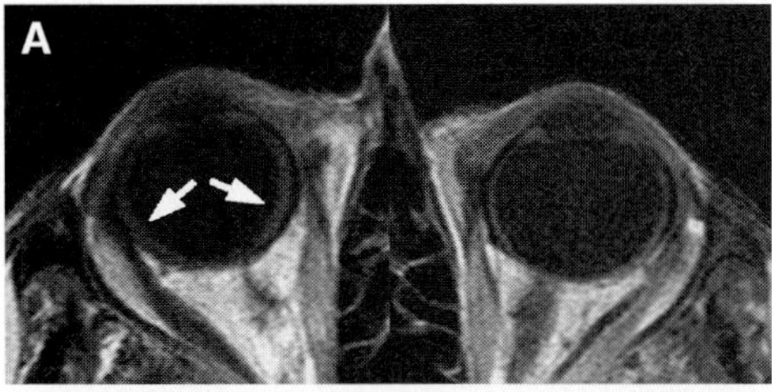


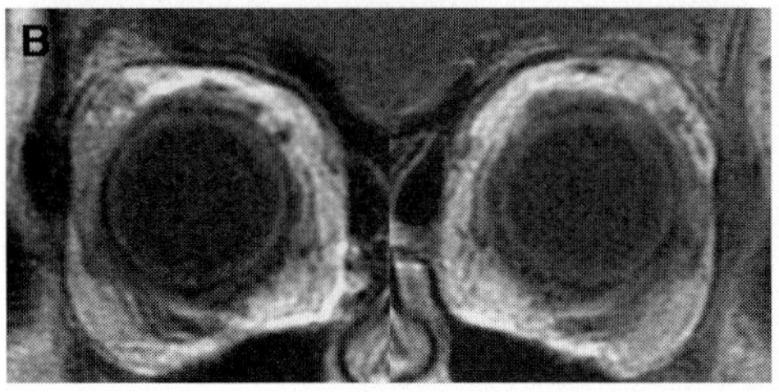


Fig. 15. Choroidal effusion (3-T MR imaging using a quadrature head coil). Enhanced axial T1W (*A*) and enhanced coronal T1W (*B*) axial T1W scans (TR/TE: 400/19 ms, 3-mm section thickness, 0.5-mm gap, 14-cm × 14-cm FOV, NEX = 4) scans show increased thickening and enhancement of uveal tract (*arrows*). The process involves both eyes.

(see Figs. 3 and 4). High-resolution FSE T2W images using a 512 × 256 or 512 × 384 matrix proved to be a real advantage of 3-T for orbital, ocular, and intracranial MR imaging. Despite prolongation of the T1 relaxation time at 3-T and a slight reduction of tissue contrast on T1W MR imaging scans, we found T1W SE images superior to 3D T1W gradient echo images, such as spoiled gradient echo sequences (SPGRs), obtained with 1-mm or isotropic voxels with 512 × 256 matrices (see Figs. 3 and 8). Although the contrast between gray and white matter is significantly greater on 3D T1W SPGRs because of lower spatial resolution, we preferred to obtain SE T1W MR imaging pulse sequences for orbital, ocular, and intracranial pathologic findings in our cases. Magnetic susceptibility effect artifacts limited the evaluation of lesions along the floor of the orbit and adjacent to hyperpneumatized posterior ethmoid and sphenoid sinuses, particularly on coronal MR imaging scans (see Figs. 4, 5, 7, and 11). Ocular imaging may be limited because of make-up artifacts, because we have found that make-up artifacts are increased at 3-T compared with 1.5-T. Early studies obtained with a quadrature head coil suffered from

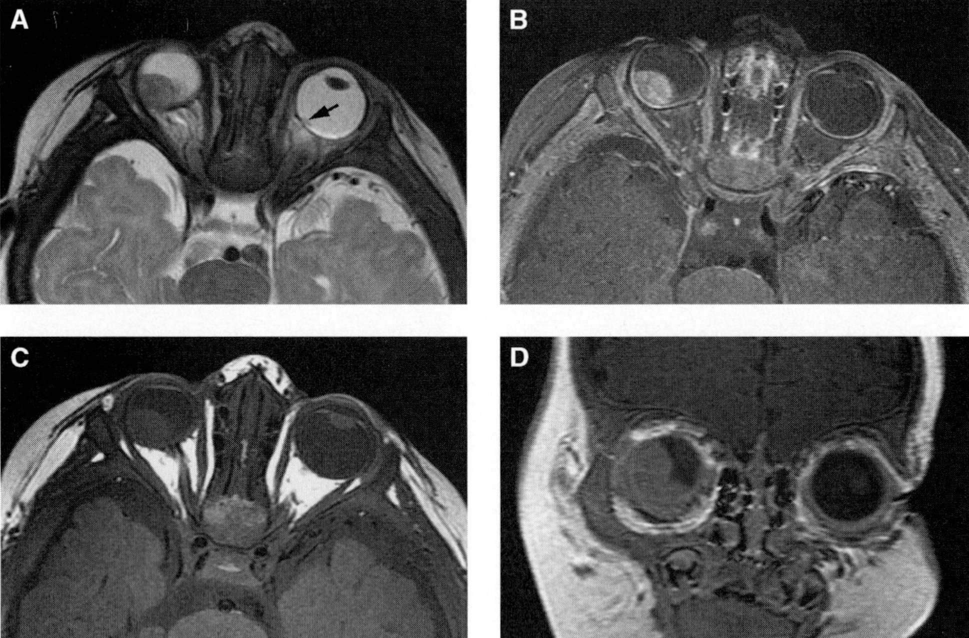


Fig. 16. Retinoblastoma (3-T MR imaging using an eight-channel head coil). (*A*) Axial FSE T2W scan (TR/TE: 5616/96 ms, 4-mm section thickness, 1-mm gap, 512 × 288 matrix, 16-cm × 16-cm FOV, NEX = 4). (*B*) Enhanced fat suppression T1W scan (TR/TE: 450/13 ms, 2.3-mm section thickness, 0.5-mm gap, 352 × 192 matrix, 16-cm × 16-cm FOV, NEX = 2). (*C*) Unenhanced T1W scan (TR/TE: 400/13 ms, 2.3-mm section thickness, 0.5-mm gap, 352 × 192 matrix, 16-cm × 16-cm FOV, NEX = 2). (*D*) Coronal enhanced three-dimensional spoiled gradient echo sequence scan (TR/TE: 10.6/2.19 ms, 1.5-mm section thickness, 512 × 192 matrix). Scans show bilateral retinoblastoma, with that on the left being extremely small (*arrow* in *A*).

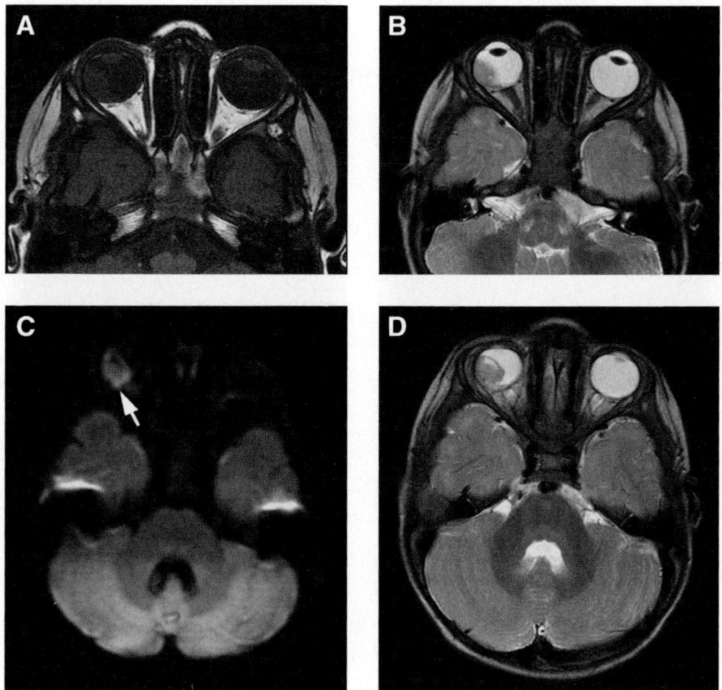


Fig. 17. Retinoblastoma (3-T MR imaging using an eight-channel head coil). Axial T1W (*A*), T2W (*B*), diffusion-weighted (DW) imaging (*C*), and axial T2W (*D*) scans show a retinoblastoma. The tumor appears hyperintense on DW imaging (*arrow* in *C*).

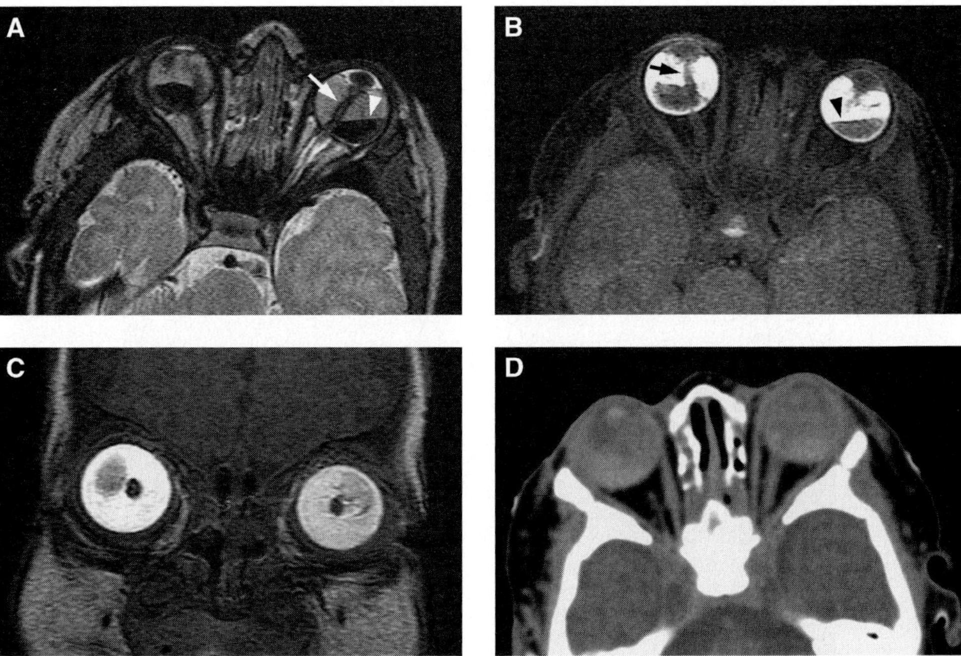


Fig. 18. Bilateral persistent hyperplastic primary vitreous (3-T MR imaging using a quadrature head coil). (*A*) Axial FSE T2W scan (TR/TE: 5000/108 ms, 1.5-mm section thickness, 140-mm × 140-mm FOV, 512 × 224 matrix, NEX = 4). (*B*) Axial unenhanced spin echo T1W fat suppression scan (TR/TE: 816/18 ms, 2-mm section thickness, 140-mm × 140-mm FOV, 384 × 192 matrix, NEX = 2). (*C*) Coronal three-dimensional spoiled gradient echo sequence scan (TR/TE: 14/2.8 ms, 1.5-mm section thickness, 140-mm × 140-mm FOV, 512 × 192 matrix, NEX = 1). (*D*) Unenhanced axial CT scan. Note the detached (congenitally nonattached) retina (*arrows* in *A* and *B*) and layered fluid (*arrowheads* in *A* and *B*), compatible with hemorrhage in the subretinal or subhyaloid space. The detached retina appears as a central hypointense image in each eye in the coronal section (*C*). The hypointensity of the sensory retina may be caused by intraretinal hemorrhage. The CT scan shows increased density of the eyes and bilateral fluid-fluid level.

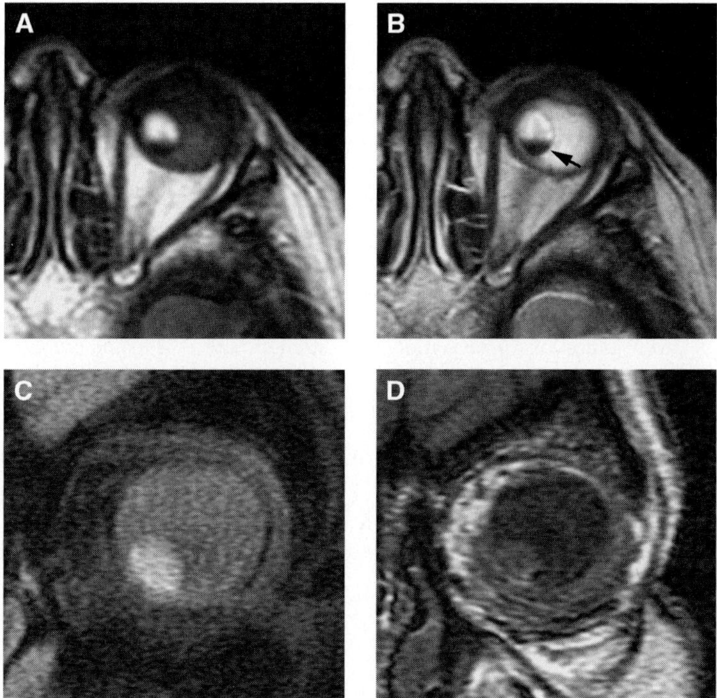


Fig. 19. Ocular cysticercosis (3-T MR imaging using a quadrature head coil). (*A*) Axial fluid-attenuated inversion recovery scan (TR/TE: 11,002/170 ms, 5-mm section thickness, 2-mm gap, 240-mm × 240-mm FOV, 320 × 192 matrix). (*B*) FSE T2W scan (TR/TE: 3500/98 ms, 5-mm section thickness, 2-mm gap, 160-mm × 160-mm FOV, 512 × 192 matrix). (*C*) Coronal spin echo T1W fat suppression scan (TR/TE: 650/22 ms, 3-mm section thickness, 160-mm × 160-mm FOV, 512 × 192 matrix). (*D*) Coronal spoiled gradient echo sequence scan (TR/TE: 13.9/2.7 ms, 1.5-mm section thickness, 220-mm × 220-mm FOV, 512 × 192 matrix). Note a heterogeneous partially cystic mass involving the nasal aspect of the left globe (*arrow* in *B*).

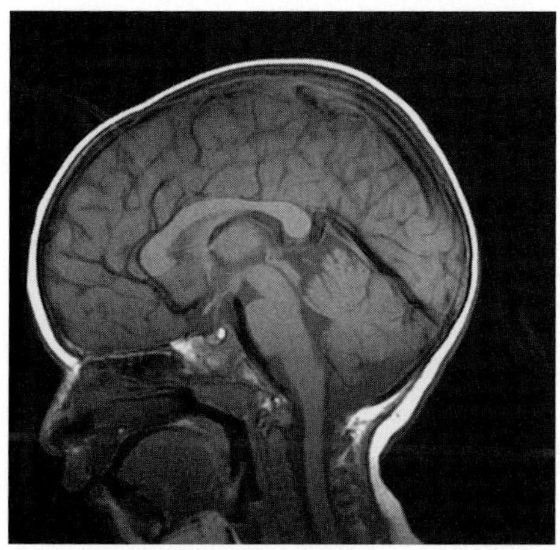

Fig. 20. Sagittal spin echo T1W scan (3-T MR imaging using an eight-channel coil). Note the uniformity of signal intensity from the vertex to craniocervical junction and the good anatomic detail of the nasopharynx nasal cavity and dorsal oral tongue.

limited cephalocaudal coverage and Z-axis uniformity of signal intensity from convexity through the base of the skull. MR imaging scans obtained at 3-T using an eight-channel head coil have proven to be similar to those obtained at 1.5-T in terms of signal intensity uniformity and anatomic details of the base of the skull and nasopharynx, infratemporal fossa, and parotid glands (Fig. 20).

## Discussion

Clinical MR imaging is mostly acquired using the current standard field strengths up to 1.5 T. Recently developed clinical 3-T MR imaging scanners have been used in many centers for better resolution and faster scanning time. Theoretically, the SNR increases linearly with increasing magnetic field ($B_o$) strength. Therefore, the SNR is doubled in 3 T in comparison to 1.5 T [22,23]. In contrast, the specific absorption rate (SAR) increases with the square root of the field strength. Therefore, the gain in the SNR is the main advantage of 3-T versus 1.5-T MR imaging. At 3 T, tumor-to-brain contrast has been found to be higher than at 1.5 T, resulting in the detection of more metastases using the same contrast dosage [22]. The T1 relaxation time increases with increasing $B_o$. Therefore, the T1 contrast between gray and white matter is reduced on T1W SE pulse sequences obtained on the 3-T unit. For this reason, IR pulse sequences are often used in conjunction with the SE sequences to improve gray-to-white matter contrast at 3-T [23]. Although prolongation of T1 relaxation times reduces the gray-to-white matter contrast, we have found that a recent technical improvement on our 3-T unit has resulted in improving clinically relevant T1W SE contrast (see Fig. 20). Conversely, prolonged T1 relaxation time of tissues has significantly improved quality of the time-of-flight (TOF) pulse sequence, as noted in our practice and others [24]. There is no question that a higher SNR significantly improves the quality of MR angiography performed at 3-T.

The effect of Gd-DTPA–based contrast medium at different field strengths depends on two basic phenomena: field-dependent relaxation of tissue and the nuclear magnetic relaxation dispersion. The nuclear magnetic relaxation dispersion or relaxivity of a paramagnetic ion to water protons decreases at higher magnetic fields [24,25]. It has been shown that after the intravenous administration of Gd-based contrast medium, the contrast between brain tumor or metastasis and the surrounding normal brain was markedly higher at 3-T compared with 1.5-T [22]. This is a result of the fact that the uptake of contrast agent produces more significant shortening of the T1 relaxation time at higher field strengths [26].

The spin resonance frequency is proportional to the $B_o$ and is determined according to the Larmor equation: $W = \gamma B_o$. The excitation frequency is doubled to 127.8 MHz at 3-T compared with 63.9 MHz at 1.5-T [23]. Accordingly, the SAR is related to the square of the proton excitation frequency and hence varies in proportion with the square of the $B_o$ field. The high excitation frequency leads to (1) higher energy absorption and increasing SAR and (2) decreased tissue penetration and thus nonhomogeneous signal intensities throughout the image [23]. Although, this is one of the disadvantages of 3-T MR imaging scanners, recent technical improvements have compensated for this problem.

In our experience, one of the major disadvantages of 3-T MR imaging in clinical practice is the increased magnetic susceptibility–induced image distortions. Magnetic susceptibility effects can be used advantageously, depicting hemosiderin in chronic hemorrhage or hemorrhage within lesions like cavernomas and providing the basis for blood oxygenation level dependent (BOLD) functional MR (fMR) imaging. Conversely, magnetic susceptibility effect also induces distortions and signal dropouts at air-bone-brain or air-bone-orbit interfaces, thus limiting the evaluation of lesions along the floor of the anterior cranial fossa, paracavernous sinuses, and floor of the orbit (see Figs. 3, 4, 7, and 14). The magnetic susceptibility effect increases with increasing field strength and is a major problem in echo planar imaging [23]. We tried to use DW imaging for some orbital pathologic findings at 3-T. Except in a few cases (see Fig. 17C), image distortion did not allow us to provide any meaningful evaluation of the lesions. Theoretically, field strength should not affect diffusion imaging properties, and the choice of b-value should not affect the degree of fluid suppression [25]. Some investigators have reported successful DW imaging at 3-T [25].

### *Safety of stents and implanted devices for the 3-T unit*

With the advent of high magnetic field strengths, there has been a resurgence of concern regarding the safety of medically implanted devices and stents. We have found that some devices, such as Dobhoff tubes, previously thought to be safe at 1.5-T have been found to undergo motion or deflection in our 3-T MR imaging unit. Therefore, it is crucial to perform ex vivo testing or the equivalent procedure on devices for which there is no safety information available at the higher field strength. This increased level of scrutiny arises from the fact that metallic objects previously shown to minimally interact with the 1.5-T field have weak ferromagnetic properties that result in a clinically significant amount of interaction at the higher field strength. Furthermore, scanner configuration, such as the traditional "long-bore" system versus the newer "short-bore" system, has been shown to alter the level of magnetic interactions of the devices at a given field strength, such as 3-T [27]. In recognition of the importance of the safety of medical devices and implants, the pertinent safety information specific for a given device must be checked for information relevant to 3-T imaging.

The use of MR scanners at higher field strength, such as 3-T, improves the SNR, providing high-resolution imaging. At least in brain imaging, however, high-field scanners have one disadvantage in that the T1 relaxation times of gray and white matter become longer, reducing the T1 contrast of brain on T1W SE pulse sequences [23,26]. IR and the use of small flip angles (even for SE imaging), however, can result in excellent gray-to-white matter contrast [23]. We have found that high-resolution T1W and particularly T2W images at 3-T are superior to those at 1.5-T in visualization of the anatomic details of the brain and orbit. MR angiography performed at 3-T is far superior to that performed at 1.5-T for visualization of dural cavernous and carotid cavernous fistulas. We were not able, however, to visualize a small intraorbital arteriovenous malformation (AVM) or an ophthalmic artery aneurysm, which were successfully depicted on standard angiography. It has been shown that contrast-enhanced MR venography at 3-T is superior to that performed at 1.5-T [28]. We have found that the three-dimensional (3D) T1W-gradient echo sequence at 1.5- and 3-T had less sensitivity for detecting orbital, optic nerve, and even pituitary pathologic findings as compared with the T1W SE pulse sequence. We have found that the intravenous administration of Gd-based contrast medium has proven to be valuable in the evaluation of orbital and ocular pathologic findings similar to its application for intracranial pathologic findings, including primary tumors and metastases [29]. We use an intravenous dose of 0.1 mmol/kg for our routine cranial and orbital MR imaging studies.

Although our experience indicates that 3-T MR imaging is clinically beneficial in assessing orbital and ocular lesions, because of increased magnetic susceptibility–induced image distortions, increased chemical shift artifacts, and prolongation of T1 at a higher field strength resulting in reduced T1 contrast on T1W SE pulse sequences, we think that an optimized imaging technique and improved pulse sequence and surface coil design are needed to advance the clinical benefit of 3-T MR imaging further. In our study, 3-T pulse sequences (T1W and T2W), including postcontrast T1W MR imaging scans, proved to be superior to 1.5-T sequences for visualization of the orbital anatomy and structures within the cavernous sinus. If the sphenoid sinuses are hyperpneumatized because of increased magnetic susceptibility effect artifacts, for example, the 3-T MR imaging scanner loses its advantage over the 1.5-T scanner.

The trochlear nerve is the smallest of the intracavernous cranial nerves (median diameter $< 1$ mm) [22]. Therefore, it is difficult to visualize at 1.5-T [30]. It can sometimes be seen on enhanced high-resolution T1W MR imaging scans obtained at 3-T, however. Images taken at 3-T are superior to those take at 1.5-T in delineating the white matter tracts, such as the optochiasmatic system, particularly on IR pulse sequences and heavily T2-weighted pulse sequences. This is desirable information for suprasellar lesions and for delineation of compressed optochiasmatic structures. Although some authors [31] prefer to use 3D T1W SPGR by obtaining 1-mm isotropic voxels with $256 \times 256$ matrices to circumvent the reduced tissue contrast on SE T1W images at 3-T, for orbital, optic nerve, optic chiasm, and sellar lesions, we prefer SE T1W images using an eight-channel head coil. Chemical shift effects increase with increasing field strength [32]. An increase in chemical shift artifact at 3-T may be a significant limiting factor in routine anatomic imaging [33]. Chemical shift effect is seen in the orbit at the fat-tissue interfaces. Despite increased chemical shift artifact at 3-T, however, we did not find this to be a significant limiting factor in our orbital and ocular MR imaging at 3-T, including FSE T2W imaging. In general, one has to be careful when using the 3-T MR imaging system in routine clinical practice because the 3-T units are more sophisticated than the 1.5-T units in terms of hardware, software, image quality, artifacts, and general clinical use [34]. As further advances in software and hardware development continue to improve image quality and reduce imaging times, there is no doubt that 3-T MR imaging is going to play an increasingly important role in diagnostic medical imaging.

## Summary

The use of clinical 3-T MR imaging scanners has gained popularity in many centers. An increased SNR is the main advantage of higher field strength, such as 3 T. This increased SNR can be used to acquire images with increased spatial resolution or to shorten acquisition time. Nevertheless, there are associated disadvantages, including changes in SAR exposure, changes in T1 and T2 relaxation times, increased sensitivity to field inhomogeneities, and increasing magnetic susceptibility effects, that render high-field MR imaging more challenging. Despite some of its disadvantages, we have found it to be useful for orbital and ocular imaging. There is still a need for developing techniques to minimize magnetic susceptibility effect artifacts, sequence parameters to improve T1W SE contrast, and improved pulse sequence and surface coil design for ocular imaging.

## Acknowledgments

The authors thank Aura Smith for her secretarial assistance and Yassir Aich for his technical assistance.

This work was approved by the Institutional Review Board of the University of Illinois at Chicago.

## References


[1] Mafee MF, Putterman A, Valvassori GE, et al. Orbital space occupying lesions: role of computed tomography and magnetic resonance imaging. An analysis of 145 cases. Radiol Clin N Am 1987;25: 529–59.

[2] Mafee MF, Goldberg MF, Valvassari GE, et al. Computed tomography in the evaluation of patients with persistent hyperplastic primary vitreous (PHPV). Radiology 1982;145:713–7.

[3] Mafee MF, Peyman GA. Choroidal detachment and ocular hypotony: CT evaluation. Radiology 1984;153: 697–703.

[4] Mafee MF, Falk ER, Langer BG, et al. Computed tomography in the evaluation of Brown syndrome of the superior oblique tendon sheath. Radiology 1985; 154:691–5.

[5] Bilaniuk LT, Shenck JF, Zimmerman RA. Ocular and orbital lesions: surface coil imaging of the orbit. Radiology 1985;156:669–74.

[6] Mafee MF, Peyman GA, McKusick MA. Malignant uveal melanoma and simulating lesions studied by computed tomography. Radiology 1985;156:403–8.

[7] Mafee MF, Peyman GA, Grisolano JE, et al. Malignant uveal melanoma and simulating lesions: MR imaging evaluation. Radiology 1986;160:773–80.

[8] Mafee MF, Peyman GA, Peace JH, et al. Magnetic resonance imaging in the evaluation and differentiation of uveal melanoma. Ophthalmology 1987;94: 341–8.

[9] Mafee MF, Linder B, Peyman GA, et al. Choroidal hematoma and effusion: evaluation with MR imaging. Radiology 1988;168:781–6.

[10] Mafee MF, Goldberg MF, Cohen SB, et al. Magnetic resonance imaging versus computed tomography of leukokoric eyes and use of in vitro proton magnetic resonance spectroscopy of retinoblastoma. Ophthalmology 1989;96(17):965–76.

[11] Mafee MF. Magnetic resonance imaging: ocular anatomy and pathology. In: Newton TH, Bilanuik LT, editors. Radiology of the eye and orbit. Modern neuroradiology, vol. 4. New York: Clavadel Press/ Raven Press; 1989. p. 2.1–3.45.

[12] Depotte P, Flanders AE, Shields JA, et al. The role of fat suppression technique and gadopentetate dimeglumine in magnetic resonance imaging evaluation of intraocular tumors and simulating lesions. Arch Ophthalmol 1994;112:340–8.

[13] Carmody RF, Mafee MF, Goodwin JA, et al. Orbital and optic pathway sarcoidosis: MR findings. American Journal of Neuroradiology 1993;15:775–83.

[14] Mafee MF, Ainbinder DJ, Hidayat AA, et al. Magnetic resonance imaging and computed tomography in the evaluation of choroidal hemangioma. Int J Neuroradiol 1995;1:67–77.

[15] Mafee MF, Inoue Y, Mafee RF. Ocular and orbital imaging. Neuroimaging Clin N Am 1996;6:291–318.

[16] Mafee MF. The eye. In: Som PM, Curtin HD, editors. Head and neck imaging. 4th edition. St. Louis: Mosby; 2003. p. 441–527.

[17] Mafee MF. The eye and orbit. In: Mafee MF, Valvassori GE, Becker M, editors. Imaging of the head and neck. 2nd edition. Stuttgart: Thieme; 2004. p. 137–294.

[18] Mafee MF, Atlas SW, Galetta SL. Eye, orbit and visual system. In: Atlas SW, editor. Magnetic resonance imaging of the brain and spine. 3rd edition. Philadelphia: Lippincott Williams & Wilkins; 2002. p. 1433–524.

[19] Mafee MF, Mafee RF, Malik M, et al. Medical imaging in pediatric ophthalmology. Pediatr Clin N Am 2003;50:259–86.

[20] Kaufman LM, Mafee MF, Song CD. Retinoblastoma and simulating lesion: role of CT, MR imaging and use of Gd-DTPA contrast enhancement. Radial Clin N Am 1998;36:1101–17.

[21] Wycliffe ND, Mafee MF. Magnetic resonance imaging in ocular pathology. Top Magn Reson Imaging 1999; 10:384–400.

[22] Trattnig S, Ba-Ssalamah A, Noebauer-Huhman IM, et al. MR contrast agent at high field MRI (3 Tesla). Top Magn Reson Imaging 2003;14:365–75.

[23] Schmitz B, Grön G, Aschoff AJ. Pitfalls in 3 Tesla MR brain imaging and how to work around them. University Hospitals Ulm, Germany. Radiological Society of North America, Chicago, Illinois, November 27–December 2, 2004.

[24] Gibbs GF, Huston III J, Bernstein MA, et al. Improved image quality of intracranial aneurysms: 3.0-T versus 1.5-T time-of-flight MR angiography. AJNR Am J Neuroradiol 2004;25:84–7.

[25] Simon JE, Czechowsky DK, Hill MD, et al. Fluid-attenuated inversion recovery preparation: not an improvement over conventional diffusion-weighted imaging at 3T in acute ischemic stroke. AJNR Am J Neuroradiol 2004;25:1653–8.

[26] Rinck PA, Fischer HW, Vander Elst D, et al. Field-cycling relaxometry: medical application. Radiology 1988;168:843–9.

[27] Shellock FG, Tkach JA, Ruggieri PM, et al. Aneurysm clips: evaluation of magnetic field interactions and translational attraction by use of "long-bore" and "short-bore" 3.T MR imaging systems. AJNR Am J Neuroradiol 2003;24:463–71.

[28] Nöbauer-Huhman IM, Ba-Ssalamah A, Mlynarik V, et al. Magnetic resonance imaging contrast enhancement of brain tumors at 3 Tesla versus 1.5 Tesla. Invest Radiol 2002;37:114–9.

[29] Reichenbach JR, Barth M, Haacke EM, et al. High resolution MR venography at 3.0 Tesla. J Comput Assist Tomogr 2000;24:949–57.

[30] Daniels DL, Pech P, Mark L, et al. Magnetic resonance imaging of the cavernous sinus. AJNR Am J Neuroradiol 1985;144:1009–14.

[31] Shapiro MD, Magee T, Williams D, et al. The time for 3T clinical imaging is now. [letter]. AJNR Am J Neuroradiol 2004;25:1628–9.
[32] Pattany RM. 3T MR imaging: the pros and cons. AJNR Am J Neuroradiol 2004;25:1455–6.
[33] Tanenbaum LN. 3T MR imaging: ready for clinical practice [letter]. AJNR Am J Neuroradiol 2004;25: 1625–7.
[34] Ross J. The high-field-strength curmudgeon. AJNR Am J Neuroradiol 2004;25:168–9.

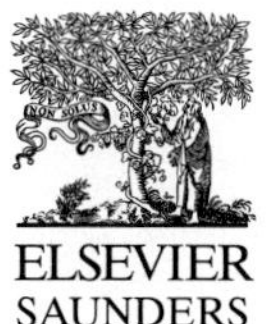

ELSEVIER
SAUNDERS

Neuroimag Clin N Am 15 (2005) 23 – 47

NEUROIMAGING
CLINICS OF
NORTH AMERICA

# Anatomy and Pathology of the Eye: Role of MR Imaging and CT

Mahmood F. Mafee, MD[a,*], Afshin Karimi, MD, PhD, JD[b], Jay Shah, BS[b], Mark Rapoport, BS[b], Sameer A. Ansari, MD, PhD[b]

[a]*Department of Radiology, University of Illinois at Chicago Medical Center, 1740 West Taylor Street, MC 931, Chicago, IL 60612, USA*
[b]*Department of Radiology, University of Illinois Hospital at Chicago, University of Illinois College of Medicine, 1801 West Taylor Street, MC 711, Chicago, IL 60612, USA*

Since the development of CT and MR imaging, significant progress has been made in ophthalmic imaging. As the technology advanced and MR imaging units improved their ability in terms of spatial resolution, the role of MR imaging in ophthalmic imaging has increased accordingly. This article considers the role of MR and CT imaging in the diagnosis of selected pathologies of the eye.

## Ocular anatomy

The globe is formed from the neuroectoderm of the forebrain (prosencephalon), the surface ectoderm of the head, the mesoderm lying between these layers, and neural crest cells [1–4]. The neuroectoderm gives rise to the retina, the fibers of the optic nerve, and smooth muscles (the sphincter and dilator papillae) of the iris [3]. The surface ectoderm on the side of the head forms the corneal and conjunctival epithelium, the lens, and the lacrimal and tarsal glands [1–4]. The surrounding mesenchyme forms the corneal stroma, the sclera, the choroids, the iris, the ciliary musculature, part of the vitreous body, and the cells lining the anterior chamber [1,4]. The eyeball (eye, globe) is made up of three primary layers (Fig. 1): (1) the sclera, or outer layer, which is composed of collagen-elastic tissue; (2) the uvea (uveal tract), or middle layer, which is richly vascular and contains pigmented tissue consisting of the choroid, ciliary body, and iris; and (3) the retina, or inner layer, which is the neural, sensory stratum of the eye. The eyeball is enveloped by a fascial sheath, known as the "fascia bulbi" or "Tenon's capsule." Tenon's capsule forms a socket for the eyeball and is separated from the sclera by Tenon's (episcleral) space [5]. Tenon's capsule is perforated near the equator by the vortex (vorticose) veins, the draining veins of the choroid and sclera [1,5]. Tenon's capsule is also perforated by the optic nerve and its sheath, the ciliary nerves and vessels. Tenon's capsule fuses with the sclera and the sheath of the optic nerve around the entrance of the optic nerve [5]. Tenon's capsule blends with the sclera just behind the corneoscleral junction and fuses with the bulbar conjunctiva [1]. The tendons of the extrinsic ocular muscles pierce Tenon's capsule to reach the sclera. At the site of perforation, Tenon's capsule is reflected back along these muscle sheaths to form a tubular sleeve [6]. The connection between the muscle fibers, sheath, and the tubular sheath is especially strong at the point where the two fuse [5,6]. For this reason, the muscles retain their attachment to the capsule and do not retract extensively after enucleation (tenotomy) [5,6].

### *Sclera*

The sclera is the outer supporting layer of the globe, extending from the limbus at the margin of the cornea to the optic nerve, where it becomes continuous with the dural sheath of the optic nerve [1]. The

* Corresponding author.
*E-mail address:* mfmafee@uic.edu (M.F. Mafee).


doi:10.1016/j.nic.2005.02.005

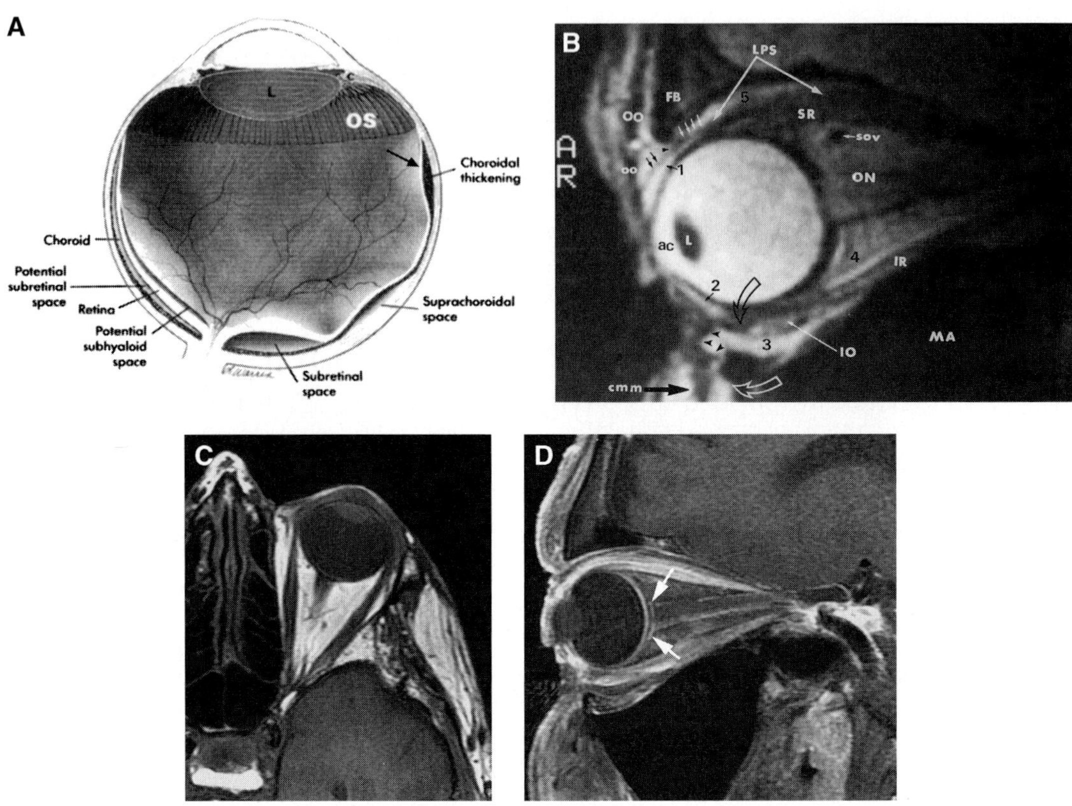


Fig. 1. (*A*) Ocular structures and various intraocular potential spaces. C, ciliary body; L, lens; OS, ora serrata. (*Modified from* Mafee MF, Inoue Y, Mafee RF. Ocular and orbital imaging. Neuroimaging Clin North Am 1996;6:292.) (*B*) Sagittal T2-weighted MR image (1.5 T) shows fibers of orbicilaris oculi (OO), frontal bone (FB), levator palpebrae superioris (LPS), extraconal fat (5), superior rectus muscle (SR), superior ophthalmic vein (SOV), optic nerve (ON), intraconal fatty reticulum (4), inferior rectus muscle (IR), maxillary antrum (MA), inferior oblique muscle (IO), extraconal fat (3), anterior wall of maxillary sinus (*white open arrow*), complex muscles of the mouth (cmm), orbital septum (*arrowheads*), presumed suspensory ligament of Lockwood (*black open arrow*), inferior (2) and superior fornices (1), anterior chamber (ac), lens (L), superior tarsal plate (*black arrows*), and the tendon of insertion of levator palpebrae superioris (*white arrows*). This tendon is an aponeurosis that descends posterior to the orbital septum (the orbital septum is depicted as an ill-defined image [*arrowhead*] in this section). The tendinous fibers then pierce the orbital septum and become attached to the anterior surface of the superior tarsal plate. Some of its fibers pass forward between the muscle bundles of the orbicularis oculi (OO) to attach to the skin. (*From* Mafee MF, Valvassori GE, Becker M, editors. Imaging of the head and neck. Stuttgart (Germany): Thieme; 2005; with permission.) (*C*) Axial T1-weighted image (566/12 ms, repetition time/echo time [TR/TE], 2.5-mm thick section, 352 × 192 matrix, 2 NEX, 160 × 160–mm field of view) obtained on a 3-T MR imaging unit, using eight-channel head coil, showing normal eye and orbit. (*D*) Sagittal fat-suppressed T1-weighted image (416/12 ms, TR/TE, 3-mm thick section, 320 × 192 matrix, 2 NEX, 140 × 140–mm field of view) obtained on a 3-T MR imaging unit using eight-channel head coil, showing normal eye and orbit. Note normal enhancement of uveoretinal coat and optic nerve meninges. Arrows point most likely to chemical shift artifact, rather than Tenon's capsule enhancement.

potential episcleral (Tenon's) space is between the outer aspect of the sclera and inner aspect of Tenon's capsule. The potential suprachoroidal space is between the inner aspect of the sclera and the outer aspect of the choroid [1,2]. In adults the sclera is 1 mm thick posteriorly, thinning at the equator to 0.6 mm. It is thinnest (0.3 mm) immediately posterior to the tendinous insertions of the rectus muscles [1,2]. The posterior scleral foramen is the site of scleral perforation by the optic nerve. At this site, the sclera is fused with the dural and arachnoid sheaths of the optic nerve. The lamina cribrosa is where the optic nerve fibers pierce the sclera.

### *Uvea (choroid, ciliary body, and iris)*

The uveal tract (from the Latin *uva* or grape) is a pigmented vascular layer that lies between the sclera and the retina (see Fig. 1). It consists of the choroid, the ciliary body, and the iris.

*Choroid*

The choroid is the section of the uveal tract that extends from the optic nerve to the ora serrata (where the sensory retina ends), beyond which it continues as the ciliary body [1,2]. The thickness of the choroid varies from 0.22 mm at the posterior pole to 0.10 mm near the ora serrata, at the optic nerve head, where it forms part of the optic nerve canal, and at the point of internal penetration of the vortex veins [1,2]. The uvea is supplied by the ophthalmic artery. The inner surface of the choroid is smooth and firmly attached to the retinal pigment epithelium (RPE). Its outer surface is roughened and is firmly attached to the sclera in the region of the optic nerve and where the posterior ciliary arteries and ciliary nerve enter the eye. It is also tethered to the sclera where the vortex veins leave the eyeball. This accounts for the characteristic shape of choroidal detachment (CD), which shows tethering at the site of the vortex veins and posterior ciliary arteries and ciliary nerves. Grossly, the choroid can be divided into four layers, extending from internally to externally as (1) Bruch's membrane, (2) the choriocapillaris, (3) the stroma, and (4) the suprachoroid [1]. Bruch's membrane (2–4 μm thick) is a rough, acellular, amorphous, bilamellar structure, situated between the retina and the rest of the choroid. Microscopically, Bruch's membrane consists of five layers: (1) the basement membrane of the RPE, (2) the inner collagenous zone, (3) a meshwork of elastic fibers, (4) the outer collagenous zone, and (5) the basement membrane of the choriocapillaris [4,7,8]. When a choroidal malignant melanoma penetrates through Bruch's membrane, it results in a characteristic mushroom-shaped (collar button) growth configuration.

*Ciliary body*

The ciliary body is continuous posteriorly with the choroid and anteriorly with the iris (see Fig. 1). The ciliary body can be considered as a complete ring that runs around the inside of the anterior sclera. The anterior surface of the ciliary body is ridged or plicated and is called the pars plicata. The pars plicata is 2 mm in length and is composed of about 70 ciliary processes arranged radially [9]. The posterior surface of the ciliary body is smooth and flat and is called the pars plana. The pars plana is 4 mm in length and is located between pars plicata and the ora serrata. The ciliary body is made up of (1) the ciliary epithelium, (2) the ciliary stroma, and (3) the ciliary muscle. The epithelium consists of two layers of cuboidal cells that cover the inner surface of the ciliary body [1,2,4,9]. The inner layer is comprised of pigmented epithelial cells, whereas the outer layer is comprised of nonpigmented epithelial cells [9]. The ciliary stroma consists of loose connective tissue, rich in blood vessels and melanocytes, containing the embedded ciliary muscle [1]. The aqueous humor is produced in the nonpigmented epithelial layer of the ciliary body [9]. The nonpigmented epithelial cells secrete mucopolysaccharide acid, one of the main components of the vitreous [9].

*Iris*

The iris forms the anterior portion of the uvea. It is a thin, contractile, pigmented diaphragm with a central aperture, the pupil (see Fig. 1). It is suspended in the aqueous humor between the cornea and the lens and divides the anterior ocular compartment (segment) into anterior and posterior chambers. The aqueous humor, formed by the ciliary processes in the posterior chamber, circulates through the pupil into the anterior chamber and exits into the sinus venous (canal of Schlemm) at the iridocorneal angle [1,2,4]. The iris consists of a stroma and two epithelial layers. The stroma consists of vascular connective tissue containing melanocytes, nerve fibers, the smooth muscle of the sphincter papillae, and the myoepithelial cells of the dilator papillae [4]. The iris pigment epithelium is continuous with the pigmented and nonpigmented layers of the ciliary body.

*Retina*

The retina is the sensory inner layer of the globe. The internal surface of the retina is in contact with the vitreous body and its external surface is in contact with the choroid. Grossly, the retina can be considered as having two layers: the inner layer, which is the sensory retina (ie, photoreceptors) and the first- and second-order neurons (ganglion cells) and neuroglial elements of the retina (Müller's cells, or sustentacular gliocytes); and the outer layer, which is the RPE, consisting of a single layer of cells whose nuclei are adjacent to the basal lamina (Bruch's membrane) of the choroid [1,10,11]. The retina is very thin, measuring 0.056 mm near the disk and 0.1 mm anteriorly at the ora serrata. It is thinnest at the fovea of the macula [1]. The sensory retina extends forward from the optic disk to a point just posterior to the ciliary body. Here the nervous tissues of the retina

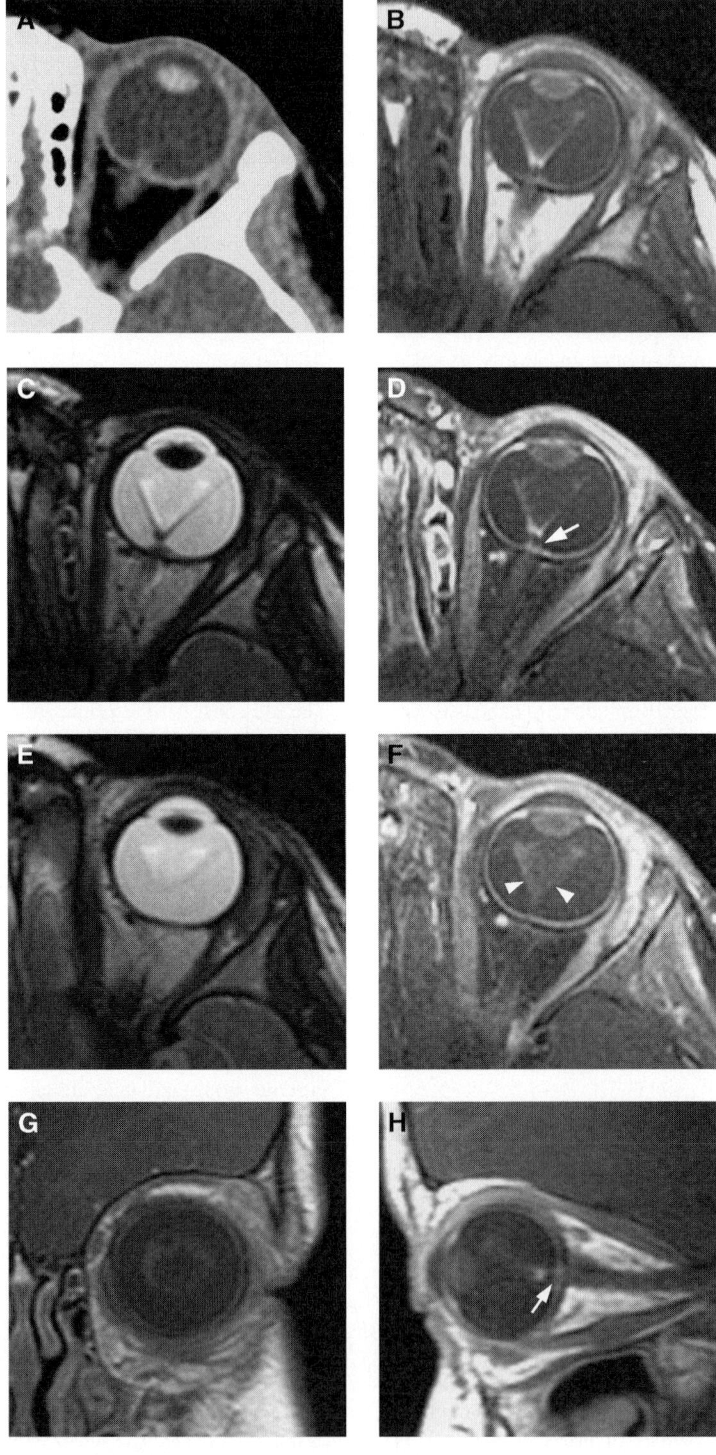
A
B
C
D
E
F
G
H

end and its anterior edge forms a crenated wavy ring called ora serrata [1]. The RPE at the ora serrata becomes continuous with the pigmented and nonpigmented cell layers of the ciliary body and its processes [1,2]. The macula, the center of the retina, lies 3.5 mm temporal to the optic disk. The retina is attached very tightly at the margin of the optic disk and at its anterior termination at the ora serrata. It is also firmly attached to the vitreous, but loosely to the RPE and it is nourished by the choroid and the RPE [1,2]. The disk is pierced by the central retinal artery and vein. At the disk, there is complete absence of rods and cones. The disk is insensitive to light and is referred to as the "blind spot." The RPE cells are joined to each other by tight junctions. This arrangement forms a barrier, the so-called "retinal blood barrier." This limits the flow of ions and prevents diffusion of large toxic molecules from the choroid capillaries to the photoreceptors of the retina. The blood supply to the retina is from two sources: the outer lamina, including the rods and cones is supplied by the choroidal capillaries (the vessels do not enter the tissues, but tissue fluid exudes between these cells); the inner parts of the retina are supplied by the central retinal artery [1,2]. The retina depends on both of these circulations, neither of which alone is sufficient [1,2,4]. Small anastomoses occur between the branches of the posterior ciliary arteries and the central retinal artery (cilioretinal artery). The central retinal vein leaves the eyeball through the lamina cribrosa. The vein crosses the subarachnoid space and drains directly into the cavernous sinus or the superior ophthalmic vein. The retina has no lymphatic vessels.

### *Vitreous*

The vitreous body occupies the space between the lens and retina and represents two thirds of the volume of the eye or approximately 4 mL [12]. All but 1% to 2% of the vitreous is water, bound to a fibrillar collagen meshwork of soluble proteins, some salts, and hyaluronic acid [1,2,10]. The clear, gel-like fluid that fills the vitreous chamber possesses a network of fine collagen fibrils that form scaffolding [1,2,4]. The vitreous body is the largest and simplest connective tissue present as a single structure in the human body [11]. Any insult to the vitreous body may result in a fibroproliferative reaction (eg, vitreoretinopathy of prematurity or diabetes), which can subsequently result in a tractional retinal detachment (RD) [10]. The vitreous body is bounded by the anterior and posterior hyaloid membranes. As one ages, the vitreous gel may undergo changes and start to shrink or thicken, forming strands or clumps inside the vitreous chamber, causing the so-called "floaters." Floaters are in fact tiny clumps of gel or cells inside the vitreous chamber. When the vitreous gel shrinks, it creates traction on the posterior hyaloid membrane, resulting in posterior vitreous detachment (Figs. 2 and 3). The vitreous body is attached to the sensory retina, especially at the ora serrata and the margin of the optic disk [4]. It is also attached to the ciliary epithelium in the region of the pars plana [4]. The attachment of the vitreous to the lens is firm in young people and weakens with age [1,2]. During the first month of gestation, the space between the lens and the retina contains the primary vitreous. It consists of the embryonic intraocular hyaloid vascular system, embryonic connective tissue, and fibrillar meshwork. Shortly, collagen fibers and a ground substance or gel component consisting of hyaluronic acid are produced. They form the secondary vitreous and begin to replace the vascular elements of the primary vitreous [1]. By the fourteenth week of gestation, the secondary vitreous begins to fill the vitreous cavity. By the sixth month of fetal development, the cavity of the eye is filled with the secondary vitreous, which is identical to the adult vitreous. The primary vitreous is reduced to a small central space, Cloquet's canal (hyaloid canal), which runs in an S-shaped course

Fig. 2. Presumed posterior hyaloid detachment. An 18-month-old child who has leukocoria of the left eye. Retinoblastoma could not be excluded on clinical evaluation. (*A*) Axial CT scan shows a noncalcified lesion, presumed to be hematoma at the left optic disk. Note a faint V-shaped linear image, extending toward the optic disk. Axial unenhanced T1-weighted (*B*), axial T2-weighted (*C*), axial enhanced fat-suppressed T1-weighted (*D*), axial T2-weighted (*E*), axial enhanced fat-suppressed T1-weighted (*F*), coronal enhanced T1-weighted (*G*), and sagittal enhanced T1-weighted (*H*) MR images showing the detached posterior hyaloid membrane (*arrowheads* in *F*). Note that the apex of the V-shaped detachment, is connected to the optic disk by a faint ill-defined linear tissue (*arrows* in *D* and *H*), representing the attached part of the vitreous to the retina at the edge of the optic disk. (A–C *from* Mafee MF, Valvassori GE, Becker M, editors. Imaging of the head and neck. Stuttgart (Germany): Thieme; 2004; with permission.)

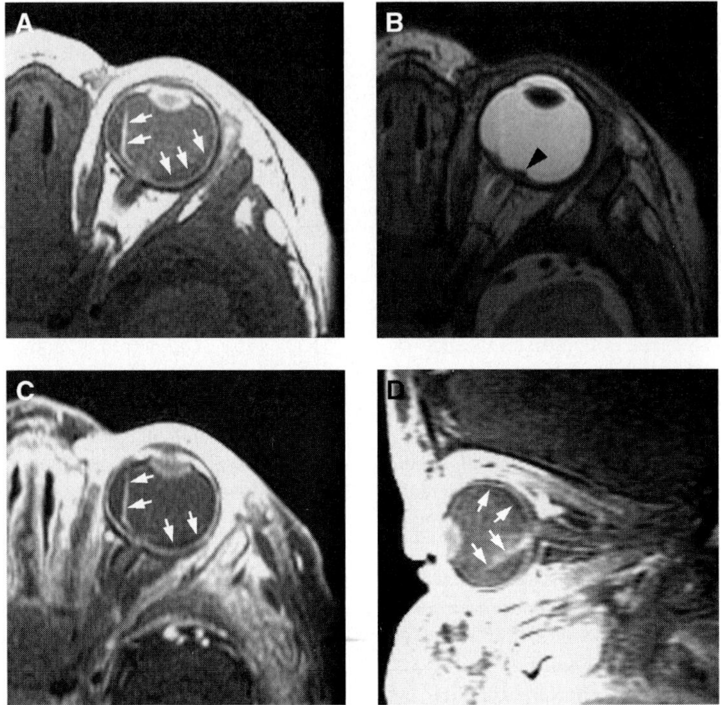


Fig. 3. Posterior hyaloid detachment. Axial unenhanced T1-weighted (*A*), axial T2-weighted (*B*), axial enhanced fat-suppressed T1-weighted (*C*), and sagittal enhanced fat-suppressed T1-weighted (*D*) MR images showing detachment of the vitreous (*arrows*). The vitreous base attachment to the retina at the optic disk is not detached. The hypointensity adjacent to the disk (*arrowhead* in *B*) is thought to be caused by hemorrhage.

between the optic disk and the posterior surface of the lens. During fetal life this channel contains the hyaloid artery. The artery disappears about 6 weeks before birth, and the canal becomes filled with liquid [4]. The vitreous body transmits lights, supports the posterior surface of the lens, and assists in holding the sensory retina against the RPE.

## Ocular pathology

### *Intraocular potential spaces and ocular detachments*

There are basically three potential spaces in the eye (see Fig. 1) that can accumulate fluid, causing detachment of various layers of the eyeball: (1) the posterior hyaloid space, the potential space between the base of the vitreous (posterior hyaloid membrane) and the sensory retina; (2) the subretinal space, the potential space between the sensory retina and the RPE; and (3) the suprachoroidal space, the potential space between choroid and the sclera. Another potential space is the episcleral or Tenon's space, which is between the outer surface of the sclera and inner surface of the Tenon's capsule.

### *Posterior hyaloid detachment*

Separation of the posterior hyaloid membrane from the sensory retina is referred to as "posterior vitreous" or "hyaloid detachment" [1,2]. In older patients, the vitreous tends to undergo degeneration and liquefaction. Extensive vitreous liquefaction leads to posterior hyaloid detachment. Accelerated vitreous liquefaction is associated with significant myopia, surgical or nonsurgical trauma, intraocular inflammation, post laser surgery of the eye, and persistent hyperplastic primary vitreous (PHPV). On CT and MR imaging, the detached posterior hyaloid membrane can be seen as a membrane within the vitreous cavity (see Fig. 2). The detached membrane is separated from the disk (or may be attached to the disk by a thin band) and attached at the level of ora serrata (see Figs. 2 and 3). There may be fluid in the retrohyaloid space, which shifts its location in the lateral decubitus position.

### *Retinal detachment*

RD occurs when the sensory retina is separated from the RPE. RD resulting from a hole or tear in the retina is referred to as "rhegmatogenous" (*rhegma* from Greek meaning to rent or rupture) RD. The sine qua non for a rhegmatogenous RD is vitreous liquefaction. Extensive vitreous liquefaction causes posterior hyaloid detachment, which in turn causes a tear at the site of vitreoretinal attachment or adhesion. The ensuing retinal break allows vitreous fluid to pass through the break into the subretinal space. Rhegmatogenous RDs are rare in pediatric patients. Most RDs in children are nonrhegmatogenous but are secondary to various ocular disease, such as retinoblastoma, PHPV, retinopathy of prematurity, Coats' disease (see Fig. 4), toxocariasis, and others. RD may be the result of retraction caused by a mass; a fibroproliferative disease in the vitreous, such as vitreoretinopathy of prematurity or vitreoretinopathy of diabetes mellitus; or accompanying an inflammatory process, such as *Toxocara* endophthalmitis [1,2]. Serous or exudative RD develops when the retinal-blood barrier is damaged. A breakdown of the retinal blood barrier with impairment of the RPE results in RD (nonrhegmatogenous RD). An increased fluid flow into the potential subretinal space (eg, in Coats' disease, scleritis, choroidal inflammation, choroidal mass, other intraocular tumor, or vitreous disease entities) may result in exudative RD. Exudative fluid may be shallow or bullous. Fluid may not extend all the way to the ora serrata (Fig. 5). In severe cases the

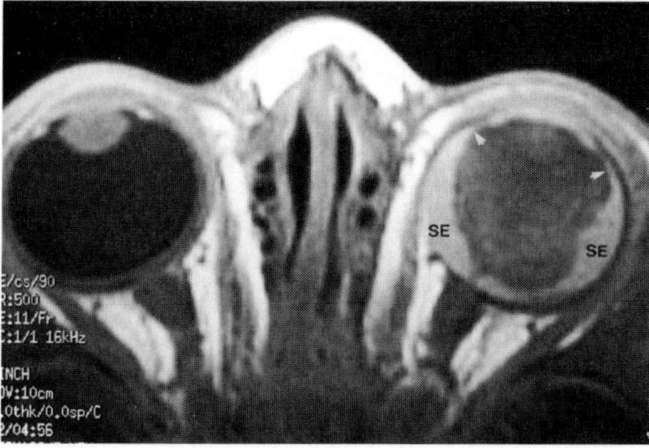


Fig. 4. Retinal detachment. Enhanced axial T1-weighted MR image in a child who has Coats' disease shows an exudative retinal detachment of the left eye. Note subretinal exudates (SE), which had the same signal intensity on unenhanced axial MR image. The detached sensory retina is limited at the ora serrata (*arrows*) and at the optic disk. The increased intensity of the left vitreous is related to protein leaking into the vitreous from abnormal retinal vessels.

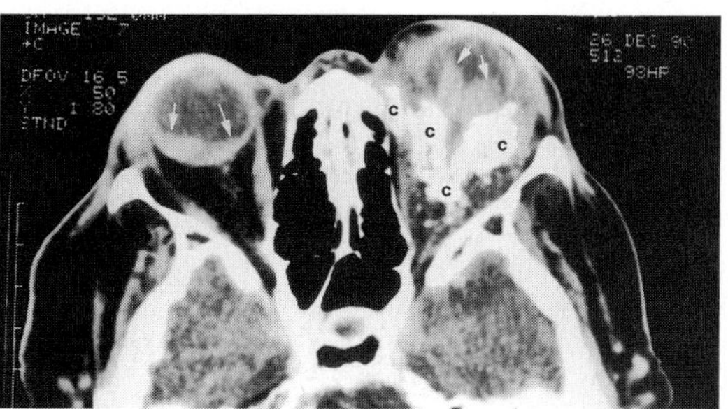


Fig. 5. Bilateral retinal detachment and orbital primary amyloidosis. Axial CT scan shows bilateral exudative retinal detachment (*arrows*). The detachment appears bullous on the left eye. The irregular calcifications (C) involving the left retrobulbar space are related to biopsy-proved amyloidosis. The cause of retinal detachment was not clear in this case.

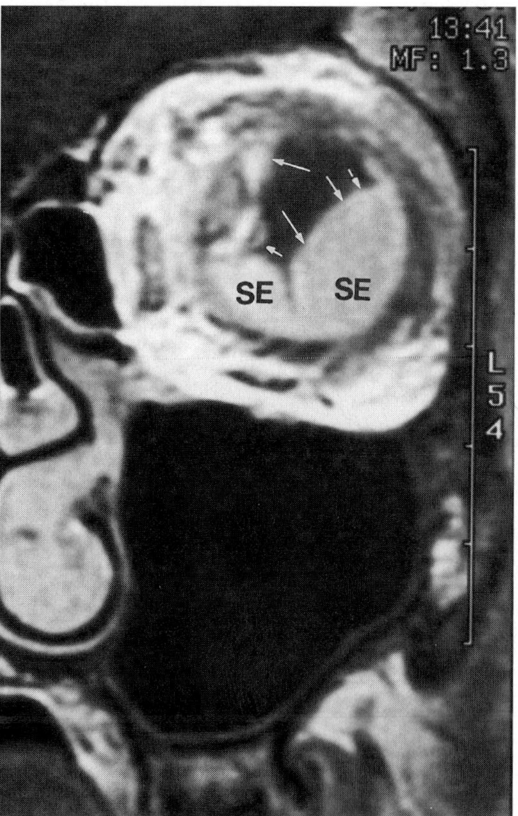


Fig. 6. Retinal detachment. Coronal enhanced T1-weighted MR image shows the characteristic corrugated retinal folds (*arrows*) on coronal view. The subretinal exudate (SE) signal was the same on unenhanced T1-weighted MR images.

**Box 1. Common and uncommon causes of serous retinal detachment**

*Common conditions*

- Coats' disease
- Retinoblastoma
- Retinopathy of prematurity
- Choroidal tumors (primary or secondary)
- Posterior scleritis
- Vogt-Koyanagi-Harada syndrome
- Exudative age-related macular degeneration
- Postsurgical (associated with choroidal detachment)
- Central serous chorioretinopathy

*Uncommon conditions*

- Orbital inflammation (pseudotumor, cellulitis)
- Infectious retinochoroiditis (toxoplasmosis, syphilis, cytomegalovirus, cat-scratch disease)
- Uveal effusion syndrome
- Vasculitis (polyarteritis nodosa, systemic lupus erythematosus, Goodpasture's syndrome)
- Acute vascular or hemodynamic compromise (hypertensive crisis, toxemia of pregnancy, nephropathy)
- Nanophthalmos (eyes with thick sclera and short axial length)
- Optic nerve pits, colobomas, and morning glory anomaly
- Familial exudative vitreoretinopathy
- Sympathetic ophthalmia
- Orbital arteriovenous malformation[a]

[a] In orbital inflammation and arteriovenous malformation the venous flow from the eye may be compromised by vascular engorgement. This results in exophthalmos and further vascular compromise. This can lead to retinal and choroidal effusion. *Modified from* Anand R. Serous detachment of the neural retina. In: Yanoff M, Duker JS, editors. Ophthalmology. St. Louis (MO): Mosby; 1999. p. 8:40.1–40.6; with permission.

detached retina may be so bullous as to contact the posterior lens surface (Fig. 6). The common and uncommon causes of serous RD are summarized in Box 1. RD typically causes decreased vision. Other visual complaints, such as pain, photophobia, redness, sudden onset of tiny floating objects (floaters), and photopsia (flashes), may be present. The presence of sudden flashes of light and sudden appearance of floaters should cause serious consideration of RD. If RD is shallow, the diagnosis can be made easily with indirect ophthalmoscopy. If the retina is bullously detached, however, the diagnosis may be difficult [13]. Ultrasound, CT, and MR imaging can be used to make the diagnosis. In the authors' experience, MR imaging is superior to other imaging techniques to demonstrate features that could differentiate different causes of RD. Exudative RD is characterized by shifting subretinal fluid, which assumes a dependent position beneath the retina. On CT and MR imaging, the appearance of RD varies with the amount of exudate, presence of hemorrhage, and organization of the subretinal materials. In a section taken at the level of the optic nerve disk, RD is seen with a characteristic V-shaped configuration with the apex at the optic disk and its extremities toward the ora serrata (see Fig. 4). When total RD is present and the entire vitreous cavity is ablated, the leaves of the detached retina may touch at the center of the eye and appear as a folding membrane extending from the optic disk to the posterior surface of the lens, simulating Cloquet's canal. The MR imaging signal intensity of subretinal fluid depends on the protein content and presence or absence of hemorrhage. The subretinal fluid of an exudative RD is rich in protein, giving higher CT attenuation values and stronger MR imaging signal intensities (on T1-weighted MR images) (see Fig. 4) than those seen in the subretinal fluid (transudate) of a rhegmatogenous detachment. In rhegmatogenous RD, produced by a retinal tear and subsequent ingress of vitreous fluid into the subretinal space, the signal of subretinal transudate is almost isointense to vitreous, making visualization of detached retina more difficult. RD is seen on coronal CT and MR images as a characteristic folding membrane, representing corrugated retinal folds (Fig. 6).

### *Choroidal detachment and choroidal effusion*

CD is caused by the accumulation of fluid (serous CD) or blood (hemorrhagic CD) in the potential suprachoroidal space [1,2,10,14–16]. Serous CD frequently occurs after intraocular surgery, penetrating ocular trauma, or inflammatory choroidal disorders [14]. Ocular hypotony is the essential underlying cause of serous CD. Ocular hypotony may be the result of ocular inflammatory diseases (uveitis, scleritis); accidental perforation of the eye; ocular surgery; or intensive glaucoma therapy. The pressure within the suprachoroidal space is determined by the intraocular pressure, the intracapillary blood pressure, and the oncotic pressure exerted by the plasma protein colloids [17]. The capillaries of the choroid are fenestrated and these openings are covered by diaphragms, which permit the relatively free exchange of material between the choriocapillaris and the surrounding tissues [18]. Ocular hypotony results in increased permeability of the choriocapillaris, and this in turn leads to the transudation of fluid from the choroidal vasculature into the uveal tissue causing diffuse swelling of the entire choroid (choroidal effusion). As the edema of the choroid increases, fluid may accumulate in the potential suprachoroidal space, resulting in serous or exudative CD [14–16]. Other causes of choroidal effusion include inflammatory disorders of the eye, myxedema, photocoagulation, retinal cryopexy, Vogt-Koyanagi-Harada syndrome, nanophthalmos, and idiopathic uveal effusion syndrome. Nanophthalmos is an autosomal-recessive disorder in which there is bilateral short axial length globes, normal-sized lenses, and thick sclerae. As a result of scleral thickening, the scleral outflow channels and transscleral passage of vortex veins become impaired. This can lead to choroidal congestion, choroidal thickening, and eventually choroidal effusion (see Fig. 7). The management of choroidal effusion in nanophthalmos and idiopathic choroidal effusion is surgical and consists of sclerotomy (scleral window operation) to decompress the vortex veins [13]. Hemorrhagic CD is a serious condition that may be associated with permanent loss of vision [19]. Both localized and massive choroidal hemorrhage may occur as a complication of most forms of ocular surgery and ocular trauma. Choroidal hemorrhage may occur in association with hemoglobinopathies, in patients receiving anticoagulant therapy, or spontaneously [19]. Intraoperative choroidal hemorrhage may progress to expulsion of intraocular tissues (expulsive choroidal hemorrhage) [19]. Clinically, the CD appears as a smooth gray–brown elevation of the choroid, extending from the ciliary body to the posterior segment [14,15]. Ophthalmoscopic visualization of the fundus may be precluded by hyphema (blood in the anterior chamber) or vitreous hemorrhage. Even when the other ocular media are clear, in pigmented eyes it is difficult to differentiate between serous and hemorrhagic CD with ophthalmoscopy [14,15]. Localized choroidal hemorrhage may be mistaken for a choroidal melanoma, particularly when it presents as a discrete, dark posterior ocular mass [19]. Ultrasonography can be very useful for the diagnosis of CD, however, ultrasonography has certain limitations in examining traumatized eyes. The appearance of serous CD and limited or diffuse hemorrhagic CD on CT has been described [14]. It appears as a smooth, dome-shaped, semilunar area of variable attenuation values. The degree of CT attenuation depends on the cause but is generally greater with inflammatory disorders of the eyeball. Hemorrhagic CD appears as either a low or high mound-like area of high density on CT. In a fresh hemorrhagic CD, the choroid and hematoma are isodense. In chronic hematoma, however, it may be possible to differentiate detached choroid and suprachoroidal fluid accumulation (see Figs. 8 and 9). Serial CT, MR imaging, and ultrasonography reveal diminishing size over a period of several weeks or months. MR imaging is an excellent method to evaluate the eye in patients who have CD, particularly if ultrasonography or CT in conjunction with the clinical examination has not provided sufficient information [1]. On MR imaging, a limited choroidal hematoma appears as a focal, well-demarcated, smooth dome-shaped or lenticular mass (Fig. 8). It is important to realize that this characteristic configuration

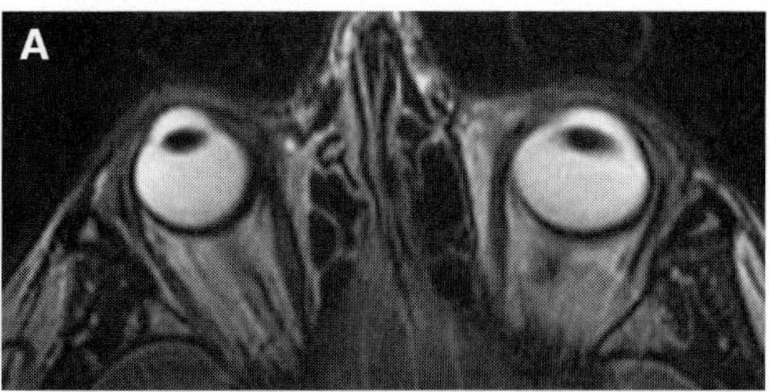


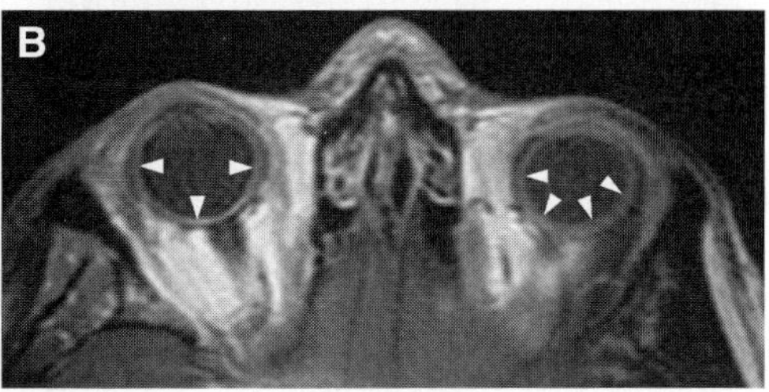


Fig. 7. Nanophthalmos and associated choroidal effusion. Axial T2-weighted (*A*) and enhanced axial T1-weighted (*B*) MR images. Note bilateral short axial length globes and marked thickened sclerae (*A*), and increased uveal enhancement (*arrowheads*), the left being greater than the right.

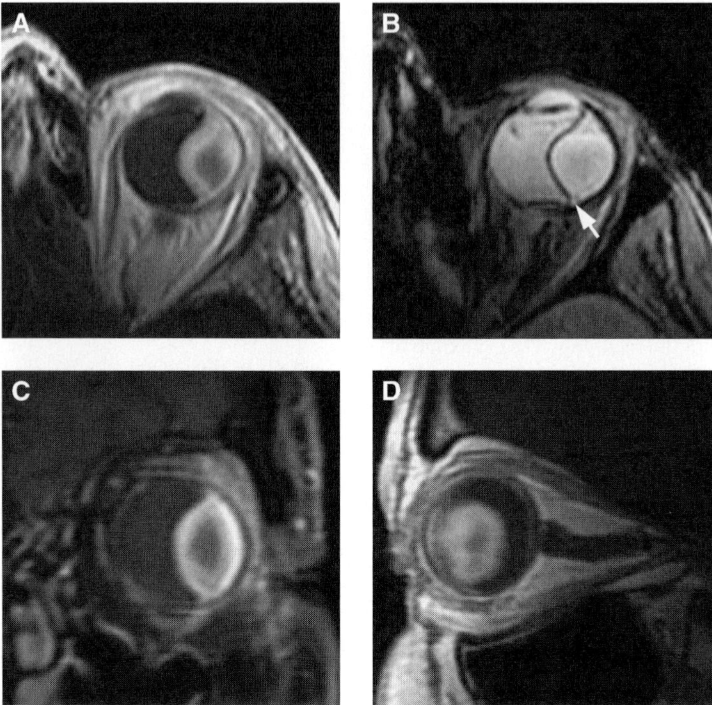


Fig. 8. Hemorrhagic choroidal detachment. Axial T1-weighted (*A*), axial T2-weighted (*B*), coronal T1-weighted (*C*), and sagittal T1-weighted (*D*) MR images showing a chronic hemorrhagic choroidal detachment. Note that the detached choroid is restricted at the expected level of the vortex vein or posterior ciliary artery (*arrow*). Note that the detached choroid extends to the ciliary body.

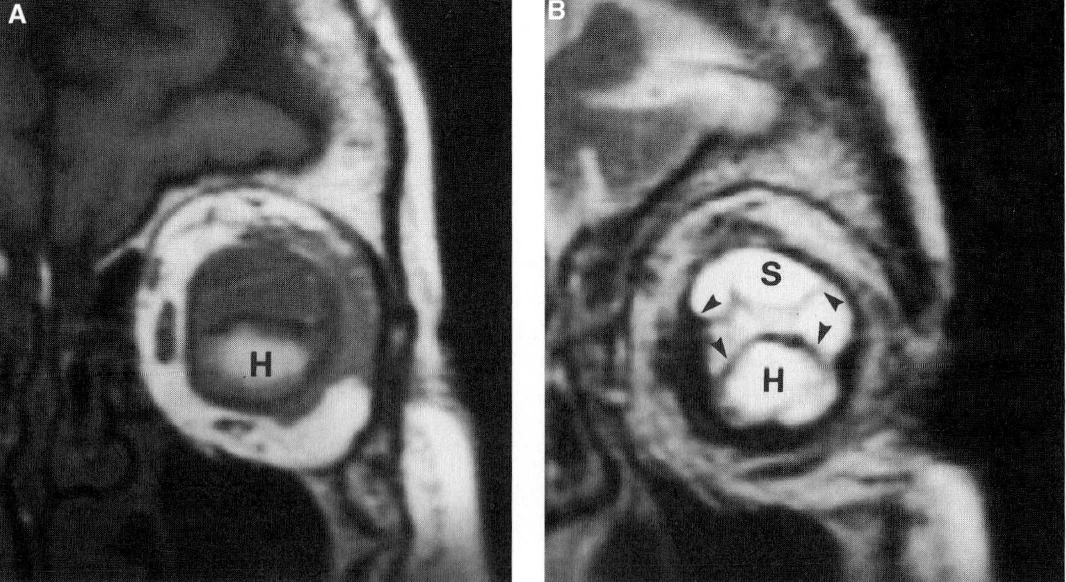


Fig. 9. Serous and hemorrhagic choroidal detachment. Coronal T1-weighted (*A*) and T2-weighted (*B*) MR images showing an inferior hemorrhagic (H) and superior serous (S) choroidal detachment. Note detached choroid (*arrows*), which is restricted at the expected level of vortex veins.

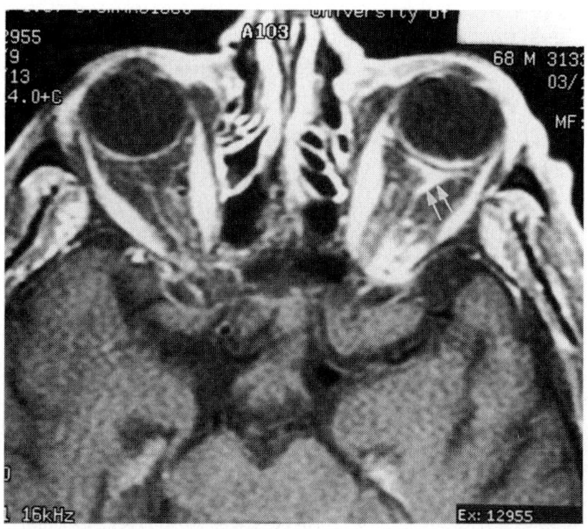


Fig. 10. Herpes zoster ophthalmitis. Axial enhanced fat-suppressed T1-weighted MR image shows abnormal enhancement along the left optic nerve sheath (*arrows*). Note also increased enhancement of left posterior globe.

usually does not change as the hematoma ages [16]. A decrease in the size of the choroidal hematoma, however, may be observed. Multiple lesions may be present (see Fig. 9). The signal intensity of choroidal hematoma depends on its age. Within the first 48 hours, the hematoma is isointense to slightly hypointense relative to the normal vitreous on T1-weighted MR images but is markedly hypointense on T2-weighted MR images. After few days, its signal intensity changes, being relatively hyperintense on T1-weighted and hypointense on T2-weighted MR images. Chronic choroidal hematoma (3 weeks or older) become hyperintense on T1-weighted and T2-weighted MR images (see Figs. 8 and 9). Serous CD and choroidal effusion have a different MR appearance compared with choroidal hematoma. The fluid in the suprachoroidal space in serous CD is often hypodense on CT, and its MR appearance is that of an exudate (Fig. 9). At times, the appearance of CD and RD may be confused. Scleral attachments of the vortex veins restrict further detachment of the choroid beyond the anchoring point of the vortex veins, however, and similarly beyond the short posterior ciliary arteries and nerves. This restriction usually results in a characteristic appearance of the leaves of the detached choroid, which unlike the detached retinal leaves do not extend to the region of the optic nerve (see Figs. 8 and 9). In addition, unlike the detached leaves of the retina, which end at the ora serrata, the detached choroid can extend to the ciliary body and also result in ciliary detachment (see Fig. 10).

## Ocular inflammatory disorders

The eye may be affected by known or idiopathic inflammatory processes. A host of infectious diseases may affect the globe. Viral infections include herpes simplex, herpes zoster (Fig. 10), cytomegalovirus (Fig. 11), rubella, rubeola, mumps, variola, varicella, and infectious mononucleosis [1]. Bacterial diseases include tuberculosis, syphilis, Lyme disease, brucellosis, leprosy, cat-scratch disease, *Escherichia coli* infection, and other agents.

Fungal infections, particularly candidiasis, may involve the globes in diabetic and immunocompromised patients [1]. Parasitic infections, particularly *Toxocara canis*, cause granulomatous chorioretinitis with an eosinophilic abscess.

### *Scleritis*

The sclera may be the site of a number of inflammatory or noninflammatory processes. Episcleritis is a relatively common idiopathic inflammation of a thin layer of loose connective tissue between the sclera and the conjunctiva. Episcleritis is usually self-limited and resolves within 1 or 2 weeks [20]. Imaging is not indicated in episcleritis. In contrast to episcleritis, scleritis is a rare condition, and a more serious disorder. Scleritis can occur as an idiopathic condition (50%) or in association with rheumatoid arthritis, other connective tissue diseases, or with a group of other disorders, such as Wegener's granulomatosis, relapsing polychondritis, inflammatory bowel disease, Crohn's disease, Cogan's syndrome, and sarcoidosis [1]. In scleritis, histopathology may demonstrate granulomatous or nongranulomatous

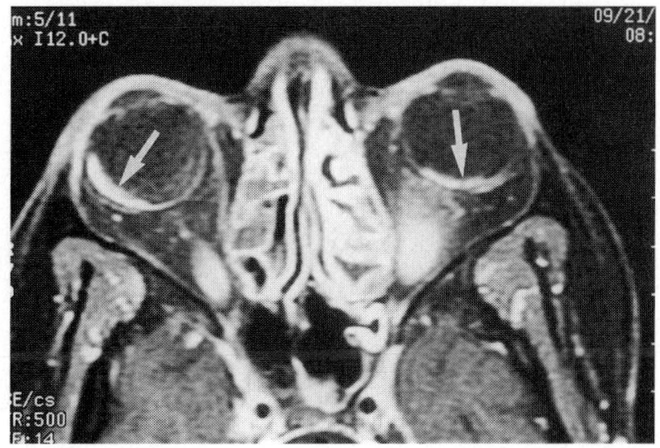


Fig. 11. Cytomegalovirus retinitis. Axial enhanced fat-suppressed T1-weighted MR image shows marked enhancement of posterior globes (*arrows*) in this immunocompromised patient who has bilateral cytomegalovirus retinitis.

inflammation, vasculitis, and scleral necrosis [20]. Histopathologically, posterior scleritis is classified into two forms: nodular and diffuse. The term "posterior scleritis" refers to scleral inflammation behind the equator. Patients who have posterior scleritis may develop exudative RD, disk swelling, and CD [20,21]. Scleritis may be associated with uveitis (iritis, choroiditis) and increased intraocular pressure. Inflammatory debris may block scleral emissary veins, resulting in elevated episcleral venous pressure and hence elevated intraocular pressure. Ciliary body detachment adjacent to active anterior scleritis may cause angle closure glaucoma. If scleritis is associated with uveitis, the trabecular meshwork may be clogged with inflammatory debris and cells, causing glaucoma. On CT scans and MR images, posterior scleritis results in thickening of the sclera (Fig. 12). There may be associated thickening of Tenon's capsule (sclerotenonitis) and secondary serous RD or serous CD. In general, it is easier to

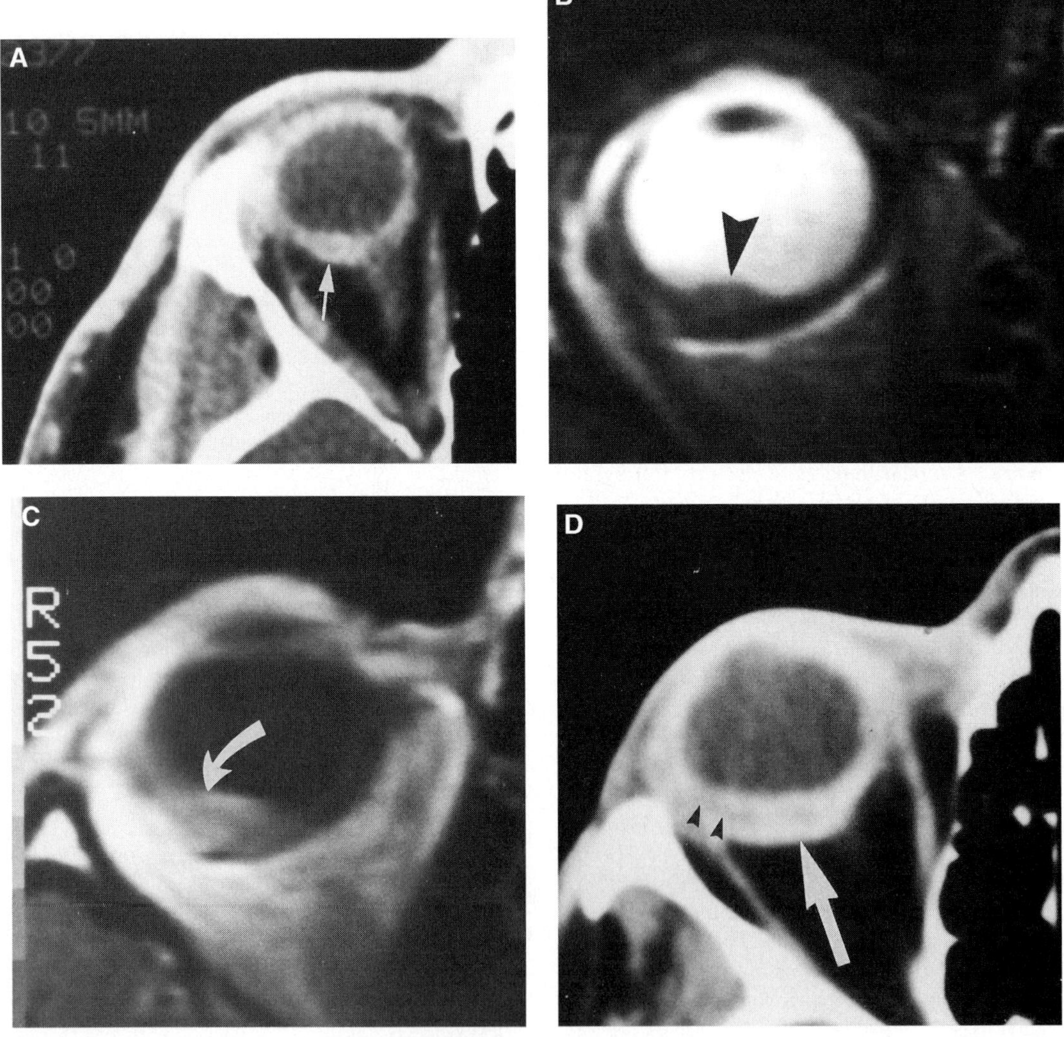


Fig. 12. Posterior nodular scleritis. (*A*) Axial enhanced CT scan shows abnormal enhancement along the posterior aspect of the right globe (*arrow*). Axial T2-weighted (*B*) and axial enhanced T1-weighted (*C*) MR images showing a mass-like lesion (*arrowhead* in *B* and *arrow* in *C*) compatible with posterior nodular scleritis. This CT and MR imaging appearance may not be differentiated from a choroidal mass. Patient responded well to a course of steroid therapy. (*D*) Enhanced axial CT scan in another patient who has necrotizing keratitis and scleritis showing thickening of the Tenon's capsule (*arrow*), fluid in the episcleral space (*arrowheads*), and marked thickening and increased enhancement of the sclera.

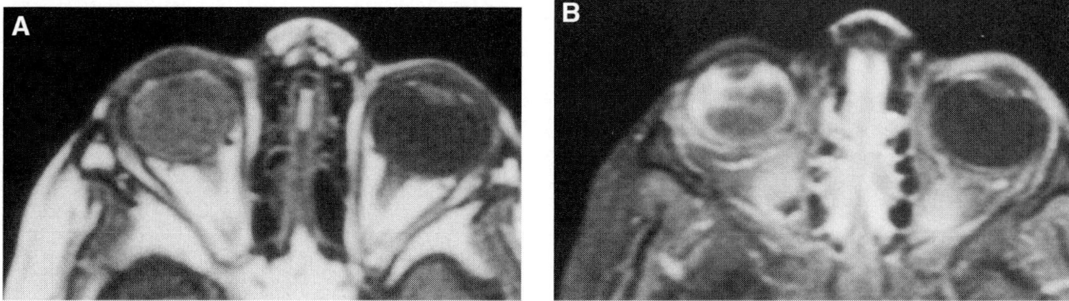


Fig. 13. Granulomatous uveitis. Axial T1-weighted (*A*) and enhanced fat-suppressed axial T1-weighted (*B*) MR images in a 3-year-old child showing marked enhancement of the right globe, predominantly adjacent to the ciliary body. Note increased intensity of the vitreous in precontrast T1-weighted image (*A*), representing leakage of protein into the vitreous or associated vitreous inflammation.

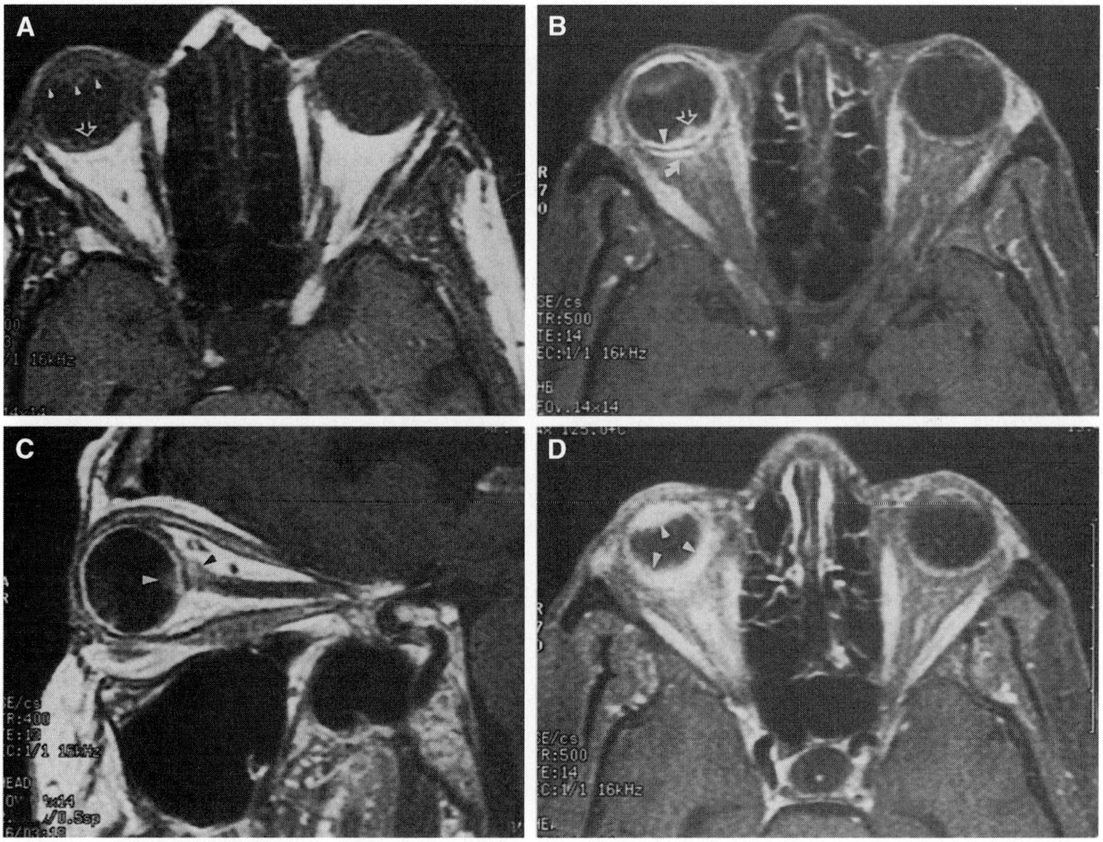

Fig. 14. Ocular sarcoidosis panuveitis. (*A*) Unenhanced axial T1-weighted (500/13 TR/TE) MR image shows nodular thickening of the posterior aspect of the right globe (*arrow*) and thickening of the anterior segment (*arrowheads*) of the right globe. (*B*) Enhanced axial fat-suppressed T1-weighted (500/13 TR/TE) MR image shows nodular enhancement of the posterior aspect of the right globe (*arrowhead* and *open arrow*) related to granulomatous involvement of the choroid. Note enhancement of the anterior segment of the right globe. Notice abnormal enhancement of Tenon's capsule (*curved arrow*). (*C*) Enhanced sagittal T1-weighted (400/13 TR/TE) MR image shows granuloma at the optic disk (*white arrowhead*) and involvement of the optic nerve (*black arrowhead*). (*D*) Enhanced axial fat-suppressed T1-weighted (500/14 TR/TE) MR image shows enhancement of markedly thickened uveal tract (*arrowheads*). (*From* Mafee MF, Dorodi S, Pai E. Saroidosis of the eye, orbit, and central nervous system. Role of MR imaging. Radiol Clin North Am 1999;37:74.)

see these changes related to posterior scleritis on CT scans rather than MR images. Posterior nodular scleritis is a focal or zonal necrotizing granulomatous inflammation of the sclera. On imaging this entity may mimic choroidal malignant melanoma or ocular lymphoma.

*Uveitis*

Inflammation of the uvea (uveitis) may be limited to the anterior uvea (iritis), ciliary body (cyclitis), the posterior uvea, or the choroid (choroiditis, posterior uveitis). Posterior cyclitis (pars planitis) is referred to as "intermediate uveitis." Inflammatory diseases of the uvea are seldom limited to this vascularized layer of the eye. The sclera and retina are usually involved [1]. Posterior uveitis may be focal, multifocal, diffuse choroiditis, chorioretinitis, or neurouveitis [22]. The etiology of uveitis is often unknown. Traumatic iridocyclitis is the most common cause of anterior uveitis. Most intermediate uveitis is idiopathic [22]. The most common causes of panuveitis are idiopathic and sarcoidosis. Uveitis may be seen in patients who have juvenile rheumatoid arthritis, seronegative spondyloarthropathies, and herpetic keratouveitis. Uveitis may be caused by a specific organism, such as *Toxoplasma*. Other causes include bacterial posterior uveitis including Whipple's disease; viral uveitis (cytomegalovirus, herpes simplex, Coxsackie virus); fungal uveitis; and parasitic uveitis. Some forms of uveitis, such as sarcoidosis, Vogt-Koyanagi-Harada syndrome, and Behçet's syndrome, have strong ethnic association. Vogt-Koyanagi-Harada syndrome is an idiopathic bilateral chronic granulomatous uveitis, with exudative choroidal effusion and nonrhegmatogenous RD associated with alopecia, vitiligo, hearing problems, meningeal signs, pleocytosis in the cerebrospinal fluid, and poliosis. Behçet's syndrome is a multisystem vasculitis of unknown cause. Patients usually present with a history of oral and genital ulcerations. Vogt-Koyanagi-Harada is a cell-mediated autoimmune disease. It is often a self-limiting disease. Sympathetic uveitis is a rare bilateral autoimmune-related uveitis that develops after penetrating injury to the eye. Larval uveitis results from ingestion of the eggs of the nematode *T canis* or *Toxocara cati*. Imaging is not indicated in classic nontraumatic anterior uveitis. Patients who have granulomatous uveitis or posterior uveitis of unclear cause may benefit from ultrasound, CT, or MR imaging to assess the degree of choroidal or scleral thickening, masses (eg, abscess), and to evaluate for the presence of RD, choroidal effusion, or intraocular foreign bodies, particularly in patients who have media opacities (Figs. 13 and 14). Optic disk enhancement on MR imaging and CT scans may be seen in patients who have pseudotumor cerebri (Fig. 15), simulating posterior uveitis, uveoneurol retinitis of cat-scratch disease, and retinal and choroidal tumors.

*Endophthalmitis*

Endophthalmitis refers to an intraocular infectious or noninfectious inflammatory process predominantly involving the vitreous cavity or anterior chamber. It is a serious complication following intraocular surgery, nonsurgical trauma, or systemic infection [23]. The visual outcome despite aggressive treatment in many cases remains poor. In exogenous endophthalmitis, the organisms gain access to eye by surgical or nonsurgical trauma (mostly from patient's lid and conjunctival flora), or may gain access to the eye hematogenously (endogenous endophthalmitis) from an infectious focus, such as endocarditis, urinary tract or bowel infections, or an infected intravenous line or shunt. A predisposing factor may be present, such as prematurity, leukemia, lymphoma, disseminated carcinoma, drug abuse, immunocompromise, and long-term use of corticosteroids [23]. Phacoanaphylactic endophthalmitis is a granulomatous infection that results from autoimmunity to exposed lens protein. In endogenous bacterial and fungal endophthalmitis, septic emboli are lodged in the choriocapillaris and retinal arterioles. Bruch's membrane is disrupted and organisms gain access into the retina and vitreous. The organisms most frequently isolated in endo-

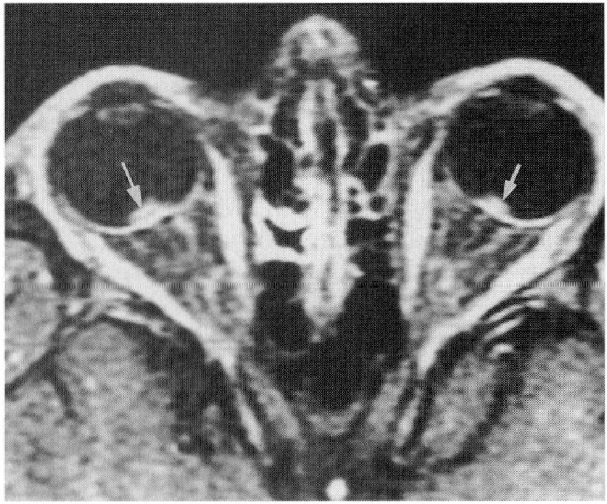

Fig. 15. Pseudotumor cerebri. Axial enhanced fat-suppressed T1-weighted MR image in a patient who has pseudotumor cerebri showing abnormal enhancement at the level of both optic discs (*arrows*).

phthalmitis are *Staphylococcus epidermidis*, *Staphylococcus aureus*, streptococcal species, and *Candida*. Parasitic granulomatosis refers to ocular inflammation as a result of infection with helminthic parasite. The most common of these are *T canis* or *T cati*, *Cysticercus cellulosae*, and microfilariae of *Onchocerca volvulus*. Toxocariasis result in granuloma formation in the posterior pole or periphery, and endophthalmitis. Cysticercosis may occur anywhere in the eye or around the eye. The CT and MR imaging findings in endophthalmitis include increased density of the vitreous on CT and increased signal intensity of the vitreous on T1-weighted and flair MR images because of increased protein from leaking retinal or choroidal vessels. The uvea may be thickened and demonstrates increased enhancement or focal enhancement (abscess) (Fig. 16). Associated CD, RD, and posterior vitreous detachment may be delineated on CT and MR imaging.

## Ocular calcifications

Calcification is commonly found in normal and abnormal ocular tissues. The presence of calcifications on CT scans can be used to correctly diagnose the type of pathology (Figs. 17–19) [24–26]. Idiopathic scleral calcification is seen in many patients older than 70 years of age. CT scan shows these calcified plaques near the insertions of lateral and medial rectus muscles. The calcified plaques may be

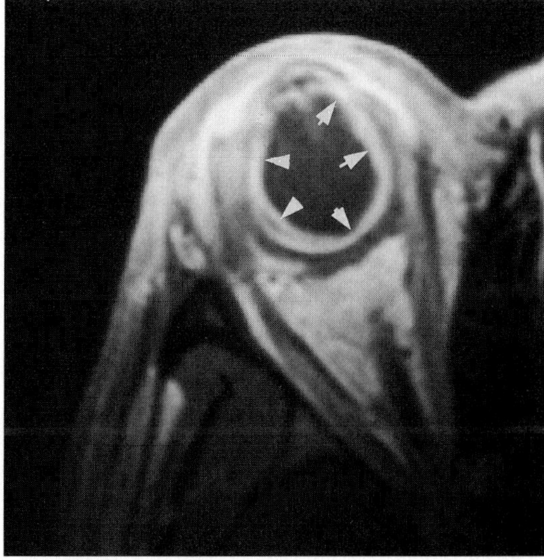

Fig. 16. Endophthalmitis. Axial enhanced T1-weighted MR image shows marked thickening and enhancement of the entire uveal tract (*arrows*).

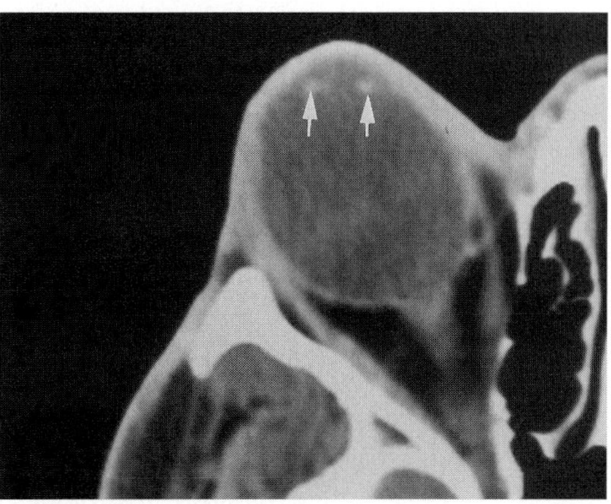

Fig. 17. Axial CT scan shows enlarged right globe caused by axial myopia. Note calcification of ciliary body (*arrows*). Lens has been removed.

in the posterior aspect of the sclera. Calcification may occur at the level of the ciliary body or in the choroid. Ciliary body calcification may be seen after trauma; after inflammation (see Fig. 17); or in teratoid medulloepithelioma of the ciliary body. Choroidal calcification often follows severe intraocular inflammation or trauma. Choroidal osteoma is an unusual but distinct cause of choroidal calcification. The osteoma is a rare, well-defined, benign tumor (choristoma) that is found mainly in otherwise healthy young women [24]. It typically arises in the choroid adjacent to the optic nerve head of one or both eyes (Fig. 18). Detection of calcification plays an important role in the diagnosis of malignant intraocular tumors, such as retinoblastoma and medulloepithelioma (see articles on retinoblastoma and medulloepithelioma elsewhere in this issue).

In published histopathologic series, calcium depositions have been seen to occur in necrotic areas of

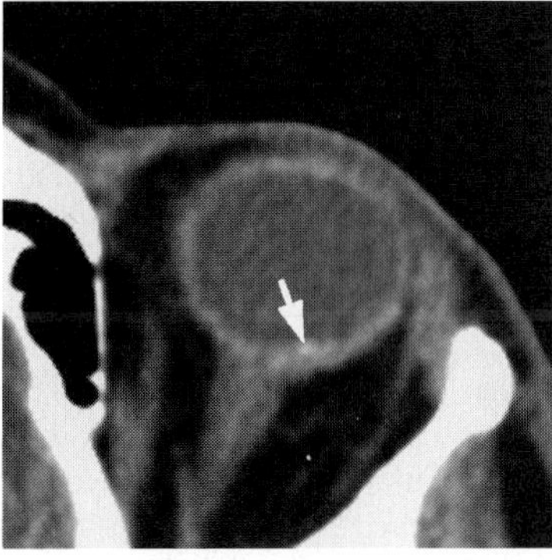

Fig. 18. Choroidal osteoma. Axial CT scan shows a calcified mass, compatible with presumed choroidal osteoma (*arrow*).

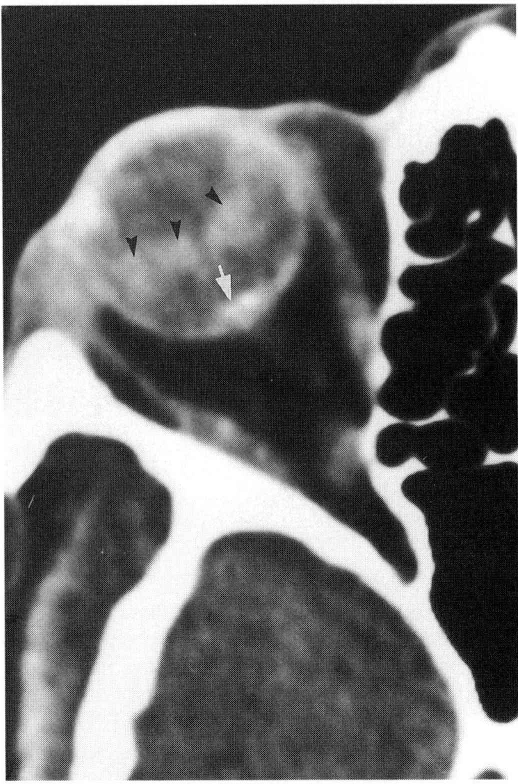

Fig. 19. Chronic retinal detachment. Axial CT scan shows retinal detachment. Note calcification at the optic disk (*arrow*). The increased thickening of the detached retina (*arrowheads*) is related to reactive retinal gliosis.

87% to 95% of retinoblastoma. CT scan demonstrates calcification in more than 90% of retinoblastoma [1,2]. CT demonstration of calcification may be helpful for differentiating retinoblastoma from PHPV, retinopathy of prematurity, Coats' disease, and a variety of other nonspecific causes of leukocoria [1,2]. In children younger than 3 years of age, CT detection of appropriate intraocular calcification suggests that retinoblastoma is the most likely diagnosis. In children older than 3 years of age, however, detection of calcification has less differential value, because some other entities including PHPV, retinopathy of prematurity, and Coats' disease can also produce calcification in older children [24]. Calcification is often absent in PHPV. In older patients, however, calcification may be found in the crystalline lens or focally in a totally detached retina. Retinopathy of prematurity is a bilateral ocular disorder resulting in abnormal proliferation of fibrovascular tissue in the retina of premature infants who previously received oxygen therapy. The abnormal tissue extends into the vitreous cavity where it causes tractional RD. Calcification in the lens, choroid, and retrolental tissue has been reported in children who have late stage of this disease [24]. Coats' disease is a unilateral exudative RD that mainly affects boys between 18 months and 18 years of age. The disease is an idiopathic congenital disorder of the retinal vessels (telangiectases). Abnormal retinal vessels can occur either in the periphery or the central retina; leakage of lipid-rich serum from telangiectatic vessels into the subretinal space results in RD (see Fig. 4). The retina may be shallowly detached or become bullously detached. Patients who have Coats' disease occasionally may have calcification in the retina. This calcification may be submacular and result from metaplasia of the RPE [2,24]. RPE is capable of metaplastic calcification or bone formation (Fig. 19). Calcification may also be detected on CT in patients who have microphthamos with or without colobomatous cyst. The calcification in these eyes most likely occurs in the choristomatous glial tissue [24]. Retinal astrocytic hamartoma is another lesion that may cause retinal calcification [2]. These hamartomas most frequently occur in tuberous sclerosis, but also may be noted in neurofibromatosis. Cytomegalovirus retinitis is a common infection in patients who have AIDS (see Fig. 11). In cytomegalovirus retinitis, calcification may be seen in the necrotic portion of the retina, or in areas of healed retina [24]. Retinal drusen is a common cause of calcification of the RPE. Drusen are well-defined excrescences that form under the RPE in aging eyes, and are often associated with age-related macular degeneration. Retinal drusen are very small and cannot be visualized by CT scanning. Subretinal neovascular membranes are fibrovascular proliferations that arise from the choroid and extend into the subretinal space, causing serous and hemorrhagic RDs. Numerous conditions may result in subretinal neovascular membranes, but age-related macular degeneration is the most common cause of subretinal neovascular membranes. Long-standing neovascular membranes may become calcified.

Drusen of the optic nerve are acellular accretions of hyaline-like material that occur on or near the surface of the optic disk. They are often seen in the prelaminar optic nerve. When drusen affect the papilla, the optic nerve head is elevated and shows blurred disk margins. Unlike retinal drusen, CT scans can readily detect optic disk drusen. Trauma in one series [24] was the single most common cause of ocular calcification. The calcification typically occurs many years after the initial trauma, when the damaged globes are in varying stages of atrophy or phthisis.

## Ocular tumors

Most primary and metastatic ocular neoplasms in adults involve the uveal tract and in particular the choroid. Malignant melanoma is the most common tumor to involve the uvea [25–30]. Most primary ocular neoplasms in children, however, involve the retina. Retinoblastoma is the most common tumor to involve the retina (see the article on retinoblastoma and simulating lesions elsewhere in this issue) [31–33]. Retinal astrocytic hamartoma is another rare lesion involving the retina. These hamartomas most frequently occur in tuberous sclerosis, but also may be found in neurofibromatosis. On pathologic examination, these hamartomas show focal benign astrocytic proliferation that usually contains calcium [24].

Medulloepithelioma is an embryonic neoplasm derived from primitive neuroepithelium, presenting as a mass behind the pupil and iris [33]. It typically arises from the ciliary body epithelium, but may also occur as a posterior mass in the retina or optic nerve (see the article on medulloepithelioma of the ciliary body and optic nerve elsewhere in this issue) [33,34].

### *Malignant uveal melanoma*

Malignant uveal melanomas are the most common primary intraocular tumor in adults. Some of these tumors may originate from pre-existing nevi [30]. Choroidal hemangioma, choroidal nevi, CD, choroidal cysts, neurofibroma and schwannoma of the uvea, uveal leiomyoma, ciliary body adenoma and adenocarcinoma, medulloepithelioma, juvenile xanthogranuloma, RD, disciform degeneration of the macula, and metastatic tumors are some of the benign and malignant lesions that may be confused with malignant uveal melanoma [27–30,34]. Because of their anatomic location, tumors of the uveal tract are not accessible to biopsy without intraocular surgery. Consequently, the diagnosis must often be made on the basis of clinical examination and judicious use of ancillary diagnostic procedures, such as fluorescein angiography, ultrasonography, CT, and MR imaging. This article only considers the role of MR imaging in the diagnosis of uveal melanoma. The MR imaging techniques for ocular lesions have been described in several prior publications [1,2,30]. The MR imaging

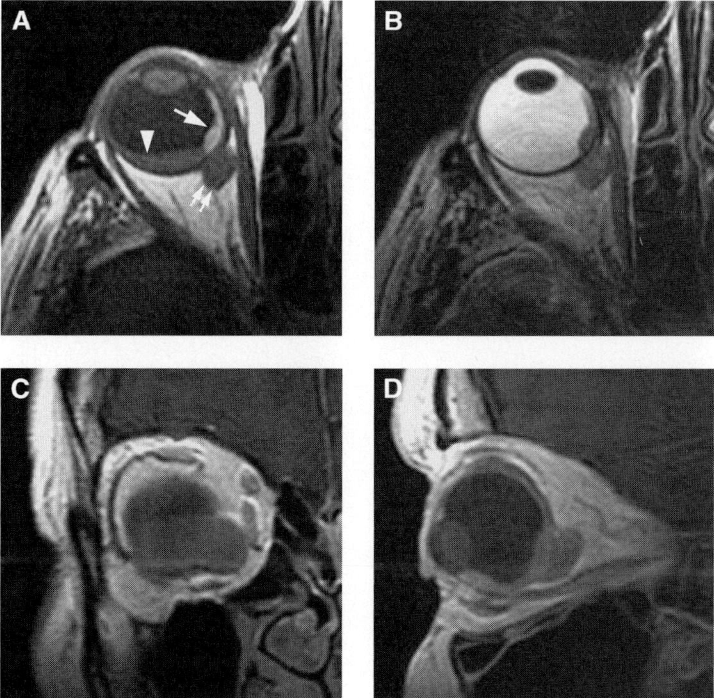


Fig. 20. Malignant choroidal melanoma. Axial T1-weighted (*A*), axial T2-weighted (*B*), coronal enhanced T1-weighted (*C*), and sagittal enhanced T1-weighted (*D*) MR images showing a plaquoid choroidal melanoma (*large arrow*), subretinal exudate (*arrowhead*), and extraocular extension of tumor (*small arrows*).

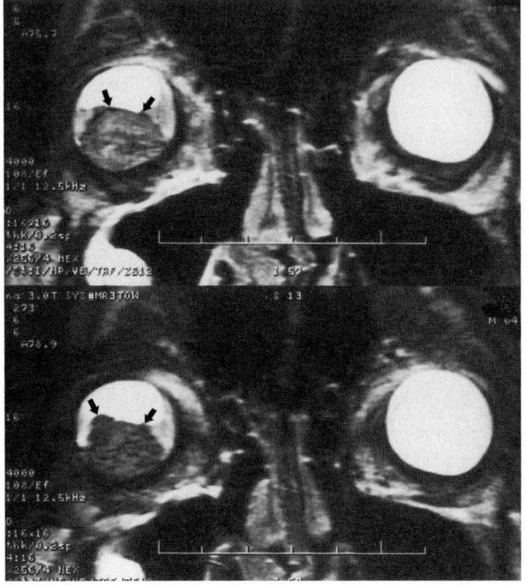

Fig. 21. Malignant choroidal melanoma. Coronal T2-weighted MR images showing a large mound-shaped choroidal melanoma (*arrows*). The MR images were obtained on a 3-T MR imaging unit using quadrature head coil.

characteristics of melanotic lesions are thought to be related to the paramagnetic properties of melanin [27]. Unlike most tumors, melanomas have short T1 and T2 relaxation time values. Most uveal melanomas appear as areas of high signal intensity on T1- and proton-weighted MR images (Fig. 20). On T2-weighted MR images, melanomas appear as areas of moderately low signal intensity (Figs. 20 and 21). The tumor may be dome-shaped (Fig. 21), mushroom-shaped, plaquoid (see Fig. 20), ring-shaped, or diffuse. Although in general the paramagnetic property of melanin plays an important role in MR imaging signal characteristics of melanomas, the histologic features of tumors undoubtedly contribute to their MR imaging features [30]. Melanomas are often arranged in tightly cohesive bundles and are highly cellular (short T2 relaxation time). Necrosis and hemorrhage are not uncommon [1,2,27,30]. At times, uveal melanomas may appear partially or completely hyperintense on T2-weighted MR images. Exudative or hemorrhagic RD may be present (see Fig. 20). Extensive extraocular extension may be present even in the presence of a small intraocular malignant melanoma (Fig. 22). Gadolinium di-

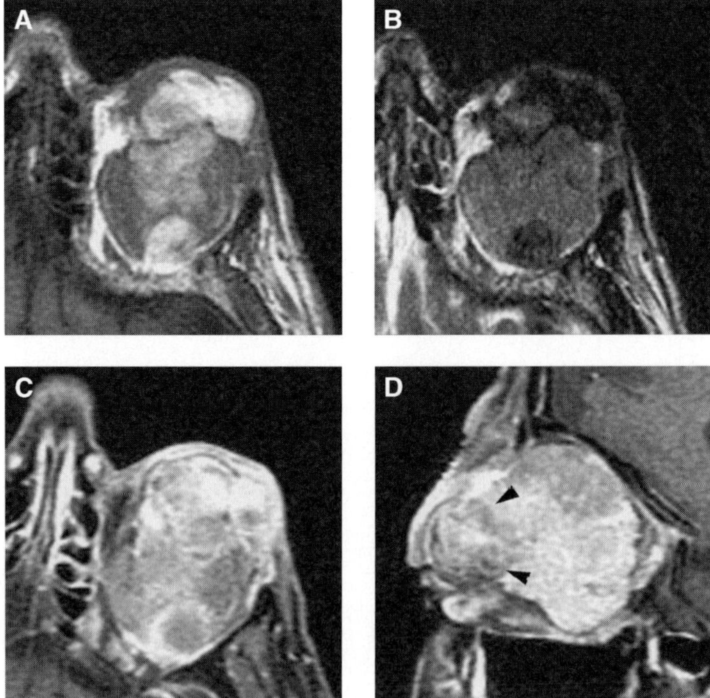


Fig. 22. Presumed ocular melanoma. Unenhanced axial T1-weighted (*A*), axial T2-weighted (*B*), enhanced axial (*C*), and sagittal T1-weighted (*D*) MR images showing an enhancing mass within the left globe (*arrowheads*) and a large retrobulbar mass. Eye examination showed a large intraocular mass. The patient was found to have multiple liver masses.

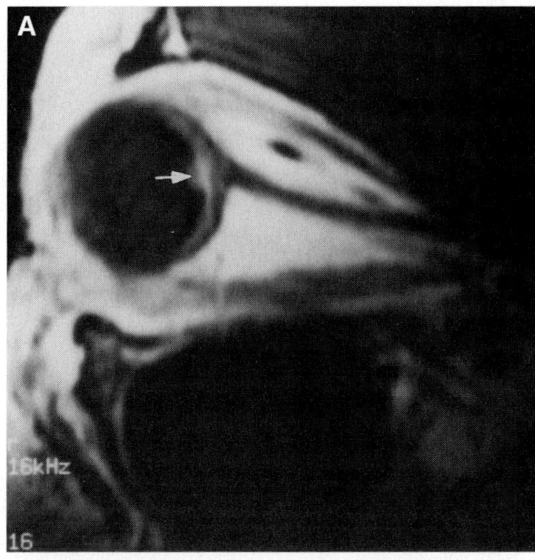


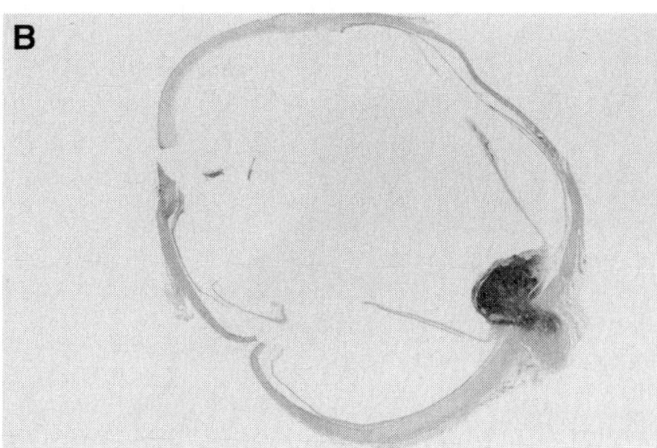


Fig. 23. Melanocytoma and melanoma of the optic disk. (*A*) Sagittal T1-weighted MR image shows a mass (*arrow*) at the optic disk. (*B*) photomicrograph of the eye showing the mass at the optic disk. This was considered to be a melanoma arising from a melanocytoma.

ethylenetriamine pentaacetic acid contrast material is very useful in the diagnosis of uveal melanomas, certain ocular pathology, and, in particular, for evaluation of optic nerve and retrobulbar extension of ocular tumors (see Fig. 20). Uveal melanomas demonstrate moderate enhancement on postgadolinium T1-weighted MR images (see Fig. 20).

Melanocytoma is a deeply pigmented benign tumor that may occur in the uvea and in the substance of the optic nerve. Approximately 50% of melanocytomas develop in blacks, whereas the incidence of malignant uveal melanoma in blacks is less than 1%. The MR imaging appearance of melanocytoma is similar to uveal melanoma (Fig. 23).

### *Choroidal hemangioma*

Choroidal hemangiomas are congenital vascular hamartomas typically seen in middle-aged to elderly individuals [35,36]. Two different forms have been reported: a circumscribed or solitary type not associated with other abnormalities; and a diffuse angiomatosis often associated with facial nevus flammeus or variations of the Sturge-Weber syndrome [1–3,6,37]. The solitary choroidal hemangioma is confined to choroid, shows distinct margins, and characteristically lies posterior to the equator of the globe [36]. It is typically seen as a tumor located in the juxtapapillary or macular region of the fundus [36]. In contrast, the hemangioma associated with Sturge-Weber syndrome is a diffuse process that may involve the choroid, ciliary body, iris, and, occasionally, nonuveal tissues, such as the episclera, conjunctiva, and limbus [37]. CT, including dynamic CT, has been shown to be useful for the diagnosis of choroidal hemangioma (Figs. 24 and 25) [36,38]. MR imaging has been shown to be superior to CT for

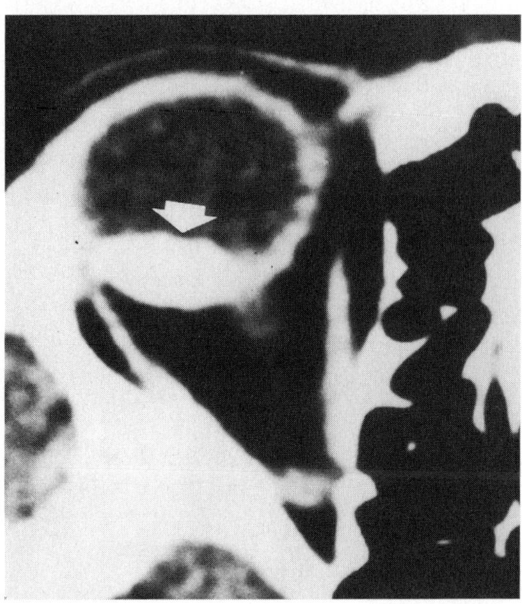

Fig. 24. Circumscribed choroidal hemangioma. Enhanced CT scan shows an intensely enhancing choroidal hemangioma (*arrows*).

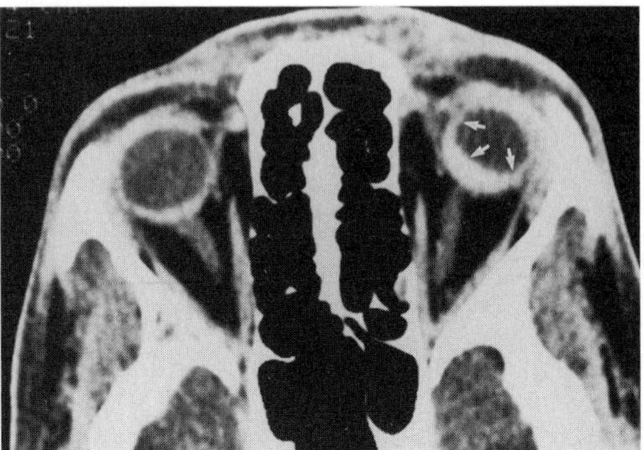

Fig. 25. Diffuse choroidal hemangioma. Enhanced CT scan shows a diffuse choroidal hemangioma (*arrows*).

evaluation of uveal melanomas, choroidal hemangioma, and simulating lesions [1,2,27,37,38]. On T1-weighted MR images, the choroidal hemangiomas appear as isointense to slightly hypertense lesions with respect to the vitreous. They appear hyperintense on T2-weighted MR images (Fig. 26), so they become isointense to vitreous on these pulse sequences. They demonstrate intense contrast enhancement on enhanced T1-weighted MR images (Figs. 26 and 27).

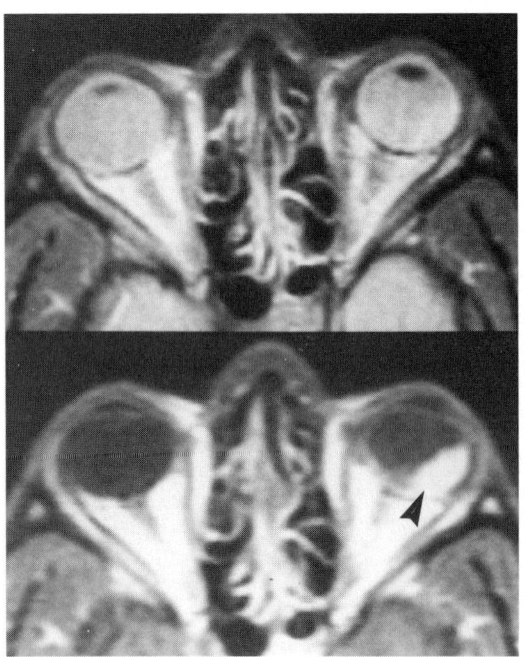

Fig. 26. Choroidal hemangioma. Proton-weighted (*top*) and enhanced T1-weighted (*bottom*) MR images showing an intensely enhancing choroidal hemangioma (*arrowhead*).

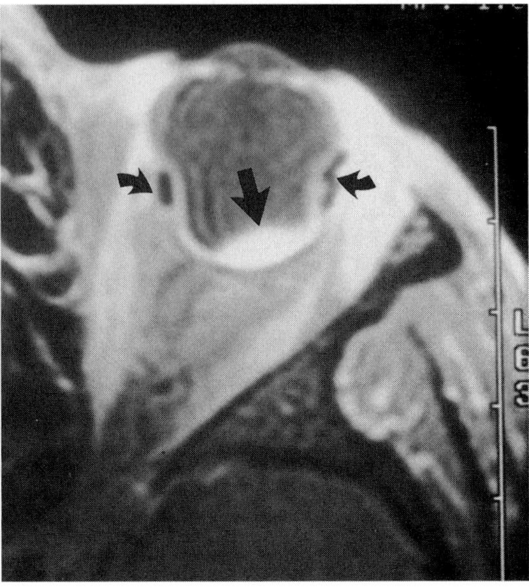

Fig. 27. Choroidal hemangioma. Axial enhanced fat-suppressed T1-weighted MR image shows an intensely enhancing choroidal hemangioma (*straight arrow*). Note scleral buckling (*curved arrows*) for the repair of retinal detachment. The cause of retinal detachment was not clear until MR imaging was performed.

### *Uveal metastases*

Uveal metastasis can be confused clinically and radiologically with uveal melanoma. Embolic malignant cells reach the globe by means of the short posterior ciliary arteries. The route of spread may be the reason why most of the metastases involve the posterior half of the globe [27]. The most common sources of secondary tumor within the eye are the breast and lung. Both eyes may be affected in about one third of the cases. Signal intensity of uveal melanomas and uveal metastases may be similar (Figs. 28 and 29).

### *Other uveal tumors*

Choroidal lymphoma and leukemic infiltration of the uveal tract can be mistaken for choroidal tumor. The process often is bilateral. On MR imaging its signal characteristics are similar to uveal melanoma [27]. Neurofibroma and schwannoma of the choroid and ciliary body, adenoma and adenocarcinoma of the ciliary body, leiomyoma of the ciliary body, and other rare lesions can also be confused with uveal melanoma on MR imaging [1,2,27].

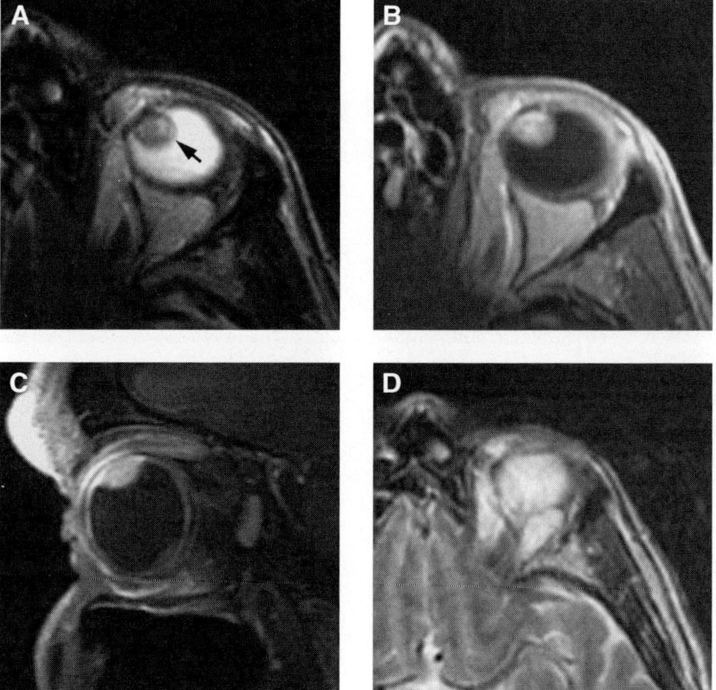


Fig. 28. Ocular metastasis. Axial T2-weighted (*A*), axial enhanced fat-suppressed T1-weighted (*B*), sagittal enhanced fat-suppressed T1-weighted (*C*), and post–proton beam treatment axial T2-weighted (*D*) MR images showing a mass (*arrow*) compatible with biopsy-proven metastatic hypernephroma. Note satisfactory response following proton beam treatment (*D*).

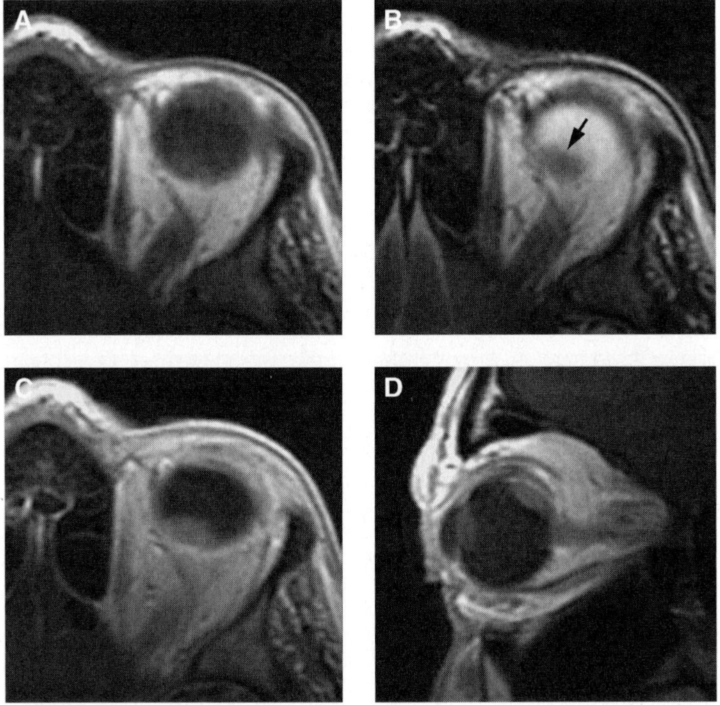


Fig. 29. Ocular metastasis. Axial T1-weighted (*A*), axial T2-weighted (*B*), enhanced axial (*C*), and sagittal T1-weighted (*D*) MR imaging showing a metastatic mass (*arrow*) from primary malignant thymoma.

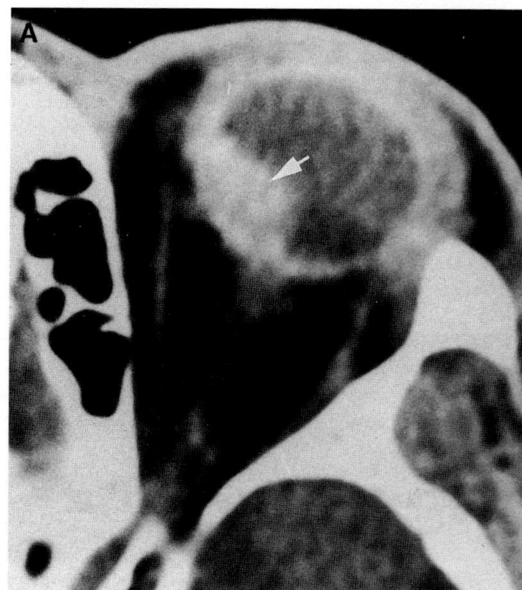


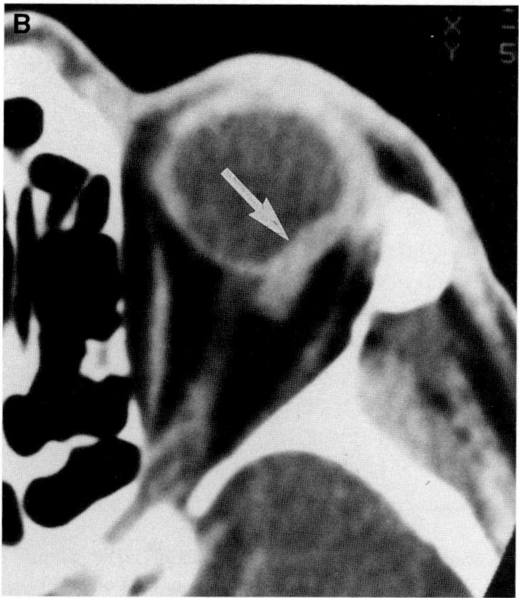


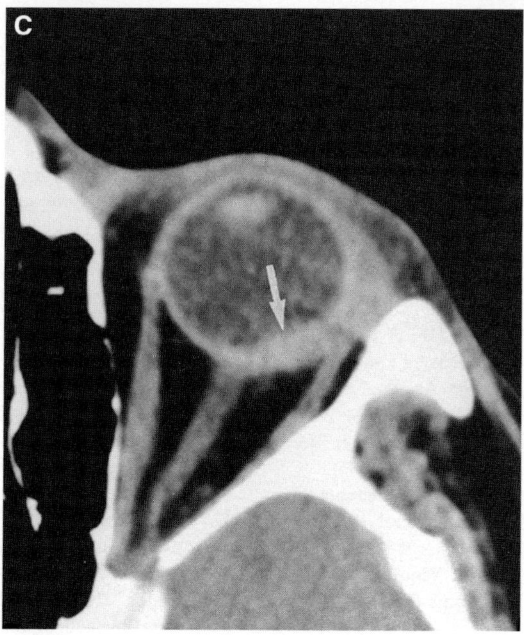


Fig. 30. Choroidal hematoma, simulating choroidal melanoma. (*A*) Axial CT scan shows a hyperdense mass (*arrow*) compatible with choroidal hematoma. (*B*) Axial CT scan shows a hyperdense mass (*arrow*) compatible with choroidal melanoma. Note extraocular extension of this melanoma. (*C*) Enhanced axial CT scan shows focal thickening of the eyeball caused by a choroidal melanoma.

*Choroidal hematoma*

Choroidal hematoma, CD (serous and hemorrhagic), and posterior scleritis may simulate choroidal melanoma, particularly on CT scans (Fig. 30).

## Summary

Since the development of CT and MR imaging, significant progress has been made in ophthalmic imaging. As the technology advanced and MR imaging units improved their ability in term of spatial resolution, the role of MR imaging in ophthalmic imaging has increased accordingly. This article considers the role of MR and CT imaging in the diagnosis of selected pathologies of the eye.

## Acknowledgments

The authors are grateful to Dr. Kiarash Mohajer for helpful literature research, Aura Smith for secretarial assistance, and Yasir Aich for technical support.

## References

[1] Mafee MF. The eye. In: Som PM, Curtin HD, editors. Head and neck imaging. 4th edition. St. Louis (MO): Mosby; 2003. p. 441–527.

[2] Mafee MF. The eye and orbit. In: Mafee MF, Valvassori GE, Becker M, editors. Imaging of the head and neck. 2nd edition. Stuttgart (Germany): Thieme; 2005. p. 137–294.

[3] Warwich R, Williams PL. Gray's anatomy. 35th British edition. Philadelphia: WB Saunders; 1973.

[4] Snell RS, Lemp MA, editors. Clinical anatomy of the eye. Boston: Blackwell Scientific; 1989.

[5] Reech MF, Wobij JL, Wirtschapter JD. Ophthalmic anatomy: a manual with some clinical applications. San Francisco: American Academy of Ophthalmology; 1981.

[6] Mafee MF, Putterman A, Valvassori GE, et al. Orbital space occupying lesions: role of computed tomography an magnetic resonance imaging. An analysis of 145 cases. Radiol Clin North Am 1987;25:529–59.

[7] Rtumin U. Fundus appearance in normal eye. I. The choroid. Am J Ophthalmol 1967;64:821–57.

[8] Nakaizumi Y. The ultrastructure of Bruch's membrane. II. Eyes with a tapetum. Arch Ophthalmol 1964;72: 388–94.

[9] Park KL. Anatomy of the uvea. In: Yanoff M, Duker JS, editors. Ophthalmology. St. Louis (MO): Mosby; 1999. p. 10:2.1–2.2.

[10] Mafee MF, Peyman GA. Retinal and choroidal detachment: role of MRI and CT. Radiol Clin North Am 1987;25:487–507.

[11] Mafee MF. Magnetic resonance imaging: ocular anatomy and pathology. In: Newton TH, Bilanuik LT, editors. Modern neuroradiology, vol. 4. Radiology of the eye and orbit. New York: Clavadel press/Raven press; 1990. p. 2.1–3.45.

[12] Mafee MF, Goldberg MF, Valvassori GE, et al. Computed tomography in the evaluation of patients with persistent hyperplastic primary vitreous (PHP's). Radiology 1982;145:713–4.

[13] Anand R. Serous detachment of the neural retina. In: Yanoff M, Duker JS, editors. Ophthalmology. St. Louis (MO): Mosby; 1999. p. 8:40.1–40.6.

[14] Mafee MF, Peyman GA. Choroidal detachment and ocular hypotony: CT evaluation. Radiology 1984;153: 697–703.

[15] Peyman GA, Mafee MF, Schulman JA. Computed tomography in choroidal detachment. Ophthalmology 1984;92:156–62.

[16] Mafee MF, Linder B, Peyman GA, et al. Choroidal hematoma and effusion: evaluation with MR imaging. Radiology 1988;168:781–6.

[17] Capper SA, Leopold IH. Mechanism of serous choroidal detachment. Arch Ophthalmol 1956;55:101–13.

[18] Siegelman J, Jakobiec FA, Eisner G, editors. Retinal diseases: pathogenesis, laser therapy and surgery. Boston: Little, Brown; 1984. p. 1–66.

[19] Kapusta MA, Lopez PF. Choroidal hemorrhage. In: Yanoff M, Duker JS, editors. Ophthalmology. St. Louis (MO): Mosby; 1999. p. 41.1–8:41.4.

[20] Goldstein DA, Tessler HH. Episcleritis, scleritis and other scleral disorders. In: Yanoff M, Duker JS, editors. Ophthalmology. St. Louis (MO): Mosby; 1999. p. 5:13.1–13.9.

[21] Chaques VJ, Lam S, Tessler HH, et al. Computed tomography and magnetic resonance imaging in the diagnosis of posterior scleritis. Ann Ophthalmol 1993;25:89–94.

[22] Forster DJ. Basic principles: general approach to the uveitis patient and treatment strategies. In: Yanoff M, Duker JS, editors. Ophthalmology. St. Louis (MO): Mosby; 1999. p. 10:3.1–3.6.

[23] Marx JL. Endophthalmitis. In: Yanoff M, Duker JS, editors. Ophthalmology. St. Louis (MO): Mosby; 1999. p. 10:21.1–21.6.

[24] Yan X, Edward DP, Mafee MF. Ocular calcification: radiologic-pathologic correlation and literature review. International Journal of Neuroradiology 1998;4:81–96.

[25] Zeffer HJ. Calcification and ossification in ocular tissue. Am J Ophthalmol 1983;101:1724–7.

[26] Bullock JD, Campbell RJ, Waller RR. Calcification in retinoblastoma. Invest Ophthalmol Vis Sci 1976;11: 252–5.

[27] Mafee MF, Peyman GA, McKusick MA. Malignant uveal melanoma and similar lesions studied by computed tomography. Radiology 1985;156:403–8.

[28] Mafee MF, Peyman GA, Grisolano JE, et al. Malignant uveal melanoma and simulating lesions: MR imaging evaluation. Radiology 1986;160:773–80.

[29] Mafee MF, Peyman GA, Peace JH, et al. MRI in the evaluation and differentiation of uveal melanoma. Ophthalmology 1987;94:341–8.

[30] Mafee MF. Uveal melanoma, choroidal hemangioma, and simulating lesions. Radiol Clin North Am 1998; 36:1083–99.

[31] Mafee MF, Goldberg MF, Greenwald MJ, et al. Retinoblastoma and simulating lesion: role of CT and MR Imaging. Radiol Clin North Am 1987;25:667–81.

[32] Mafee MF, Goldberg MF, Cohen SB, et al. Magnetic resonance imaging of leukokoric eyes and use of in

vitro proton magnetic resonance spectroscopy of retinoblastoma. Ophthalmology 1989;96:965–76.

[33] Kaufman LM, Mafee MF, Song CD. Retinoblastoma and simulating lesions: role of CT, MR imaging and use of Gd-DTPA contrast enhancement. Radiol Clin North Am 1998;36:1101–17.

[34] Chavez M, Mafee MF, Castillo B, et al. Medulloepithelioma of the optic nerve. J Pediatr Ophthalmol Strabismus 2004;41:48–52.

[35] Enochs SW, Petherick P, Bogdanova A, et al. Paramagnetic metal scavenging by melanin: MR imaging. Radiology 1997;204:417–23.

[36] Mafee MF, Ainbinder DJ, Hidayat AA, et al. Magnetic resonance imaging and computed tomography in the evaluation of choroidal hemangioma. International Journal of Neuroradiology 1995;1:67–77.

[37] Mafee MF, Atlas SW, Galetta SL. Eye, orbit, and visual system. In: Atlas SW, editor. Imaging of the brain and spine. 3rd edition. Philadelphia: Lippincott Williams & Wilkins; 2002. p. 1433–524.

[38] Mafee MF, Miller MT, Tan W, et al. Dynamic computed tomography and its application to ophthalmology. Radiol Clin North Am 1987;25:715–31.

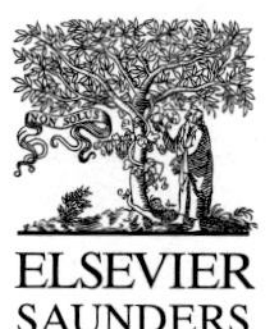
ELSEVIER
SAUNDERS

Neuroimag Clin N Am 15 (2005) 49 – 67

NEUROIMAGING
CLINICS OF
NORTH AMERICA

# Retinoblastoma and Simulating Lesions: Role of Imaging

Michael A. Apushkin, MD[a], Marsha A. Apushkin, MD[b], Michael J. Shapiro, MD[b], Mahmood F. Mafee, MD[c,*]

[a]*Department of Radiology, University of Illinois at Chicago, Chicago, IL, USA*
[b]*Department of Ophthalmology and Visual Science, University of Illinois at Chicago, Chicago, IL, USA*
[c]*Department of Radiology, University of Illinois at Chicago Medical Center, 1740 West Taylor Street, MC 931, Chicago, IL 60612, USA*

Retinoblastoma (Rb) is a malignant tumor of childhood that was first described in the sixteenth century [1]. Now, it is the most common intraocular tumor in children [2,3] and accounts for 3% of the all cancers occurring in children younger than 15 years of age [4]. Rb occurs in 1 of 18,000 to 30,000 live births worldwide [5]. In the United States alone, 200 children are diagnosed annually [2–5]. No racial or sexual preference for the development of this cancer was found [6,7]. More than 95% of the children with Rb are diagnosed before the age of 5 years [3,8]. In the United States, the average age at diagnosis is 13 months [9].

Rb may present in a familial or sporadic form. The hereditary pattern of the disease is autosomal dominant, and the hereditary form includes patients with a positive family history and those who have sustained new germline mutations. Rb occurs as a result of a mutation in both alleles in the tumor suppressor oncogene (Rb1 gene) located on chromosome 13q14 [10–13]. This gene encodes a 110-kd nuclear phosphoprotein (pRb) that regulates the cell cycle. Its deletion results in a loss of cell cycle control and abnormal cell division.

Hereditary Rb presents as bilateral disease in 85% of cases and as unilateral disease in 15%. Children with the germline form of Rb are at risk of "trilateral Rb." Trilateral Rb [14] describes the presentation of bilateral Rb accompanied by an intracranial primitive neuroectodermal tumor (PNET) along the midline of the brain, most commonly found in the pineal gland (pinealoblastoma), suprasellar, or parasellar region [15,16]. It causes 50% of the deaths from Rb in the first 5 years of life. Screening patients with germline mutations for intracranial trilateral Rb using MR imaging may improve treatment outcome as a result of early diagnosis and onset of the treatment. Therefore, children with hereditary Rb should be screened by MR imaging every 6 months after diagnosis for 4 years [17]. Patients with the hereditary form of Rb are also at a lifelong risk of developing second malignancies. They account for a significant reduction in longevity in this group, with a 26% occurrence rate within 40 years of diagnosis [18].

It is important to recognize Rb in early stages when the lesion is limited to the globe, because the response to therapy at this stage shows a survival rate of greater than 90% over a 5-year period [19]. Untreated Rb is uniformly fatal. To apply efficient therapy, Rb must be differentiated from other intraocular lesions presenting with leukocoria (Box 1) [20–22]. Clinical and imaging studies are particularly important in Rb because it is one of the few human cancers for which the decision about definitive treatment is made based on findings of the clinical examination and radiologic studies and without a confirmed histopathologic diagnosis [20,22].

## Pathologic features

In nineteenth century, Virchow [23] proposed a glial origin of Rb. Almost a century later, Popoff and

* Corresponding author.
*E-mail address:* mfmafee@uic.edu (M.F. Mafee).

1052-5149/05/$ – see front matter 
doi:10.1016/j.nic.2005.02.003

**Box 1. Leukocoria and lesions simulating retinoblastoma**

*Intraocular mass and mass-like lesions*

- Medulloepithelioma
- Retinal astrocytoma
- Combined hamartoma of the retinal pigment epithelium and retina
- Von Hippel-Lindau retinal angiomatosis
- Choroidal hemangioma
- Juvenile xanthogranuloma
- Mesoectodermal leiomyoma
- Intraocular foreign body
- Choroidal osteoma
- Retinal gliosis

*Loss of red reflex because of media opacities*

- Congenital cataract
- Infantile glaucoma
- Hyphema
- Hypopyon
- Cornea opacity
- Vitreous hemorrhage
- Uveitis
- Endophthalmitis
- Toxocariasis
- Myiasis

*Leukocoria from retinal detachments (major syndromes only)*

- Coats disease
- PHPV
- ROP
- Incontinentia pigmenti
- Familial exudative vitreoretinopathy
- X-linked retinoschisis
- Retinal dysplasia
- Organized subretinal hemorrhage
- Rhegmatogenous retinal detachment
- Developmental retinal cyst
- Stickler syndrome

*Leukocoria from retinal white-appearing pathologic findings without mass or retinal detachment*

- Myelinated nerve fibers
- Papillitis
- Optic nerve head drusen
- Chorioretinal coloboma
- Optic disc coloboma
- Morning glory disc
- Staphyloma of the optic disc
- Staphyloma of the posterior pole
- Subretinal neovascular membrane

Ellsworth [24] and Tso [25] described Rb as a tumor of neuroectodermal cells, which become retinal photoreceptors under normal conditions. A characteristic finding of Rb on light microscopy is a presence of Flexner-Wintersteiner rosettes, which are composed of cells arranged in a circular fashion around a well-defined lumen [24–27]. Of interest, the presence of rosettes was independently discovered and described in nineteenth century by two investigators, Flexner [28] and Wintersteiner [29]. The tumor cells can be poorly differentiated, undifferentiated, or well differentiated. Poorly differentiated tumors are composed of small round cells with a high nuclear-cytoplasmic ratio and hyperchromatic nuclei. More differentiated tumors contain rosettes or florets [26,27]. Necrosis with focal areas of calcification is another typical histopathologic finding of Rb. Some tumors show areas of glial differentiation [26,27].

## Clinical presentation

The most common presenting sign of Rb is the presence of a white or white-yellow pupillary reflex known as leukocoria (Fig. 1) [7,20]. Normally, the retina has a red reflex that can be seen at the pupil when a bright light is shown directly into the eye. Frequently, the abnormal pupil reflex is identified by family and friends and noted in flash photography. Howard and Ellsworth showed [30] that of 500 children with leukocoria, 235 (47%) were diagnosed with Rb. The white reflex at the pupil is dependent on the size, location, and pigmentation of the intraocular pathologic findings. Leukocoria in a patient with Rb is caused by reflection of the light from the white tumor (Fig. 2) or the associated exudative retinal detachment. The red retinal reflex may also be

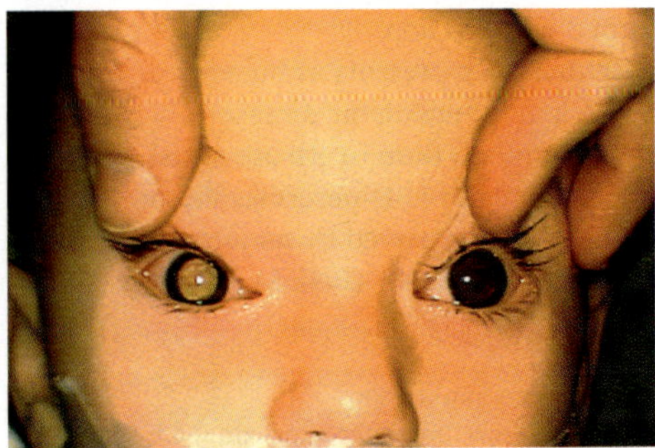

Fig. 1. Leukocoria is mostly discovered by the parents while obtaining photographs with a flash camera.

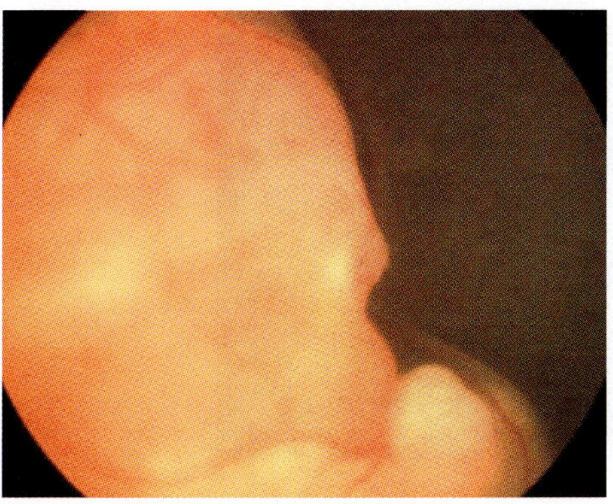

Fig. 2. Large tumor responsible for clinical picture of a patient presenting with leukocoria.

obscured by opacification of the vitreous with blood, inflammatory exudate, or tumor cells (Fig. 3) or by nonexudative retinal detachment unrelated to Rb. Typical Rb presenting with leukocoria has central tumors that are large (Figs. 4–6).

Strabismus is the second most common presenting sign of Rb. It is a result of macular involvement by the tumor. The macula is temporal to the optic nerve and the part of the retina responsible for high-resolution vision; therefore, tumors extending into the macula reduce vision in the affected eye. These tumors disrupt the sensory input needed to maintain ocular alignment, thus resulting in strabismus. Interestingly, vision often returns after treatment if the regressed tumor shrinks away from the macula. Rb may also present with findings like vitreous hemorrhage, retinal detachment, angle-closure glaucoma, hyphema, pseudohypopyon, iris heterochromia, proptosis, and pseudo-orbital cellulites. Although Rb is a relatively rare disease, high suspicion for this tumor must be present during the evaluation of any child younger than 5 years of age with leukocoria, strabismus, or unexplained vision loss.

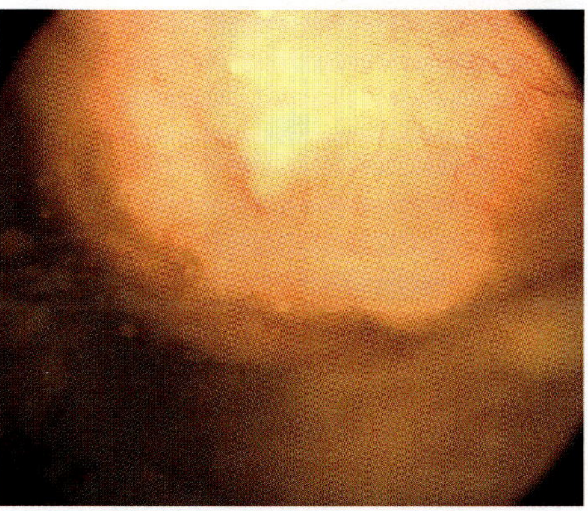

Fig. 3. Massive endophytic tumor with clumps of free-floating tumor seeds in the vitreous.

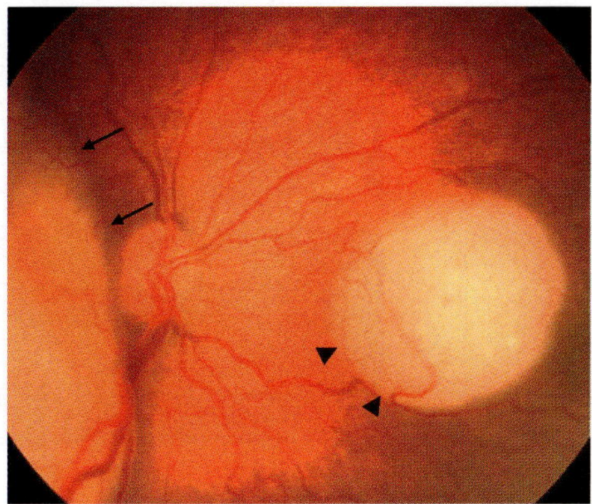

Fig. 4. Fundus photograph of the right eye shows two tumors (*arrows* and *arrowheads*). One is located in the macula and is responsible for reduced visual acuity as well as for the patient's presentation with leukocoria.

Rb was classified into five groups by Reese and Ellsworth [31] to provide a prognosis for local cure and vision of eyes treated with external beam radiotherapy (EBT) (Box 2). More recently, an international classification for intraocular Rb (ABC) has been created for the purpose of clinical trials using chemotherapy (Box 3) [32]. It reflects the prognosis for salvage of the eye with standard chemotherapy. Generally early evaluation is important, because early diagnosis and treatment improve the prognosis for vision and may also spare the patient side effects and complications associated with radiation or chemotherapy.

## Diagnostic imaging

Although most Rb cases are diagnosed by ophthalmoscopic examination, imaging studies should be used in all patients to help confirm the diagnosis; to determine the extent of the ocular disease; and to detect retrobulbar spread, the presence of intracranial metastasis, or trilateral Rb [33–35]. Additionally, imaging is critical in cases of children less than 5 years of age with media opacity or leukocoria for which ophthalmoscopy is not adequately diagnostic. Aside from evaluation for Rb in eyes with a poor ophthalmoscopic view, imaging also provides infor-

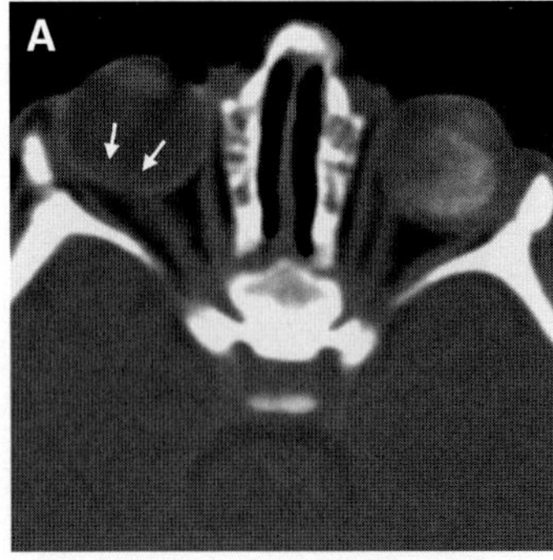


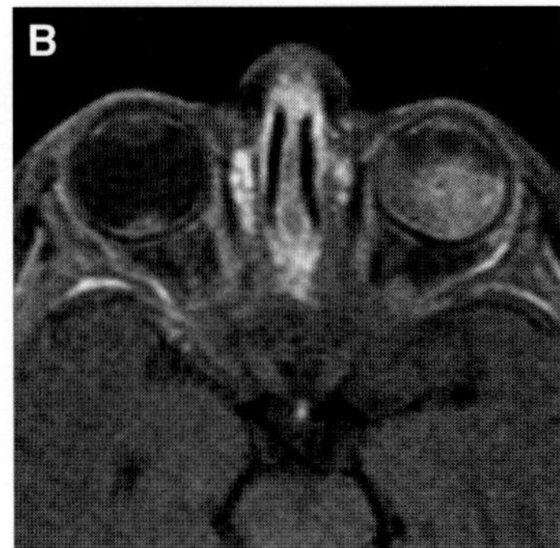


Fig. 5. Patient with bilateral Rb. (*A*) Nonenhanced CT scan demonstrates a large calcified mass in the posterior pole of the left eye and smaller lesions in the right eye located just lateral to the optic disc (*arrows*). (*B*) Enhanced T1-weighted MR image with fat saturation (TR/TE: 650/14 ms) shows enhancing masses in both eyes and confirms the diagnosis of Rb.

mation about the status of the retina before cataract surgery, vitrectomy, or repair of the retina.

Ultrasonography, CT, and MR imaging are the most useful imaging techniques in the evaluation of Rb. Ultrasonography is relatively simple to perform and is available at most ophthalmology offices in the United States. It is a modality that lacks ionizing radiation. Sedation is rarely required for this study. Intraocular masses and calcification can be detected by ultrasonography in cases in which direct visualization of the retina is complicated or not possible. Ultrasonographic imaging can also detect retinal

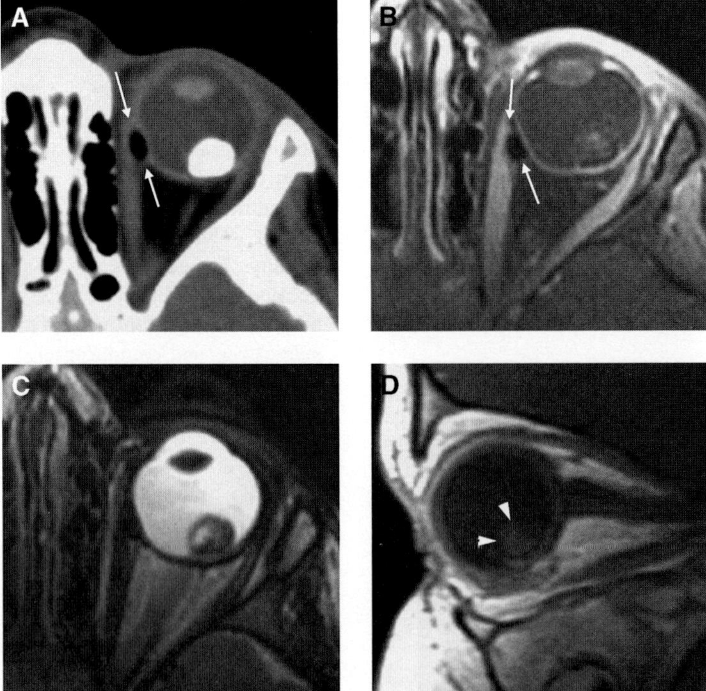


Fig. 6. Same patient as in Fig. 5. after chemotherapy and laser treatment. (*A*) Nonenhanced CT scan shows a shrunken and densely calcified tumor indicating a good response to therapy. Note a silicone sponge of the scleral buckle (*arrows*); the patient developed retinal detachment requiring buckling. (*B*) Enhanced T1-weighted MR image (TR/TE: 600/9 ms) demonstrates a significant decrease in the size of the primary tumor. The arrow on this image also points to the scleral buckle. Axial T2-weighted MR image (TR/TE: 4000/105 ms) (*C*) and parasagittal enhanced T1-weighted MR image (*D*) depict shrunken Rb (*arrowheads*).

**Box 2. Classification of retinoblastoma by Reese and Ellsworth**

1. Extremely favorable prognosis: multiple or solitary tumors less than 4 disc diameters (DDs) in size and located posterior to the equator
2. Favorable prognosis: multiple or solitary tumors less than 10 DD in size located posterior to the equator
3. Doubtful prognosis: any tumor at or anterior to the equator, a tumor larger than 10 DD in size, or a tumor extending to the ora serrata
4. Unfavorable prognosis: multiple tumors with some larger than 10 DD in size or any lesions extending anterior to the ora serrata
5. Extremely unfavorable prognosis: massive tumors involving more than half of the retina or the presence of vitreous seeding.

*From* Reese A, Ellsworth R. Evaluation and current concept of retinoblastoma therapy. Trans Am Acad Ophthalmol Otolaryngol 1963;67:164–72; with permission.

detachment and persistent fetal vasculature, and it frequently eliminates Rb from the differential diagnosis. The ultrasonographic units commonly available do not reliably image the anterior segment, ciliary body, or extreme anterior retina. In cases of tumors with small subtle calcification, sonography is less sensitive at detecting calcification than CT. Finally, ultrasonography is not useful in identification of tumor extent beyond the globe into the orbit or optic nerve or in identification of the presence of a PNET in the brain [36]. Generally, MR imaging and CT are more effective choices of imaging studies for evaluation of Rb.

CT is the best imaging modality for detection of intraocular calcifications [33,37]. Foci of calcification are present in more than 90% of Rb cases, and calcium deposits are highly characteristic for this tumor, especially in children younger than 3 years of age [22]. Calcium deposits result from the formation of complexes with DNA that is being released from necrotic neoplastic cells. Only a few pathologic conditions show calcium deposits in extremely young children. These include microphthalmos with and without colobomatous cysts [22,38,39]. In children older than 3 years of age, several additional lesions, such as astrocytoma of the retina, retinopathy of prematurity (ROP), cytomegalovirus (CMV) retinitis, toxocariasis, medulloepithelioma, and optic nerve drusen, may have calcifications, thus mimicking the appearance of Rb [22,33]. Thin-section (1.5-mm) CT scans are extremely important for detection of small foci of calcium (Fig. 7) and precise determination of tumor extent [33,38,39]. Even with its relatively fast acquisition time, sedation is still required for a diagnostic CT examination. Currently, imaging of the intraocular tumor has shifted toward baseline MR imaging. If MR imaging is not an option, however, CT of the orbits and brain with contrast offers good results in depicting the primary tumor with high-

**Box 3. International classification system for intraocular retinoblastoma (ABC)**

Group A: small tumors ($\leq$ 3 mm) confined to the retina, more than 3 mm from the fovea, and more than 1.5 mm from optic disc

Group B: tumors more than 3 mm in size confined to the retina in any location, clear subretinal fluid 6 mm or less from the tumor margin

Group C: localized vitreous or subretinal seeding ($\geq$ 6 mm in total from the tumor margin); no tumor masses, clumps, or snowballs in the vitreous or subretinal space

Group D: diffuse vitreous and/or subretinal seeding ($\geq$ 6 mm in total from tumor margin), subretinal fluid more than 6 mm from the tumor margin

Group E: No visual potential or presence of any one or more of the following:
- Tumor in the anterior segment
- Tumor in or on the ciliary body
- Neovascular glaucoma
- Vitreous hemorrhage obscuring the tumor or significant hyphema
- Phthisical or prephthisical eye

*Data from* Protocol from Children's Oncology Group. International classification system. National Cancer Institute. Available at: http://www.cancer.gov. Accessed March 10, 2005.

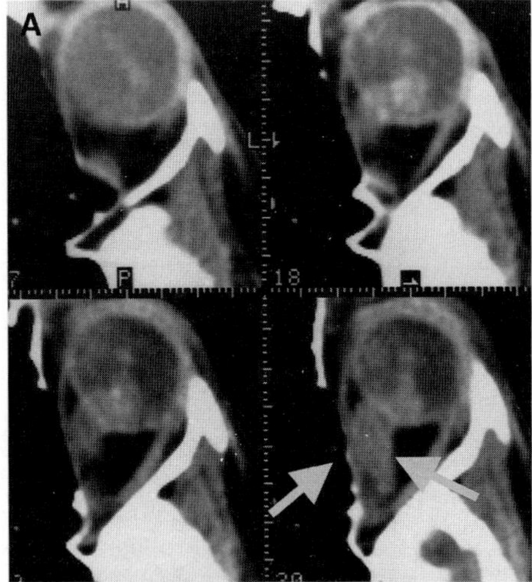

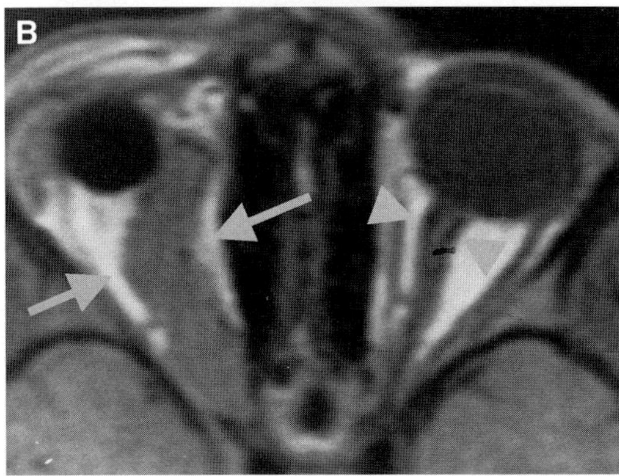

Fig. 7. Patient with Rb and massive involvement of the optic nerve. (*A*) Nonenhanced serial axial CT scans of the orbit demonstrate a calcified mass at the posterior pole of the eye and marked thickening of the intraorbital portion of the optic nerve (*arrows*). (*B*) Postcontrast axial proton density MR image (TR/TE: 2000/20 ms) of the orbits in another patient with recurrent Rb after enucleation of the right eye. There is marked thickening and enhancement of the right optic nerve (*arrows*) indicating tumor recurrence. Note the normal appearance of the left optic nerve (*arrowheads*).

quality images (see Fig. 7), its extent and intracranial spread, and the presence of concurrent tumors. Again, CT is the best modality to document the presence of intratumoral calcifications and is being widely used for this purpose in questionable MR imaging cases. At our institution, we only use CT in selected cases requiring identification of calcifications.

We suggest the following protocol for evaluation of Rb patients: 1.5-mm axial sections with a small field of view (FOV) through both orbits before and after administration of intravenous contrast (2 mL/kg of body weight of iohexol [Omnipaque; Amersham Health, Cork, Ireland] 300 mgI/mL). Direct coronal images should be obtained if a lesion at the upper or lower pole of the globe is suspected and for detailed visualization of the optic nerve. If CT is performed in conjunction with MR imaging, administration of intravenous contrast is not necessary.

At the present time, MR imaging is preferred over CT because of its superior tissue contrast, demonstration of the entire visual pathway, multiplanar capabilities, and absence of known biologic side effects. Contrast-enhanced MR imaging is the modality of choice and should be used whenever possible to answer the key clinical questions [40] and to evaluate an intraocular mass or masses, determine the extent of the tumor, involvement of the optic nerve (Figs. 8 and 9) and retrobulbar space, presence of leptomeningeal spread (Fig. 10), or existence of a second neoplasm [33,41]. Masses with a diameter as little as 3 mm can be detected on MR imaging examinations [33]. MR imaging, however, poorly demonstrates characteristic calcifications of Rb (Figs. 11 and 12).

We perform MR imaging of Rb patients on 1.5- and 3-T Signa magnets (General Electric, Milwaukee, WI) with the use of head coils and, when clinically feasible, surface coils. The 3-T magnet studies use only the head coil. For a complete description of our experience with imaging of the eye and orbit using a 3-T magnet, it is suggested that the reader refer to the article by Mafee et al in this issue. Examinations performed with the head coil only using either magnet strength (1.5 or 3 T) result in high-quality diagnostic images and seem to be the most practical approach for evaluation of Rb. The head coil study protocol includes small FOV sequences through the orbits as well as large FOV images of the entire brain. This allows a good depiction of the entire globe, orbit, and intracranial contents. The use of the surface coil improves the signal-to-noise ratio (SNR) of the images, thus allowing higher resolution and thinner slice thickness. These additional imaging sequences, however, prolong imaging and anesthesia time.

With development of newer eye-preserving treatment options, MR imaging is becoming an increasingly important tool for monitoring focal response to therapy (Figs. 13 and 14) and development of recurrent tumors. For practical purposes, even with the use of a surface coil, MR imaging can only reliably detect lesions larger then 2 to 3 mm. Retinal masses can be adequately monitored by ophthalmoscopic examination in most cases. When it comes to monitoring of the disease process outside the globe or intracranially, however, the cross-sectional imaging modalities, such as MR imaging or CT, are the only

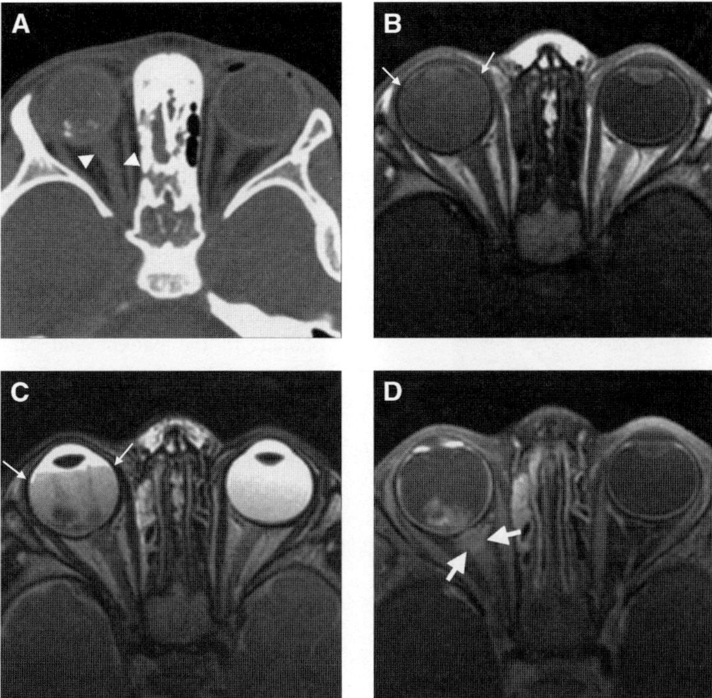


Fig. 8. Patient with Rb. (*A*) Nonenhanced CT scan demonstrates foci of calcium in the posterior pole of the right eye and a thickened right optic nerve (*arrowheads*). (*B*) T1-weighted MR image (TR/TE: 450/14 ms) shows abnormally high signal in the right eye (complete retinal detachment). Note that the subretinal space is limited by the ora serrata (*arrows*). The tumor is inconspicuous on this image. T2-weighted MR image (*C*) and enhanced T1-weighted MR image (*D*) with fat saturation (TR/TE: 4000/107 ms and 700/14 ms, respectively) confirm the presence of an enhancing mass of the posterior pole of the right eye. The right optic nerve is irregular and shows enhancement (*large arrows*), thus indicating invasion by the tumor. Small arrows on the image in *C* also point to the ora serrata, which limits the subretinal space.

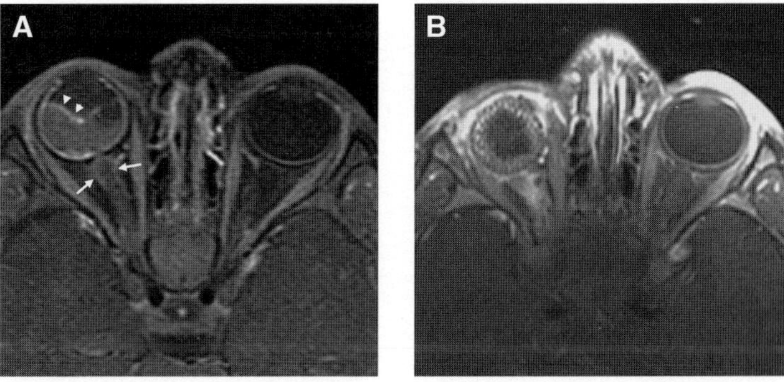


Fig. 9. Posttreatment imaging of the patient presented in Fig. 8. (*A*) Enhanced T1-weighted MR image with fat saturation (TR/TE: 566/9 ms) demonstrates a persistent right optic nerve irregularity and abnormal enhancement (*arrows*); in addition, note the enhancing material along the detached sensory retina (*arrowheads*). Both findings indicate the presence of residual tumor. (*B*) Later study after enucleation of the right eye. Postcontrast T1-weighted MR scan with fat saturation shows increased enhancement around the right orbital implant and enhancement along the right optic nerve. This enhancement within the implant is caused by the presence of neovascularization. The abnormal enhancement of the right optic nerve is also an indication of reactive gliosis or tumor recurrence.

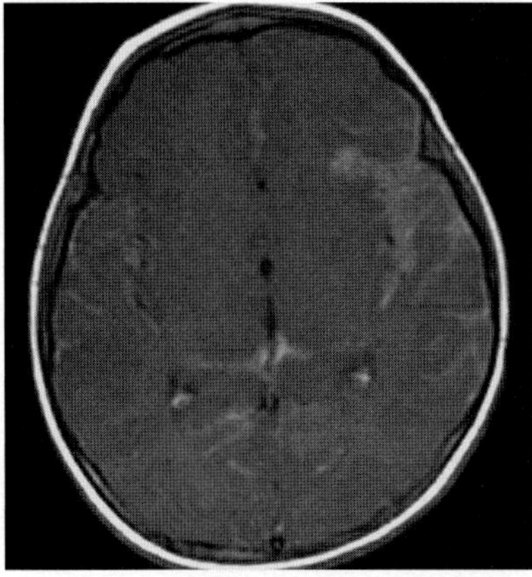

Fig. 10. MR image of the brain of the patient presented in Figs. 3 and 9. The disease had progressed despite continued treatment. An enhanced T1-weighted MR image (TR/TE: 500/14 ms) depicts diffuse leptomeningeal enhancement reflecting seeding of the subarachnoid space by the tumor.

possible options. Imaging of the entire brain is of special importance in patients with hereditary Rb, with the goal of early detection of trilateral Rb (Fig. 15).

Several imaging protocols have been described for Rb patients; however, alteration and additional imaging are commonly required to answer specific clinical questions or to fit a particular clinical situation.

A high-quality MR imaging examination requires the full cooperation of the patient and his or her parents. The procedure needs to be carefully explained to the patient and family members. Conscious sedation is used in most cases. As a rule, oral chloral hydrate (75–100 mg/kg of body weight) provides an adequate level of sedation in infants and children 4 years of age and younger. When chloral hydrate administration is inadequate, a one-time dose of intramuscular diphenhydramine (Benadryl, 1.0 mg/kg) or midazolam (Versed, 0.05–0.08 mg/kg) may be added for children from 5 to 8 years of age.

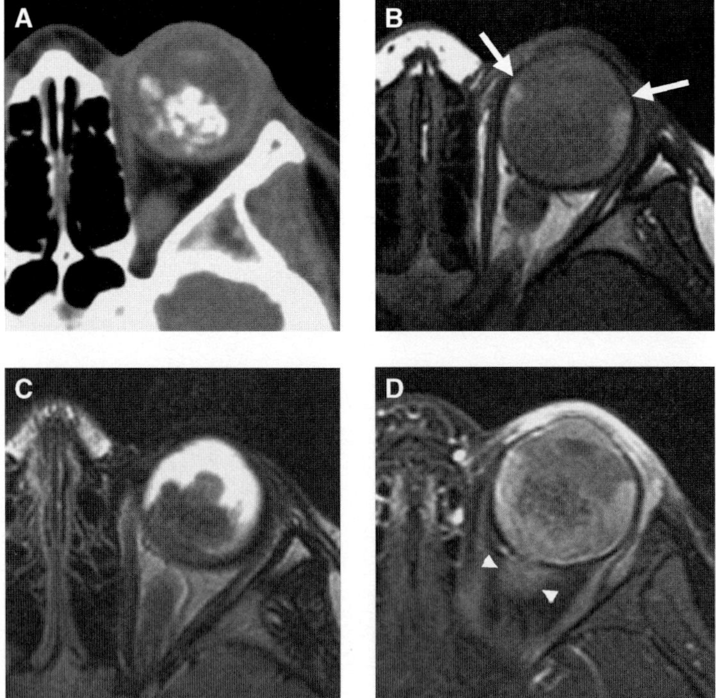


Fig. 11. Patient with Rb. (*A*) Nonenhanced CT scan of the left orbit shows chunky calcifications in the left eye. Dense material in the subretinal space represents exudated fluid. High density fluid in the subretinal space is present in the image. (*B*) Nonenhanced T1-weighted MR image (TR/TE: 450/20 ms) confirms the presence of subretinal exudated fluid. The ora serrata limits the subretinal space anteriorly (*arrows*). T2-weighted MR image (*C*) and enhanced T1-weighted MR image (*D*) with fat saturation (TR/RE: 4000/107 ms and 650/20 ms, respectively) confirm the presence of an enhancing mass with low T2 signal intensity. This appearance is typical for Rb. The optic nerve is thick and also demonstrates abnormal enhancement, indicating involvement by the tumor (*arrowheads*).

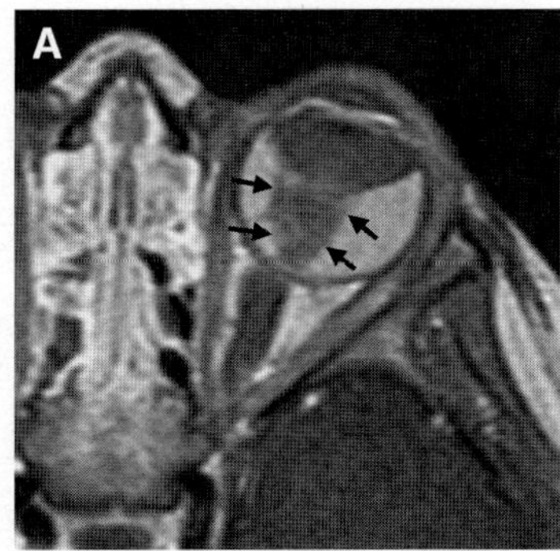


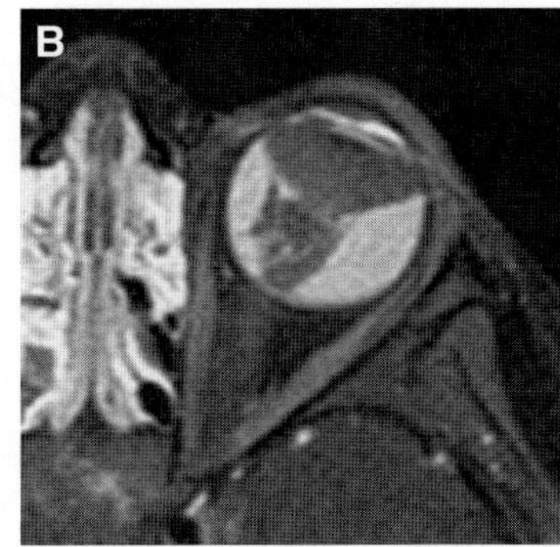


Fig. 12. The same patient as in Fig. 11. Axial enhanced T1-weighted MR images without (*A*) and with (*B*) fat saturation (TR/TE: 400/14 ms and 600/14 ms, respectively) after chemotherapy show a contracted primary mass (*arrows*) and increased subretinal exudate. The optic nerve appears normal in this study.

Challenging studies may require intravenous sedation or the use of general anesthesia. Sedated patients require continuous monitoring by means of pulse oximetry. Each hospital has its procedures for approving and certifying conscious sedation protocols, including patient monitoring by MR imaging center nurses or physicians. General anesthesia is provided by the anesthesia service with the use of MR imaging–compatible monitoring and ventilation equipment. If possible, an attempt should be made to combine the imaging examination with an ophthalmoscopic examination while the patient is under anesthesia.

Below we present our ocular MR imaging protocol with the use of a head coil and/or surface coil for the evaluation of Rb and allied conditions that occur in young children:

- Fast T2-weighted axial view: repetition time (TR) of 4000 milliseconds and echo time (TE) of 80 to 120 milliseconds, with a 256 × 192 matrix, 12- to 16-cm FOV, 3-mm slice thickness with 0.3 spacing, number of excitations (NEX) equalling 2, and no phase wrap (NP)
- Precontrast axial view: TR of 500 milliseconds and TE of 20 milliseconds, with a 256 × 192 matrix, 12- to 16-cm FOV, 3-mm slice thickness with 0.3 spacing, 2 to 3 NEX, and NP
- Postcontrast axial and coronal views: TR of 500 milliseconds and TE of 20 milliseconds, with a 256 × 192 matrix, 12- to 16 -mm FOV, 3-mm slice thickness with 0.3 mm spacing, 3 NEX, and NP
- Postcontrast axial and coronal views with fat saturation: TR of 500 milliseconds and TE of 20 milliseconds, with a 256 × 192 matrix, 12- to 16-cm FOV, 3-mm slice thickness with 0.3 mm spacing, 3 NEX, and NP
- Postcontrast images of the brain using the head coil: TR of 500 milliseconds and TE of 20 milliseconds, with a 256 × 192 matrix, 22- to 24-cm FOV, 5-mm slice thickness with 1.5 mm spacing, 1 NEX, and NP

Parasagittal postcontrast images with fat saturation are usually obtained (they are parallel to the long axis of the optic nerve). Additional sequences may also be obtained according to specific findings seen on the routine scan.

### *CT and MR appearance of retinoblastoma*

The typical appearance of Rb on CT is that of an enhancing mass with calcifications of different number, size, and shape (see Figs. 7, 8A, and 11A). Associated subretinal and vitreous hemorrhage presents as nonenhancing areas of hyperdensity, sometimes extending to the posterior aspect of the lens. On MR imaging, Rb usually demonstrates intermediate T1 and low T2 signal intensity (see Fig. 8) and shows moderate enhancement after contrast media infusion (Fig. 16). The MR imaging appearance is not as specific as that of CT because of the inability of MR imaging to show calcifications.

Note that focal thickening or irregularity of the choroid may indicate focal spread of the tumor. Normal choroid has fine uniform linear enhancement as shown in Fig. 8D.

In cases of optic nerve involvement, the optic nerve appears thickened with an irregular outline (see Fig. 7). Abnormally high enhancement is seen within and around the affected nerve (see Figs. 8 and 9). An

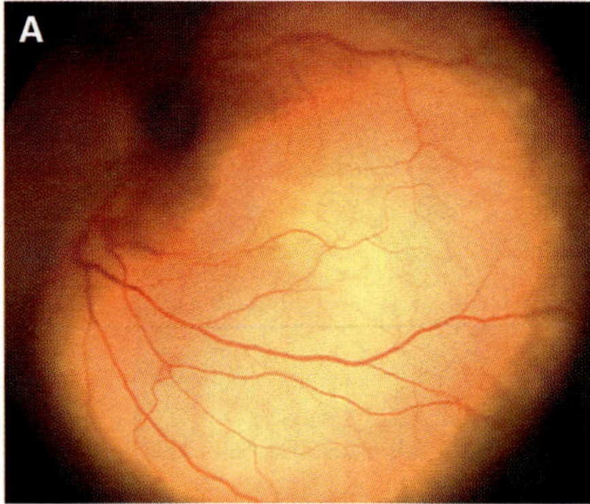


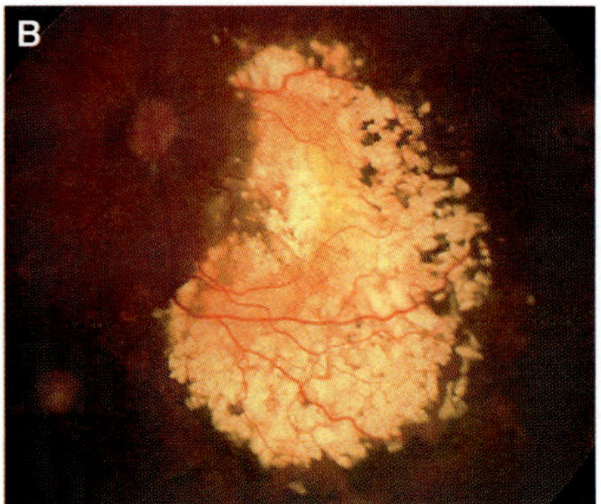


Fig. 13. A 10-month-old white female child with bilateral Rb. (*A*) Fundus photograph of the left eye shows a large tumor with exophytic and endophytic components and associated retinal detachment. (*B*) Fundus photograph of the same eye after treatment with chemotherapy (vincristine, etoposide, and carboplatin) demonstrates a significant reduction of the tumor and resolution of the retinal detachment.

intracranial PNET, as in trilateral Rb, is an avidly enhancing mass with low T1 and intermediate to high T2 signal intensity on precontrast images (see Fig. 15). Associated hydrocephalus may be observed. We have also observed benign enlargement of the pineal gland in several patients, with the pineal gland remaining stable in size on multiple follow-up studies (Fig. 17).

Cerebrospinal fluid (CSF) seeding by Rb commonly presents with diffuse leptomeningeal enhance-

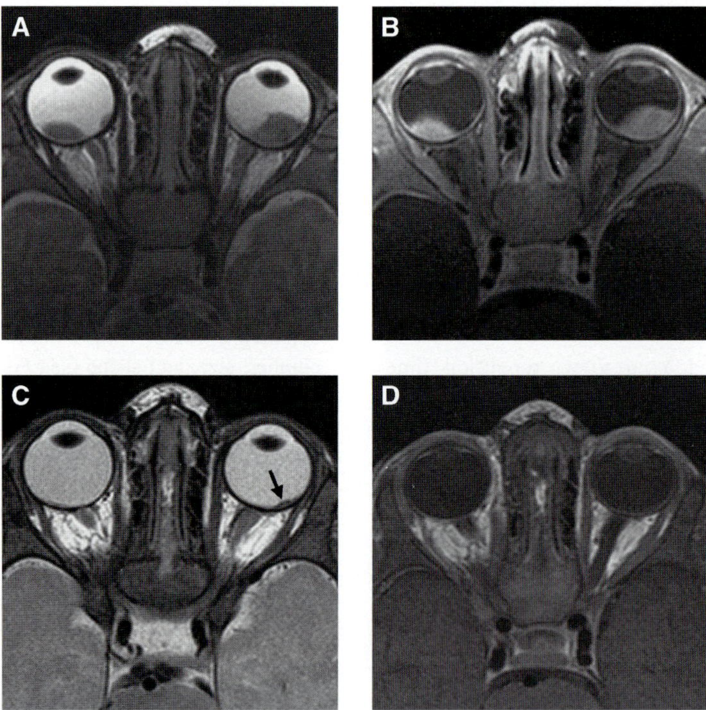


Fig. 14. Same patient as in Fig. 13. Pretreatment T2-weighted MR image (*A*) and enhanced T1-weighted MR image (*B*) with fat saturation (TR/TE: 2800/98 ms and 600/9 ms, respectively) show a large enhancing retinal mass in the left globe and at least two masses in the right globe. T2-weighted MR image (*C*) and enhanced T1-weighted MR image (*D*) (TR/TE: 3000/82 ms and 366/9 ms, respectively) after five cycles of chemotherapy demonstrate a small residual retinal thickening in the left eye (*arrow*) and no radiographically detectable tumor in the right eye.

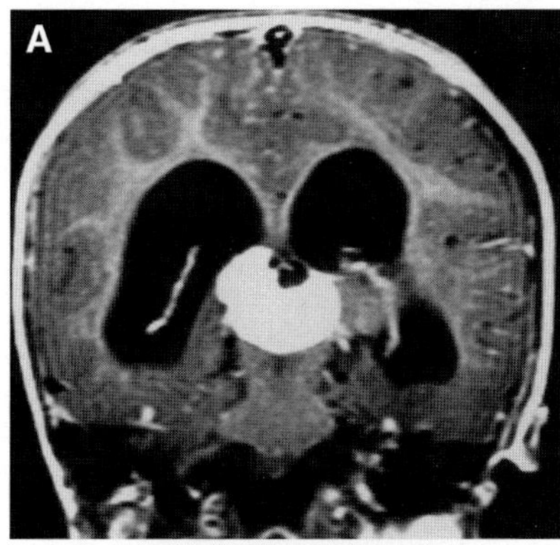


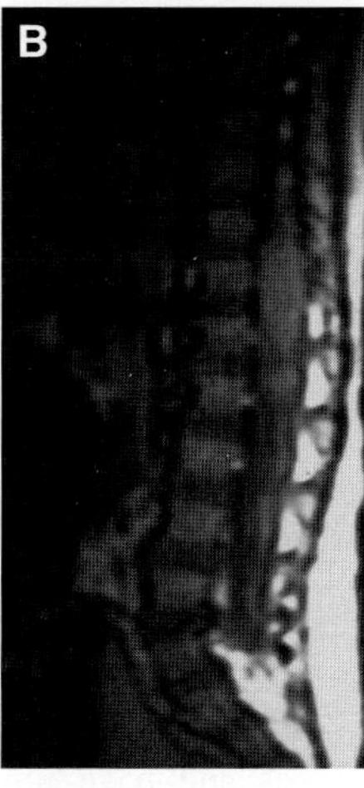


Fig. 15. Pinealoblastoma in a patient with bilateral Rb. (*A*) Enhanced coronal T1-weighted MR image (TR/TE: 600/20 ms) demonstrates a strongly enhancing mass of the pineal gland, which is compatible with pinealoblastoma and associated massive dilation of the lateral ventricles. (*B*) Enhanced sagittal T1-weighted MR image of the thoracolumbar spine shows diffuse abnormal intrathecal enhancement consistent with diffuse CSF spread and leptomeningeal seeding by pinealoblastoma/Rb tumor cells.

ment in the subarachnoid and intrathecal spaces (see Figs. 10 and 15B).

*Ocular oncology perspective of the diagnosis of retinoblastoma*

Radiographic, MR, and ultrasonographic images are important diagnostic tools for Rb; however, the ophthalmoscope remains the most powerful tool for the diagnosis and observation of intraocular Rb. Fine details as small as 50 μm can be observed ophthalmoscopically. Once expertise is obtained, high levels of diagnostic accuracy are achieved with the ophthalmoscopic examination alone. Experts use imaging mainly for evaluation of tumor extension and brain involvement and diagnosis of non-Rb cases in infants with leukocoria to discover treatable pediatric retinal conditions. CT and MR imaging are used for diagnosis in a few cases with uncertainty arising from an obscured view or an atypical appearing tumor that overlaps with other diagnoses. Imaging may also help less experienced ophthalmologists to reach the diagnosis of Rb. Because the treatment of Rb requires a high level of multidisciplinary expertise, we believe that immediate referral to an experienced physician benefits the patient. We use ophthalmoscopy and photography to monitor the response to treatment and watch for recurrence (Fig. 18) and the development of new tumors, which is the general rule for germline disease. The response typically shows a rapid reduction in volume, loss of vascularity, and replacement of tumor with calcification (see Fig. 6). Recurrent tumors are detected by observing the tumor margins using ophthalmoscopy and photography whenever available at monthly intervals.

Rb has a number of ophthalmoscopic appearances. The appearance relates to the size; pattern of growth; and presence of retinal detachment, tumor seeds, and blood. To avoid confusion, it is also important to recognize the secondary alterations caused by glaucoma, inflammation, scleral erosion, and optic nerve and orbital involvement.

All tumors begin intraretinally as a small opalescent mound of retina that protrudes from the surface. As the tumor grows, it appears more opaque white and gains a visible blood supply. Continued rapid growth shows an increasingly prominent blood supply as well as flecks of intense white calcification reflecting the necrosis of parts of the tumor that have

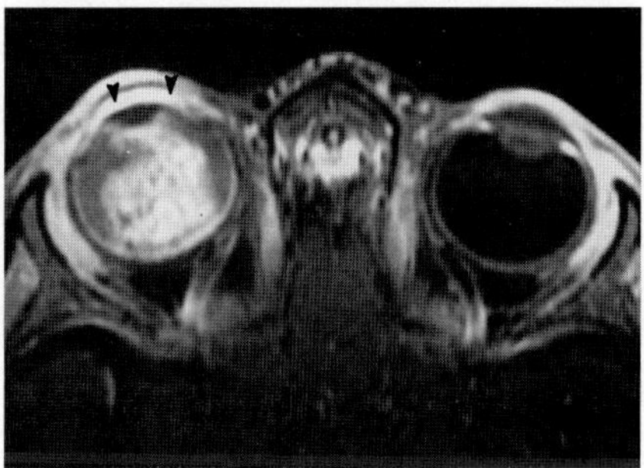

Fig. 16. Patient with Rb. Enhanced T1-weighted MR image (TR/TE: 500/14 ms) with fat saturation shows a large and markedly enhanced mass in the right eye, which is consistent with a diagnosis of Rb. Note the abnormal enhancement of the anterior chamber (*arrowheads*). This enhancement is not caused by tumor involvement or seeding and was thought to represent impairment of the ocular blood barrier.

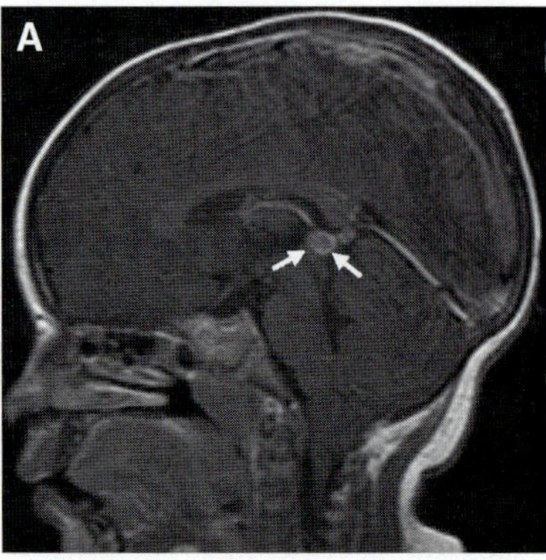


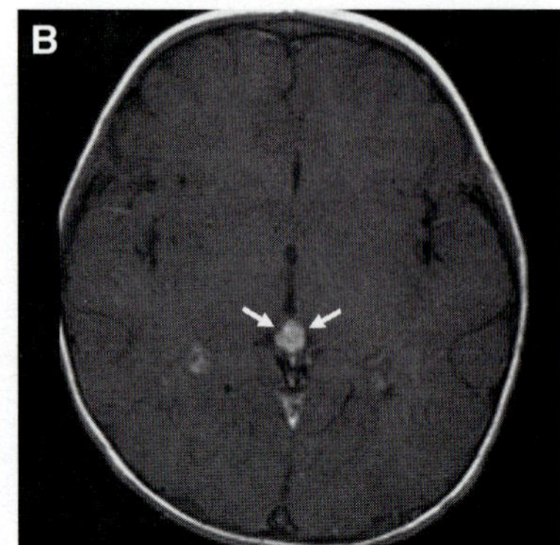


Fig. 17. Benign enlargement of pineal gland (*arrows*). (*A*) Prominent pineal gland measured at 8 mm was discovered on an MR image. No foci of calcification were seen within the gland, and follow-up scans demonstrated no further pineal enlargement. No malignant cells were found in the CSF. This represents benign hypertrophy of the pineal gland and is not a pineoblastoma (trilateral Rb). (*B*) Similar abnormality seen in another patient with bilateral Rb. The size (7 mm) of the pineal gland in this patient also remained stable.

grown beyond their vascular supply. Increasing growth and blood flow through leaky blood vessels cause an exudative retinal detachment (see Fig. 8). The detachment may increase until it elevates to just behind the lens (Fig. 19). In larger tumors, pieces of the tumor may break off and float as clouds or clumps of tumor seeds in the subretinal or vitreous space (see Fig. 3). Some tumors may invade beyond the retina into the optic nerve, choroid, or ciliary body. Seeds of tumor may spread into the anterior segment, with development of a pseudohypopyon. Secondary neovascularization (see Fig. 9), inflammation, and glaucoma may also occur. Untreated, the tumor grows into the orbit and meninges and further into the central nervous system (CNS) (see Fig. 10).

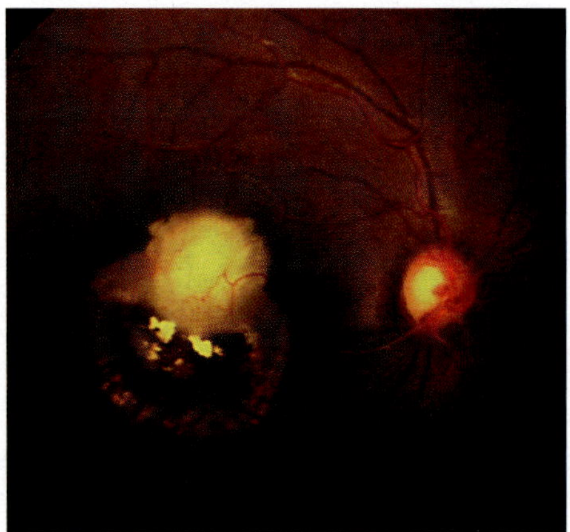

Fig. 18. Fundus photograph of the right eye treated with chemotherapy shows new growth at the superior margins of treated Rb.

Three patterns of tumor growth have been identified [20,22]:

1. Endophytic growth, when the tumor breaks through the internal limiting membrane of the retina into the vitreous. These masses often extend from intraretinal or exophytic tumors. They are chalky white with a scant vessel pattern. Over time, clumps of cells break off and float freely in the vitreous. They are called vitreous seeds and have important prognostic importance.
2. Exophytic growth, when the tumor proliferates outside the retina into the subretinal space. The overlying vessels become engorged. With time, the tumor exudates from incompetent vessels and an exudative retinal detachment may form. Clumps of cells may break free, and they are termed "subretinal seeds."
3. Diffuse infiltrating growth, when the mass spreads within the retina and has the appearance of a placoid mass. This is rare, and diagnosis is typically late. This form is a diagnostic challenge for ophthalmologists as well as radiologists because of its atypical clinical presentation and a lack of tumor calcification [42].

The diagnosis of Rb was achieved by ophthalmoscopy alone in more than 90% of the cases that we have seen. After the diagnosis is determined, imaging plays a key role for staging. In other cases of leukocoria with an obscure retina or complete retinal detachment without specific physical findings and neither a family history nor a history of prematurity,

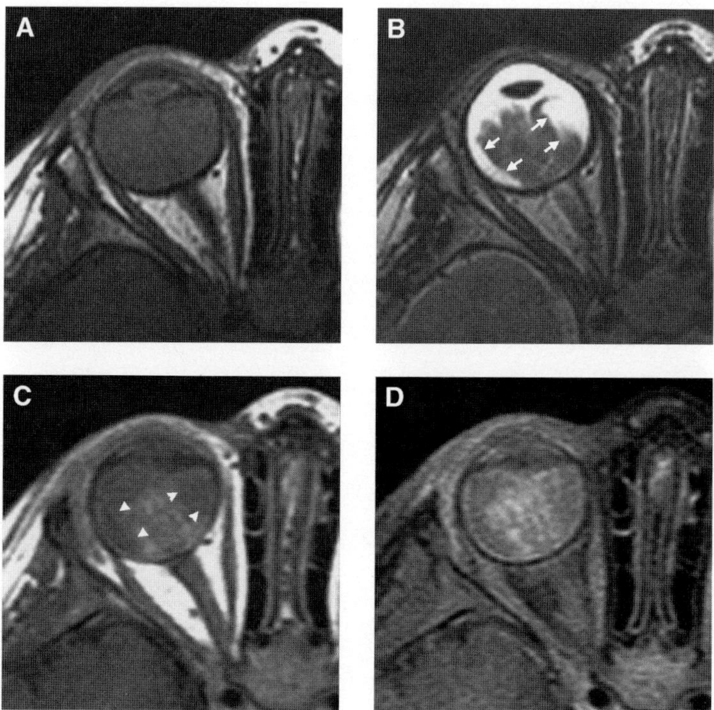


Fig. 19. Patient with unilateral Rb. (*A*) T1-weighted MR image (TR/TE: 483/14 ms) demonstrates a large mass in the right eye. (*B*) T2-weighted MR image (TR/TE: 4000/108 ms) shows peripheral areas of high signal (*arrows*) consistent with subretinal exudates and a tumor mass of low signal intensity. Contrast-enhanced T1-weighted MR images without (*C*) and with (*D*) fat saturation (TR/TE: 400/14 ms and 650/9 ms, respectively) reveal an enhancing mass and nonenhancing subretinal exudates (*arrowheads*).

ultrasonography and MR imaging have been quite useful not in excluding the diagnosis of Rb but rather in identifying findings of the so-called "simulating" lesions. These conditions are found in a group of patients who share only one finding with Rb—leukocoria, a white pupil. In fact, this level of confusion with Rb may exist only for the least expert physicians unable to examine the eye. Nonetheless, a diagnosis is required for all these patients, and most are made by a pediatric ophthalmologist. Others require an expert in pediatric retinal diseases or in ocular oncology. The use of imaging defines most situations. In a few atypical cases, tumors are observed for progression or regression and, rarely, biopsy is required.

## Intraocular conditions simulating retinoblastoma

### *Persistent hyperplastic primary vitreous*

Persistent hyperplastic primary vitreous (PHPV) results from arrested development, the failed regression of the fetal vascular system with subsequent proliferation of the associated embryonic connective tissue [43]. PHPV is the second most frequent cause of leukocoria after Rb [44]. Clinical examination may reveal microphthalmia, a shallow anterior chamber, angle-closure glaucoma, and a fibrovascular stalk between the optic disc and posterior capsule of the lens. The ophthalmoscopic examination is often incomplete because of cataract or retrolental tissue. Ultrasonography, MR imaging, and CT are useful for visualization of the posterior segment of the eye and for differentiation from other lesions producing leukocoria [22,33,45–47].

The CT findings of PHPV include microphthalmia, an absence of calcifications within or outside the globe, and increased attenuation of the entire vitreous body as a result of hemorrhagic exudates in the subretinal and/or subhyaloid space (Fig. 20) [45,46]. The value of CT or MR imaging is significantly increased by administration of intravenous iodinated contrast, which may reveal enhancing tissue within the vitreous compartment, which is tubular, cylindrical, or triangular (Fig. 21) [46,47]. Differentiation

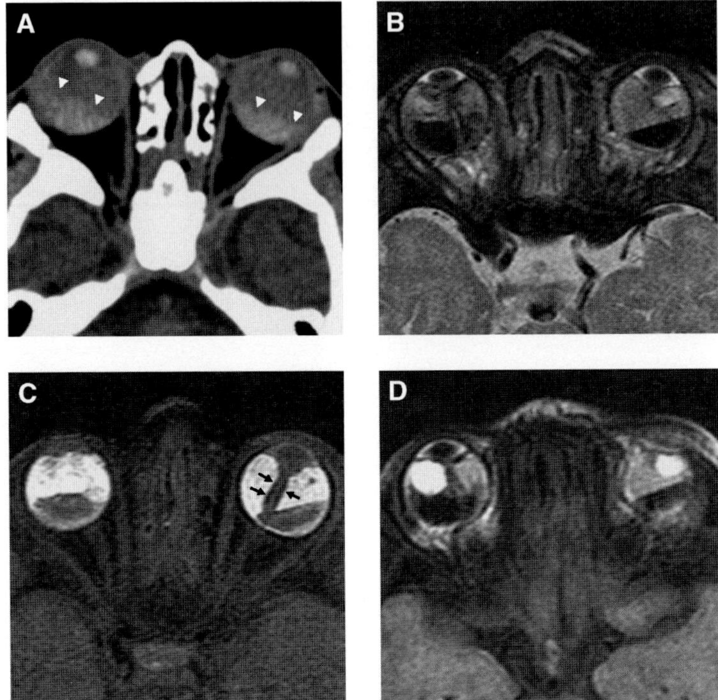


Fig. 20. Patient with bilateral PHPV. (*A*) Nonenhanced CT scan demonstrates hyperdense masses in the posterior segments of both globes (*arrowheads*) consistent with exudate or hemorrhage in the subhyaloid or subretinal space. T2-weighted MR image (*B*), nonenhanced T1-weighted MR image with fat saturation (*C*), and fluid-attenuated inversion recovery (FLAIR) MR image (*D*) (TR/TE: 5000/108 ms, 816/18 ms, and 10,000/175 ms, respectively) reveal typical subretinal exudates with fluid-fluid levels in both eyes. Arrows in *C* point to a tubular structure traversing the globe, which was thought to represent congenitally nonattached retina.

between PHPV and Rb is not always possible by CT. In these instances, MR imaging may be useful. Fluid-fluid levels may be seen on MR imaging and CT, which result from a sedimentation effect within subretinal and subhyaloid hemorrhagic exudates. The appearance of PHPV on MR imaging has a wide spectrum and is sometimes difficult to differentiate from ROP (Fig. 22). The typical patient with ROP has a history of short gestation, usually less than 30 weeks, and shows evidence of disease by ophthalmoscopic examination of the other eye.

### *Tractional retinal detachment associated with retinopathy of prematurity, familial exudative vitreoretinopathy, and Norrie disease*

ROP is retinal vascular disease that forms because of arrested vasculogenesis associated with premature birth. In familial exudative vitreoretinopathy (FEVR) and Norrie disease, this arrest is genetic. Abnormal fibrovascular proliferation may occur at the junction of the vascular and avascular retina, with retinal detachment in severe cases. There is a spectrum of tractional retinal detachment configurations, and the most common is the funnel-shaped retinal detachment. The eyes may be small or normal in size. In the most extreme cases, a retrolental mass, collapsed anterior chamber, glaucoma, and subretinal blood may be seen. The fibrosis of the retrolental mass shows a radiating vascular pattern of blood vessels and is connected to the optic nerve disc by the detached retina. The disease is usually bilateral and fairly symmetric. Calcifications are rare but may be present in the advances stages of ROP.

### *Coats disease*

Coats disease, retinal telangiectasia, is a congenital disorder that usually occurs unilaterally in boys [48]. Diagnosis is made based on the presence of abnormal telangiectatic vessels commonly seen in the temporal quadrant of the retina. Exudative retinal detachment often results from the abnormal vascular leakage (Fig. 23) [49]. Because large exophytic Rb

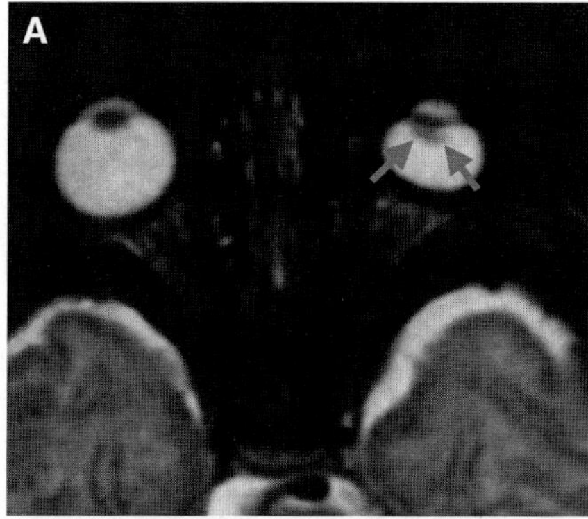


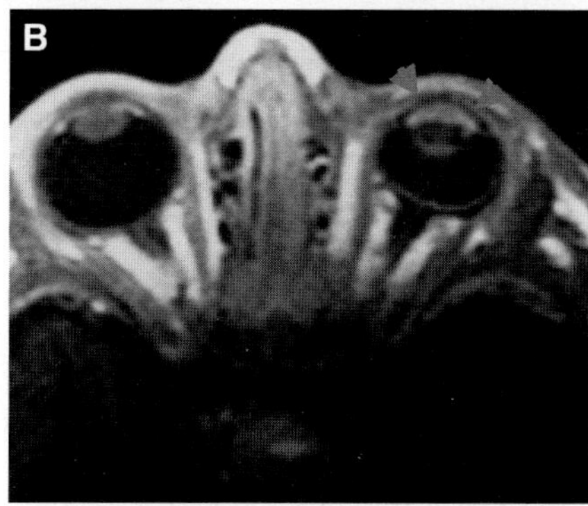


Fig. 21. Patient with PHPV. (*A*) Axial T2-weighted MR image shows left microphthalmia. Note the mass with low signal intensity (*arrows*) at the posterior pole of the lens. (*B*) Axial enhanced T1-weighted MR image demonstrates abnormal signal of the left lens, enhancement of the retrolental mass, and increased enhancement of the anterior chamber (*arrowheads*). The latter is related to leakage of gadolinium contrast from elongated ciliary processes, which is commonly seen in patients with PHPV.

and Coats disease are both accompanied by advanced exudative detachment on funduscopic examination, imaging studies are useful. The presence of classic telangiectatic vessels is not a part of Rb, and a tumor mass is not part of Coats disease. Therefore, most cases of Coats disease are readily diagnosed with ophthalmoloscopy and ocular ultrasonography. Bleeding may obscure the diagnostic vessels ophthalmoscopically or add confusion to the ultrasound.

CT and MR imaging characteristics of Coats disease are based on the main pathophysiologic presentation: leakage of a large amount of fluid with high cholesterol and protein content from immature telangiectatic retinal vessels. This fluid accumulates in the subretinal space, causing retinal detachment. Early stages of Coats disease may not be apparent on CT or MR imaging studies; however, the late stage of the disease is marked by thickening of the retina with or without extensive retinal detachment, which presents as homogeneous hyperdensity on CT and as high T1 and T2 signal material on MR imaging [33,47].

Calcifications are rare findings. Contrast enhancement is of utmost importance in the differentiation of Coats disease from Rb. Fluid does not enhance, nor does the apparent mass in patients with Coats disease. Some enhancement may be seen along the retina or border between the vitreous remnant and subretinal exudates, which corresponds to the presence of telangiectatic retinal blood vessels. At times, MR imaging may detect intrinsic irregularity of the subretinal fluid, which usually corresponds to hemorrhage or fibrosis as a result of organized hematoma.

### *Toxocariasis*

Ocular toxocariasis is a chorioretinitis caused by an inflammatory response to the nematode *Toxocara canis* [50]. Ocular toxocariasis is usually unilateral and is seen in older children. Clinically, it presents as endophthalmitis with a vitreous haze (Fig. 24) from a

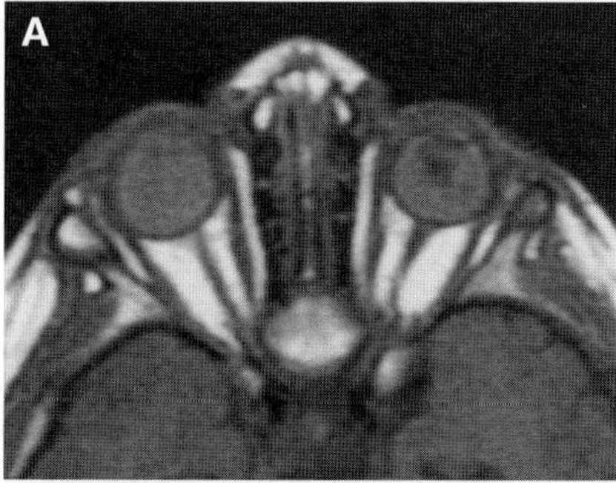


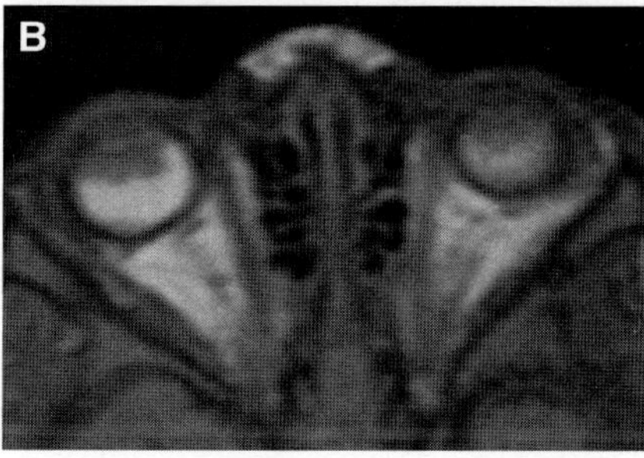


Fig. 22. Patient with ROP. (*A*) Axial nonenhanced T1-weighted MR image (TR/TE: 400/15 ms) shows bilateral microphthalmia. Note the increased signal intensity in both globes, which is related to bilateral total retinal detachment. (*B*) Axial proton density weighted MR (TR/TE: 2000/20 ms) in another patient with ROP demonstrates increase signal intensity in both globes. This also represents bilateral retinal detachment.

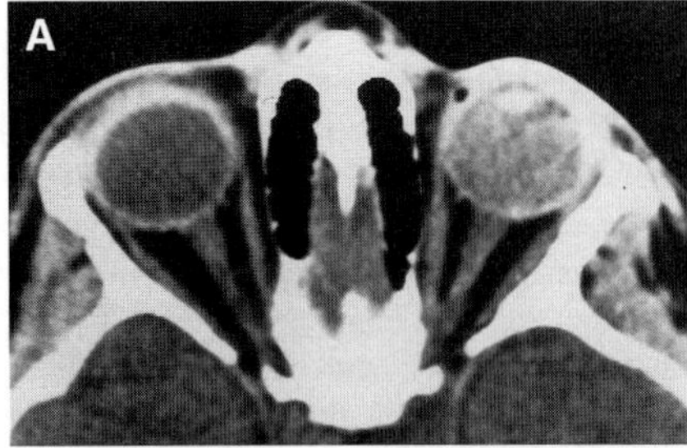


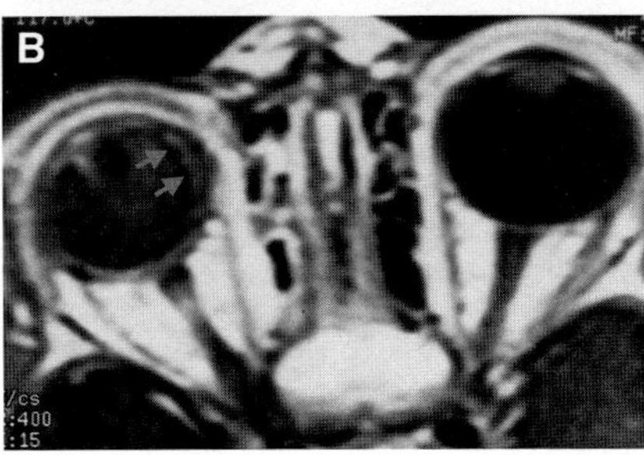


Fig. 23. Patient with Coats disease. (*A*) Axial nonenhanced CT scan shows increased density of the left eye as a result of total retinal detachment. (*B*) Enhanced T1-weighted MR image (TR/TE: 400/15 ms) without fat saturation in another patient with Coats disease. Note the increased thickening of the detached sensory retina, which is related to intraretinal exudate. Also note the enhancement of the detached sensory retina (*arrows*), reflecting increased vascularity (telangiectasia), the underlying cause of Coats disease.

profound inflammatory response (granulomatous inflammation surrounding the dead larvae, consisting of eosinophils, epithelioid cells, lymphocytes, and plasma cells) or as a posterior or peripheral retinal granuloma [51], which appears as a white elevated mass in the retina and may have associated adherent vitreous bands, vitreous tractions, tractional retinal detachment, and dragging of the retina and optic disc. The inflammation is responsive to steroids, the granuloma does not look like Rb, and the associated retinal detachment is usually tractional rather than exudative. Nevertheless, because both conditions are rare, a granuloma in the posterior pole may be confused with Rb [52].

### *Medulloepithelioma*

Medulloepithelioma is a congenital slowly growing tumor that arises from the ciliary body epithelium and typically presents as a mass behind the pupil or iris, although reports of retina and optic nerve involvement have been published (see the article by Vajaranant et al elsewhere in this issue) [53]. Patients usually present with leukocoria, pain, poor vision, or angle-closure glaucoma. The tumor is more dense in appearance and less vascular than Rb. Calcifications are common; however, it tends to appear in larger volumes rather than as the flecks seen in Rb (Fig. 25). The survival rate is excellent, because the tumor tends to stay localized within the eye. Patients with medulloepithelioma usually present at a later age than Rb patients, and it is discussed in elsewhere in this issue.

### *Retinal astrocytoma*

Retinal astrocytoma is a rare, benign, yellow-white retinal tumor that may present as an isolated

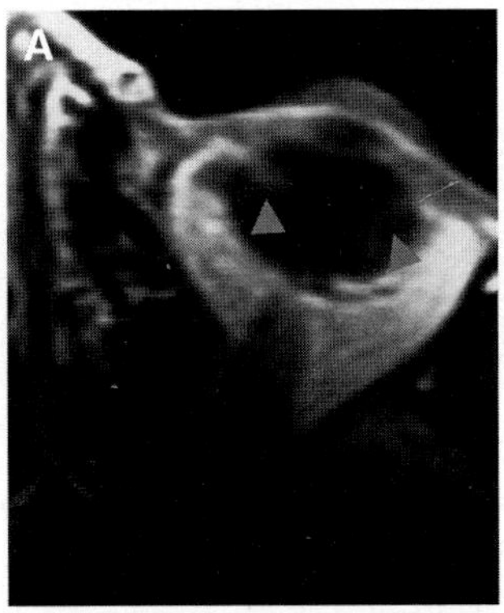


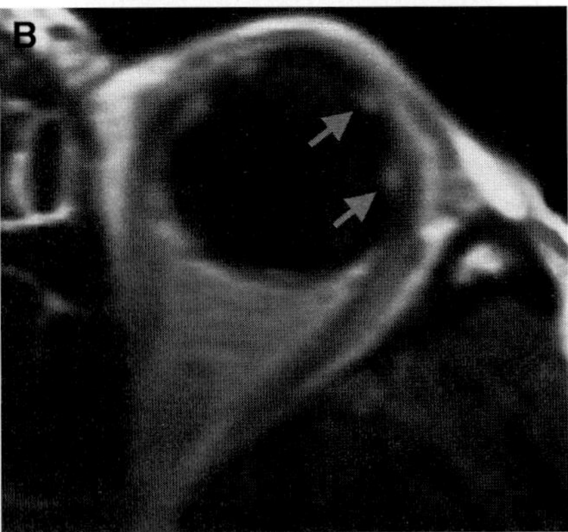


Fig. 24. Patient with *Toxocara* infection of the left eye. (*A*) Enhanced axial T1-weighted MR image without fat saturation (TR/TE: 400/20 ms) through the lower aspect of the orbits demonstrates intravitreal bands (*arrowheads*), which are related to *Toxocara* endophthalmitis. (*B*) Enhanced axial T1-weighted image without fat saturation (TR/TE: 400/20 ms) of the left eye at a higher level in the same patient shows multiple enhancing choroidal granulomas (*arrows*).

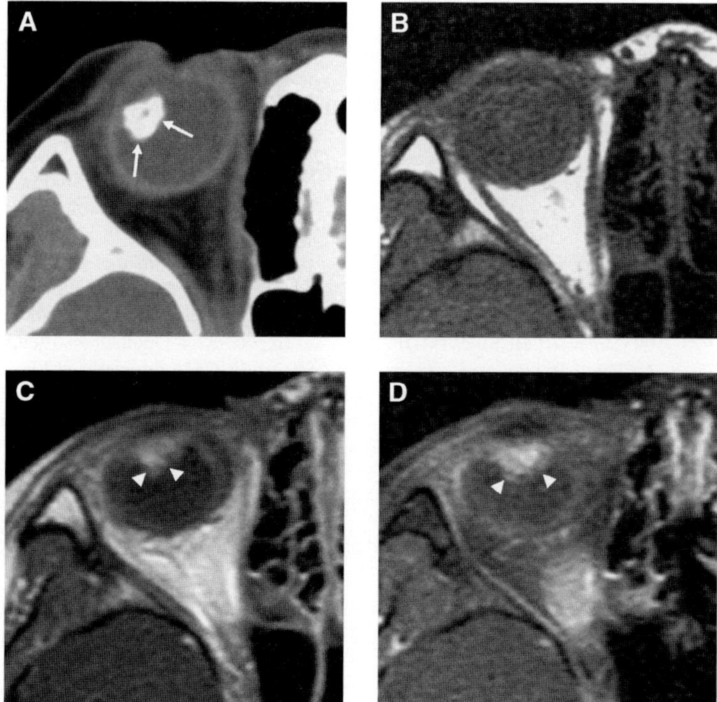


Fig. 25. Patient with teratoid medulloepithelioma of the ciliary body. (*A*) Nonenhanced CT scan of the right orbit demonstrates a mass with calcification (*arrows*) at the lateral aspect of the ciliary body of the right eye. Axial nonenhanced image (*B*) and enhanced T1-weighted MR images without (*C*) and with (*D*) fat saturation (TR/TE: 400/9 ms) confirm the presence of an enhancing mass in the same location.

ocular pathologic finding or in association with tuberous sclerosis or neurofibromatosis [54]. It is usually small, thin, and translucent near the optic nerve. It may also be more dense, multilobulated, and minimally vascular. It may be associated with an exudative retinal detachment, hemorrhage, and calcification. Unlike Rb, it rarely grows and then only modestly.

### *Optic nerve head drusen*

Optic nerve head drusen are the result of axonal degeneration and are composed of acellular concentric laminations that become calcified [55]. Drusen are mostly found accidentally on fundus examination as nodular glistening structures arising from the surface of the optic disc. Most cases are idiopathic; however, autosomal dominant transmission of this condition has been observed [56]. Occasionally, drusen are associated with ocular diseases, such as retinitis pigmentosa [57].

## Summary

Although the diagnosis of Rb is made primarily by means of clinical examination, CT and MR imaging are very helpful to confirm the diagnosis, determine the extent of the intraocular tumor, and exclude extraocular or intracranial involvement. They are also valuable in differentiating Rb from lesions that simulate Rb.

## References

[1] Dunphy EB. The story of retinoblastoma. Am J Ophthalmol 1964;58:539–52.
[2] Francois J. Hereditary of malignant tumors of the eye. Congenital anomalies of the eye. In: Symposium on Surgical and Medical Management of Congenital Anomalies of the Eye, New Orleans, 1967. Congenital anomalies of the eye; transactions. St. Louis: CV Mosby; 1968. p. 199–246.
[3] Devesa SS. The incidence of retinoblastoma. Am J Ophthalmol 1975;80:236–65.

[4] Shields CL, Honavar SG, Meadows AT, et al. Chemoreduction plus focal therapy for retinoblastoma: factors predictive of need for treatment with external beam radiotherapy or enucleation. Am J Ophthalmol 2002;133(5):657–64.

[5] Pendergrass TW, Davis S. Incidence of retinoblastoma in the United States. Arch Ophthalmol 1980;98: 1204–10.

[6] National Cancer Institute (US). National Institute of Health (US), Surveillance, Epidemiology and End Results. Retinoblastoma. In: Cancer incidence and survival among children and adolescents: United States SEER Program. 1975–1995 [Internet]. Bethesda (MD): The Institute. p. 73–8. Available at: http://seer.cancer.gov/publications/childhood/.

[7] Abramson DH. Retinoblastoma: diagnosis and management. Cancer J Clin 1982;32:130–40.

[8] Lennox EL, Draper GJ, Sanders BM. Retinoblastoma: a study of natural history and prognosis of 268 cases. BMJ 1975;3:731–4.

[9] Ellworth RM. The management of retinoblastoma. Trans Am Ophthalmol Soc 1969;67:462–534.

[10] Knudson AG. Mutation and cancer: statistical study of retinoblastoma. Proc Natl Acad Sci USA 1971;68: 820–3.

[11] Knudson AG. Retinoblastoma: a prototype heredity neoplasm. Semin Oncol 1978;5:57–60.

[12] Francke U. Retinoblastoma and chromosome 13. Cytogenet Cell Genet 1976;16:131–4.

[13] Knudson AG, Meadows AT, Nichols WW, et al. Chromosomal deletion and retinoblastoma. N Engl J Med 1976;295:1120–3.

[14] Jakobiec FA, Tso MO, Zimmerman LE, et al. Retinoblastoma and intracranial malignancy. Cancer 1977;39: 2048–58.

[15] Bader JL, Meadows AT, Zimmerman LE, et al. Bilateral retinoblastoma with ectopic intracranial retinoblastoma: trilateral retinoblastoma. Cancer Genet Cytogenet 1982;5:203–13.

[16] Bader JL, Miller RW, Meadows AT, et al. Trilateral retinoblastoma. Lancet 1980;2:582–3.

[17] Kivelä T. Trilateral retinoblastoma: a meta-analysis of hereditary retinoblastoma associated with primary ectopic intracranial retinoblastoma. J Clin Oncol 1999; 17(6):1829–37.

[18] Wong FL, Boice JD, Abramson DH, et al. Cancer incidence after retinoblastoma. Radiation dose and sarcoma risk. JAMA 1997;278(15):1262–7.

[19] Abramson DH, Ellsworth RM, Tretter P, et al. Treatment of bilateral groups I through III retinoblastoma with bilateral radiation. Arch Ophthalmol 1981;99: 1761–2.

[20] Haik BG, Saint Louis L, Smith ME, et al. Magnetic resonance imaging in the evaluation of leukokoria. Ophthalmology 1985;92:1143–52.

[21] Kaufman LM, Mafee MF, Song CD. Retinoblastoma and simulating lesions. Role of CT, MR imaging and use of Gd-DTPA contrast enhancement. Radiol Clin N Am 1998;36:1101–17.

[22] Mafee MF, Goldberg MF, Greenwald MJ, et al. Retinoblastoma and simulating lesions: role of CT and MR imaging. Radiol Clin N Am 1987;25:667–81.

[23] Virchow R. Die kranhaftergeschwalste, vol. 2. Berlin: August Hirschwald; 1864. p. 151–69 [in German].

[24] Popoff NA, Ellsworth RM. The fine structure of retinoblastoma, in vivo and in vitro observations. Lab Invest 1971;25:389–402.

[25] Tso MOM. Clues to the cells of origin of retinoblastoma. Int Ophthalmol Clin 1980;20:191–210.

[26] Tso MOM, Fine BS, Zimmerman LE, et al. Photoreceptor elements in retinoblastoma: a preliminary report. Arch Ophthalmol 1969;82:57–9.

[27] Tso MOM, Zimmerman LE, Fine BS. The nature of retinoblastoma: 1. Photoreceptor differentiation: a clinical and histopathologic study. Am J Ophthalmol 1970;69:339–49.

[28] Flexner S. A peculiar glioma (neuroepithelioma?) of the retina. Bull Johns Hopkins Hosp 1891;2:115–9.

[29] Wintersteiner H. Das Neuroepithelioma Retinae. Eine Anatomische und Klinische Studie. Vienna: Franz Deuticke; 1897.

[30] Howard GM, Ellsworth RM. Differential diagnosis of retinoblastoma: a statistical survey of 500 children. I. Relative frequency of the lesions which simulate retinoblastoma. Am J Ophthalmol 1965;60:610–8.

[31] Reese A, Ellsworth R. Evaluation and current concept of retinoblastoma therapy. Trans Am Acad Ophthalmol Otolaryngol 1963;67:164–72.

[32] Protocol from Children's Oncology Group. International classification system. National Cancer Institute. Available at: http://www.cancer.gov.

[33] Mafee MF. Eye and orbit. In: Valvassori's imaging of the head and neck. 2nd edition. New York: Thieme; 2005. p. 137–294.

[34] Badley LJ, Hurst RW, Zimmerman RA, et al. Imaging in the trilateral retinoblastoma syndrome. Neuroradiology 1996;38:166–70.

[35] DePotter P, Shields CL, Shield JA. Clinical variations of trilateral retinoblastoma: a report of 13 cases. J Pediatr Ophthalmol Strabismus 1994;31:26–31.

[36] Goldberg BB, Kotter MN, Ziskin MD. Diagnostic uses of ultrasound. New York: Grune & Stratton; 1975. p. 100–76.

[37] Danziger A, Prince MI. CT findings in retinoblastoma. AJR Am J Roentgenol 1979;133:695–702.

[38] Maffee MF, Maffee RF, Malik M, et al. Medical imaging in pediatric ophthalmology. Pediatr Clin N Am 2003;50:259–86.

[39] Maffee MF. The eye. In: Som PM, Curtin HD, editors. Head and neck imaging. St. Louis (MO): Mosby; 2003. p. 453–89.

[40] Kaufman L, Maffee MF, Song DC. Retinoblastoma and simulating lesions. Role of CT, MR imaging and use of Gd-DTPA contrast enhancement. Radiol Clin N Am 1998;36(6):1101–17.

[41] Schulman JA, Peyman A, Mafee MF, et al. The use of magnetic resonance imaging in the evaluation of retinoblastoma. J Pediatr Ophthalmol Strabismus 1986;23:144–7.

[42] Bhatnagar R, Vine AK. Diffuse infiltrating retinoblastoma. Ophthalmology 1991;98:1657–61.

[43] Manshot WA. Persistent hyperplastic primary vitreous: special reference to preretinal glial tissue as a pathologic characteristic and to the development of the primary vitreous. Arch Ophthalmol 1958;59:188–203.

[44] Goldberg MF. Persistent fetal vasculature (PVF): an integrated interpretation of signs and symptoms associated with persistent hyperplastic primary vitreous (PHPV). LIV Edward Jackson Memorial Lecture. Am J Ophthalmol 1997;124:587–626.

[45] Mafee MF, Goldberg MF, Valvassori GE. CT in the evaluation of patients with PHPV. Radiology 1982; 145:713–7.

[46] Mafee MF, Goldberg MF. PHPV: role of CT and MR imaging. Radiol Clin N Am 1987;25:683–92.

[47] Edward DP, Mafee MF, Garcia-Valenzuella E, et al. Coats' disease and persistent hyperplastic primary vitreous: role of MR imaging and CT. Radiol Clin N Am 1998;36(6):1119–31.

[48] Morgales AG. Coats' disease: natural history and results of treatment. Am J Ophthalmol 1965;60:855–64.

[49] Haik BG. Advanced Coats' disease. Trans Am Ophthalmol Soc 1991;89:371–476.

[50] Zinkman WH. Visceral larva migrans: a review and reassessment indicating two forms of clinical expression: visceral and ocular. Am J Dis Child 1978;132: 627–33.

[51] Wilder HC. Nematode endophthalmitis. Trans Am Acad Ophthalmol Otolaryngol 1950;55:99–109.

[52] Shields JA. Ocular toxocariasis: a review. Surv Ophthalmol 1984;28:361–81.

[53] Broughton WL, Zimmerman LE. A clinicopathologic study of 56 cases of intraocular medulloepithelioma. Am J Ophthalmol 1978;85:407–18.

[54] Gass JDM. New observations concerning choroidal osteomas. Int Ophthalmol 1979;1:71–84.

[55] Tso MOM. Pathology and pathogenesis of drusen of the optic nerve head. Ophthalmology 1981;88:1066–79.

[56] Apple DJ, Rabb MF, Walsh PM. Congenital anomalies of the optic disc. Surv Ophthalmol 1982;27:3–41.

[57] Puck A, Tso MOM, Fishman GA. Drusen of the optic nerve associated with retinitis pigmentosa. Arch Ophthalmol 1985;103:231–4.

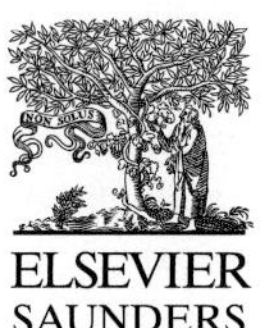
ELSEVIER
SAUNDERS

Neuroimag Clin N Am 15 (2005) 69 – 83

NEUROIMAGING
CLINICS OF
NORTH AMERICA

# Medulloepithelioma of the Ciliary Body and Optic Nerve: Clinicopathologic, CT, and MR Imaging Features

Thasarat S. Vajaranant, MD[a], Mahmood F. Mafee, MD[b], Rashmi Kapur, MD[a], Mark Rapoport, BS[c], Deepak P. Edward, MD[a,*]

[a]*Department of Ophthalmology and Visual Sciences, University of Illinois at Chicago, 1855 West Taylor Street, M/C 648, Chicago, IL 60612, USA*

[b]*Department of Radiology, University of Illinois at Chicago Medical Center, 1740 West Taylor Street, MC 931, Chicago, IL 60612, USA*

[c]*Department of Radiology, University of Illinois College of Medicine, 1801 West Taylor Street, MC 711, Chicago, IL 60612, USA*

Medulloepitheliomas are nonhereditary unilateral embryogenic neoplasms derived from primitive neuroepithelium [1–4]. Medulloepithelioma is the most common congenital tumor of the nonpigmented ciliary epithelium [2] In rare cases, the neoplasm can arise from the retina and the optic nerve [1–6]. Familiarity with the clinical presentation and radiologic findings of medulloepitheliomas is crucial for diagnosing this rare tumor. In this review, we discuss the imaging features, including CT and MR imaging of medulloepitheliomas of the ciliary body and the optic nerve and correlate these findings with the histopathologic changes seen in such eyes.

## Medulloepithelioma of the ciliary body

### *Clinical presentation*

Medulloepitheliomas of the ciliary body are usually diagnosed in the first decade of life, at a mean age of 4 years [2,3]. Rarely, these tumors can present in adults [1,7,8]. There is no racial or sexual predilection [1]. The right and left eyes are equally affected [1]. The common clinical presentations include a ciliary body mass, lens coloboma, lens subluxation, cataract, cyclitic membrane (a fibrovascular membrane across the ciliary processes), and glaucoma [1–3].

On clinical examination, the tumor often shows characteristic cystic lesions with an irregular surface in 60% of cases [3]. In some cases, spherical free-floating cysts containing hyaluronic acid can be observed [1–3]. Calcification with chalky opacity confined to the ciliary body is suggestive of medulloepithelioma [3]. Definitive diagnosis is made by histopathologic examination.

### *Histopathologic features*

On gross examination, medulloepitheliomas appear as fleshy tan or white masses located in the ciliary body region. The tumor surface is characteristically cystic [1–4]. Chalky gray-white deposits are often found within the tumor. These deposits are histologically composed of hyaline cartilage or bone. The tumors may extend anteriorly into the iris or posteriorly into the vitreous cavity involving the retina. In advanced cases, the entire eye may be filled with tumor, mimicking other intraocular tumors like retinoblastoma. Funnel-shaped retinal detachment that occasionally can be associated with medulloepitheliomas may imitate persistent hyperplastic primary vitreous (PHPV) [2,9]. In case of optic nerve in-

This article was supported in part by National Eye Institute Core Grant for Vision Research EY01792 (Bethesda, MD), an unrestricted grant from Research to Prevent Blindness (New York, NY), and a gift from Mrs. Doris Semmler.

* Corresponding author.
*E-mail address:* deepedwa@uic.edu (D.P. Edward).

1052-5149/05/$ – see front matter 
doi:10.1016/j.nic.2005.02.008

volvement, the patients may present with disc edema and diffuse thickening of the orbital portion of the optic nerve.

By microscopy, medulloepitheliomas are characterized by folded multilayered sheets and cords of poorly differentiated neuroepithelium [1]. These cells histologically resemble embryonic retina and ciliary epithelium [1]. Under low magnification, the connected sheets and cords with cystic spaces in between give a net-like appearance (dyktomatous pattern). The characteristic rosette-like structure, Homer-Wright and Flexner-Wintersteiner rosettes, may be observed [1]. Zimmerman classified medulloepitheliomas into nonteratoid (so-called "diktyoma") and teratoid types [1,3]. In addition to the proliferating cords and sheets of ciliary epithelium observed in nonteratoid tumors, teratoid medulloepitheliomas are composed of heteroplastic tissue elements, such as cartilage, skeletal muscle, and brain-like tissue. The teratoid form accounts for 30% to 50% of cases [1,3]. Therefore, on radiologic examination, the presence of intraocular masses with tissue characteristics resembling such structures should help in making a diagnosis. Medulloepitheliomas may be benign or malignant. The criteria for malignancy include poor cellular differentiation, cellular pleomorphism, sarcomatous changes, and invasion of surrounding ocular tissues [1]. Most reported cases were malignant. Broughton and Zimmerman [1] reported a rate of 66% malignancy in their series, whereas Shields et al [3] reported that 9 of 10 cases in their series were malignant.

*Management*

In the absence of extraocular involvement, treatment includes local resection for limited lesions or enucleation for extensive lesions [1–3]. In the presence of extraocular extension, exenteration, radiation, and chemotherapy are options. The prognosis is favorable in cases that do not have extraocular extension [1–3]. Compared with acquired epithelial tumors of the ciliary epithelium, such as adenoma or adenocarcinoma of the ciliary body, medulloepitheliomas have a high recurrence rate after local resection [4].

*Ancillary tests*

In clinical ophthalmology practice, ultrasonography is a readily available diagnostic tool. It can be helpful in detecting cystic appearance and calcification in some cases [3,10]. Other echographic features included irregular high internal reflectivity, irregular tumor surface, molding around intraocular structures, and internal vascularity [10]. The classic calcification of the ciliary body mass detected on ultrasonography may help to distinguish teratoid medulloepithelioma from retinoblastoma [3]. The involvement of the ciliary body in retinoblastomas is rare and may occur if the tumor is anteriorly located in older children [11].

*Characteristics of CT and MR imaging*

In addition to ultrasonography, CT and MR imaging are beneficial in distinguishing medulloepitheliomas from other intraocular tumors. CT and MR imaging provide better resolution compared with ultrasonography, and the extent of the tumor can be further evaluated. Radiation exposure during a CT scan is often a concern, especially in the pediatric population. In contrast to CT, MR imaging is considered a noninvasive technique with no known biologic side effects [12]. In current practice, these investigations are routine, and the findings from both modalities complement each other. Information from such imaging is often crucial not only for diagnosis but for developing a treatment plan. In one study, the sensitivity of detecting an intraocular tumor larger

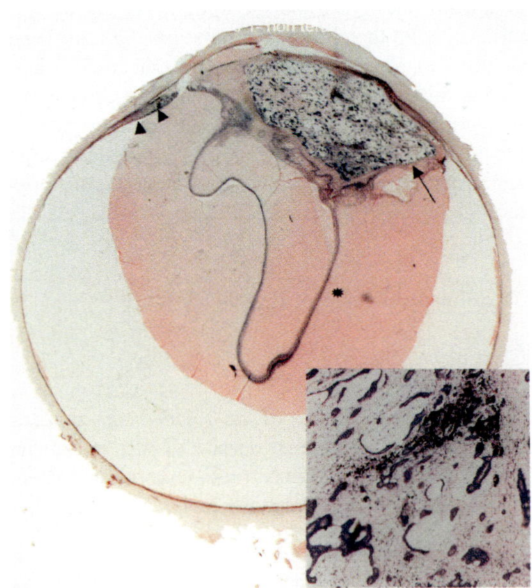

Fig. 1. Histopathologic findings of nonteratoid medulloepithelioma of the ciliary body show a mass arising from the ciliary body region (*arrow*) with associated retinal detachment (*). Note the normal ciliary body on the opposite side (*arrowheads*). High magnification (hematoxylin–eosin [H & E] stain, original magnification ×20) shows connected sheets and cords in a loose matrix giving a net-like appearance (dyktomatous pattern).

than 2 mm in precontrast study was 78% compared with 81% in postcontrast studies [13]. In general, a CT scan has the advantage of detecting calcification, which can be helpful in the differential diagnosis of intraocular tumors [12–14]. In contrast, MR imaging gives better soft tissue resolution and provides more precise information in determining the specific tissue characteristics [12–14]. This ability of MR imaging is particularly useful in case of intraocular tumors.

The following sections discuss imaging features seen in the different histopathologic variants of ocular medulloepitheliomas. The differential diagnoses of each category are further reviewed.

*Nonteratoid medulloepithelioma of the ciliary body*

On CT scans, nonteratoid medulloepithelioma appears as a dense noncalcified mass in the region of the ciliary body, with moderate to marked enhancement [12,15]. The histopathologic findings of medulloepithelioma of the ciliary body are shown in Fig. 1. Compared with CT, MR imaging provides better soft tissue resolution. Medulloepithelioma appears as a slightly to moderately hyperintense mass on T1-weighted MR imaging (Fig. 2A) and hypointense on T2-weighted MR imaging (Fig. 2B) with respect to the vitreous [12,13]. After intravenous gadolinium-based contrast infusion, T1-weighted MR imaging shows moderate to marked contrast enhancement (Fig. 2C). The enhancement is typically homogeneous; however, because of cystic changes, it may also be heterogeneous [12].

The differential diagnosis of hyperintense signal compared with vitreous signal on T1-weighted images and hypointense signal on T2-weighted images in children includes anteriorly located retinoblas-

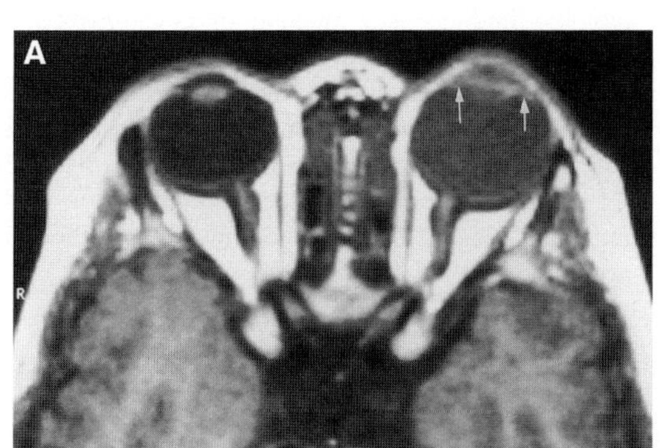


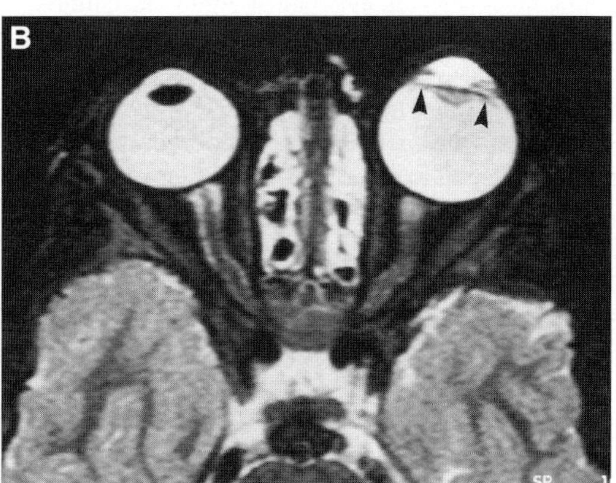


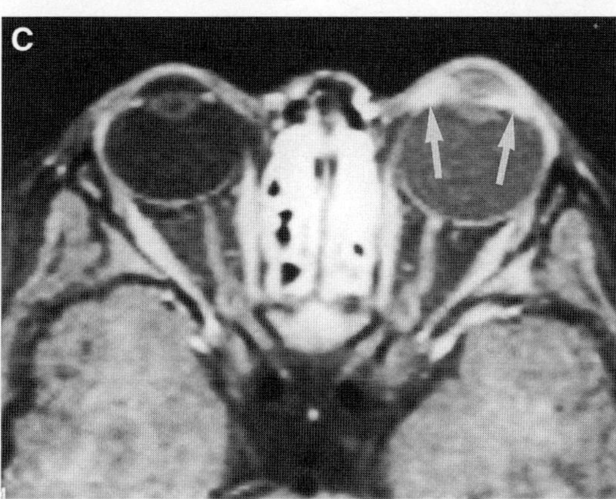


Fig. 2. Medulloepithelioma of the ciliary body. Axial T1-weighted (*A*), axial T2-weighted (*B*), and enhanced axial T1-weighted (*C*) MR imaging scans in a child show an infiltrative process compatible with medulloepithelioma invading the ciliary body (*arrows*) of the left eye. The enlarged size of the left eye is a result of secondary glaucoma. (Courtesy of S. Lingawi, MD, Saudi Arabia.)

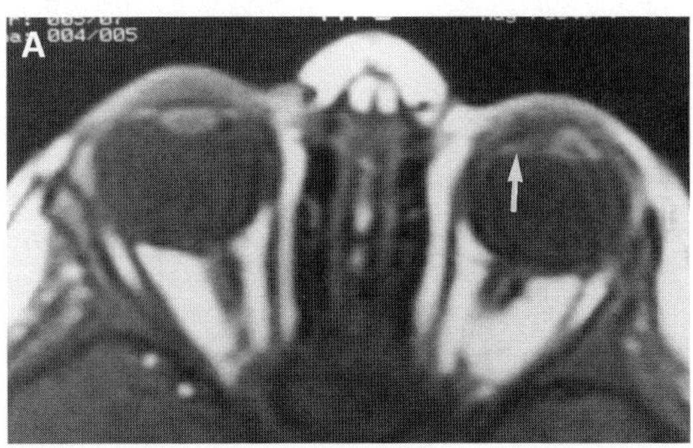


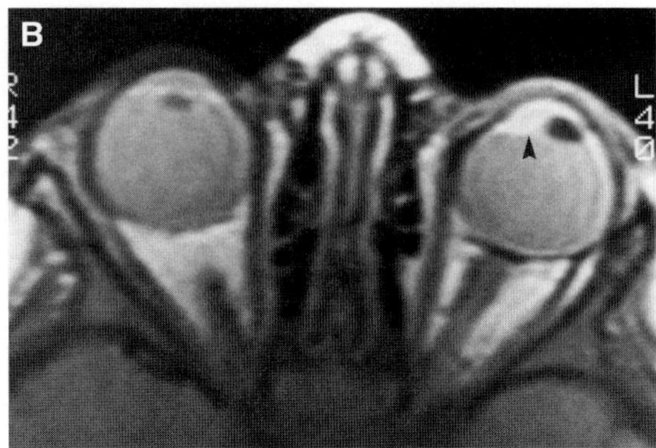


Fig. 3. MR imaging findings of a ciliary body cyst. Axial T1-weighted (*A*) and T2-weighted (*B*) MR imaging scans show a ciliary body cyst (*arrow* in *A, arrowhead* in *B*).

toma, mesoectodermal leiomyoma, a ciliary body cyst (Fig. 3), and xanthogranuloma of the ciliary body [13,16]. Retinoblastoma is the most common and highly malignant intraocular tumor in children, with a mean age of 13 months [17]. Most tumors are characteristically calcified. Only approximately 5% of cases show no calcification [17]. On clinical presentation, this anteriorly located retinoblastoma is more common in older pediatric patients compared with typical cases that arise from the posterior retina in younger children [11]. In addition, the anteriorly located retinoblastoma usually infiltrates the iris, causing increased intraocular pressure. Fig. 4 shows the histopathologic findings of an anteriorly located retinoblastoma without calcification. Leiomyomas of the ciliary body are extremely rare and appear as well-defined masses in the iris, the ciliary body, or the choroid [4,17]. Fig. 5 shows the histopathologic findings and imaging of a leiomyoma of the ciliary body. Xanthogranuloma of the ciliary body is a benign histiocytic lesion affecting the uveal tissues, retina, and optic nerve. The infiltrative nature of the tumor may cause hyphema or uveitis [17]. Fig. 6 demonstrates the histopathologic findings and imaging of a xanthogranuloma of the ciliary body.

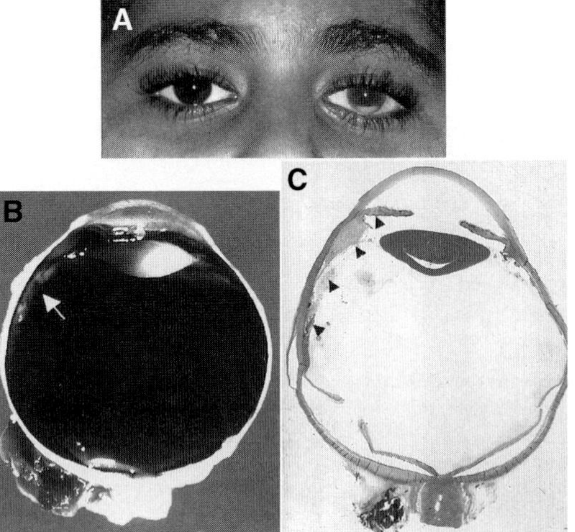


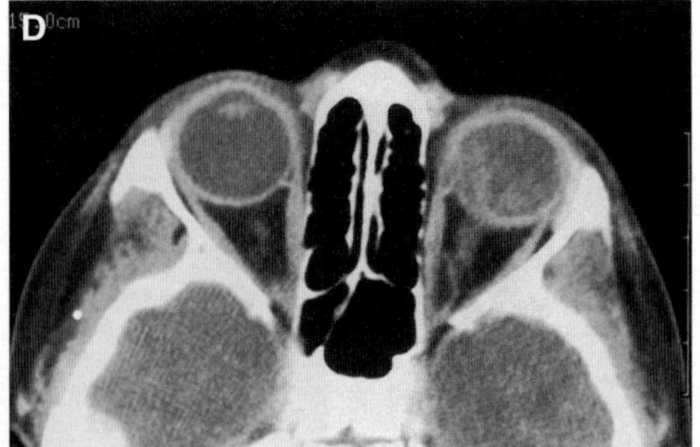


Fig. 4. Anteriorly located retinoblastoma without calcification. (*A*) Hypopyon in the left eye on clinical examination. (*B*) Gross examination shows thickening of the retina with tumor cells invading the ciliary body region (*arrow*). (*C*) Microscopic examination shows tumor infiltration resulting in thickening of the iris, ciliary body, and retina (*arrowheads*) without areas of calcification (H & E stain). (*D*) CT scan in another patient shows a diffuse noncalcified retinoblastoma involving the left eye in this 7-year-old boy.

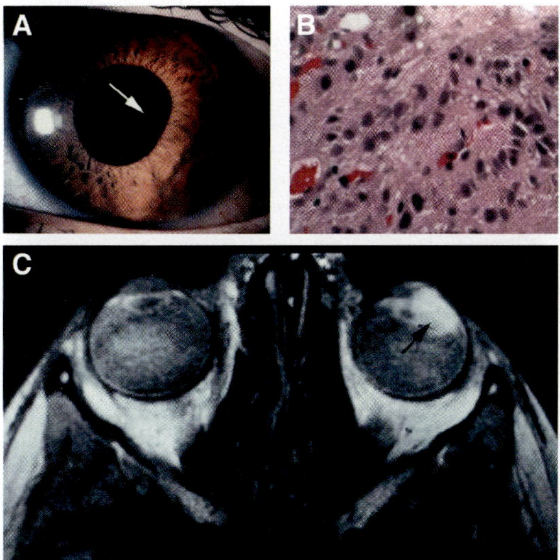


Fig. 5. Mesoectodermal leiomyoma of the ciliary body. (*A*) Clinical appearance of mass arising from the ciliary body region (*arrow*). (*B*) Histopathologic examination shows vascularized tumor with spindle-shaped cells and oval neuroid cells (HE stain, original magnification ×40). (*C*) Axial PW proton-weighted MR imaging scan shows the medulloepithelioma (*arrow*).

### *Teratoid medulloepithelioma of the ciliary body*

Approximately 30% of teratoid medulloepitheliomas show cartilage [3]. The cartilaginous tissue within the tumors may demonstrate dystrophic calcification; therefore, CT may be valuable in the diagnosis of teratoid tumors. The calcification can be detected even if the area is as small as 2 mm [12]. Teratoid medulloepitheliomas with cartilaginous differentiation and associated calcification appear as a dense irregular calcified mass in the region of ciliary body. Fig. 7 illustrates the clinical appearance and gross examination and the histopathologic findings of a teratoid medulloepithelioma of the ciliary body. Fig. 8 shows MR imaging and CT findings of the same case. This presence of calcification may also occur in anteriorly located retinoblastomas that occur in older children and may be difficult to differentiate from medulloepithelioma. Fig. 9 shows the histopathologic findings and imaging of retinoblastoma with calcification. Anteriorly located retinoblastomas may show diffuse iris invasion and vitreous seeding, findings that are not usually seen in medulloepitheliomas. Of note, masses that are localized mainly in the ciliary body are more suggestive of medulloepithelioma [3]. In advanced medulloepithelioma involving the vitreous cavity and the retina, other causes of intraocular calcified lesions cannot be excluded. Intraocular calcification simulating retinoblastoma and teratoid medulloepithelioma include cytomegalovirus (CMV) chorioretinitis (Fig. 10), *Toxocara* endophthalmitis, retinopathy of prematurity (ROP), choroidal osteoma, and retinal astrocytoma [12,17].

Although calcification may be detected by MR imaging, it is inferior to ultrasonography and CT. In one series, MR imaging demonstrated 54% sensitivity in detecting intraocular calcified lesions [13]. On MR imaging, calcification most often appears as a hypointense signal on T1- and T2-weighted images without enhancement [13]. Fig. 8 demonstrates the MR imaging findings of a case of teratoid medulloepithelioma.

### *Other simulating intraocular lesions*

Retinal detachment is an associated finding seen in advanced cases of medulloepithelioma. Similar to medulloepitheliomas, other intraocular lesions with retinal detachment or subretinal fluid can present with leukocoria or a retrolental mass. The differential diagnosis in this category includes Coat's disease, PHPV, ROP, and secondary subretinal fluid from metastasis [2,9,13]. This subretinal fluid exudate appears hyperintense in T1- and T2-weighted images without enhancement [13]. Improved soft tissue resolution on MR imaging may help to identify the associated solid tumors. Imaging features of these lesions have been described elsewhere in this issue in an article by Apushkin and his colleagues.

## Medulloepithelioma of the ciliary body in adults

Medulloepitheliomas of the ciliary body are extremely rare in adults. Carrillo and Streeten hypothesized that these cases represented asymptomatic benign lesions in childhood with malignant transformation later in adult life [7,8]. Based on a review of cases in adults ranging in age from 28 to 69 years, they were classified as malignant in five of six cases and teratoid in three of six cases [8]. Clinically, these lesions mimic malignant melanoma of the ciliary body [8,16]. On MR imaging, adult medulloepitheliomas are hyperintense on T1-weighted imaging and hypointense on T2-weighted imaging, similar to which are the MR imaging findings in ocular melanoma [13]. Fig. 11 demonstrates the his-

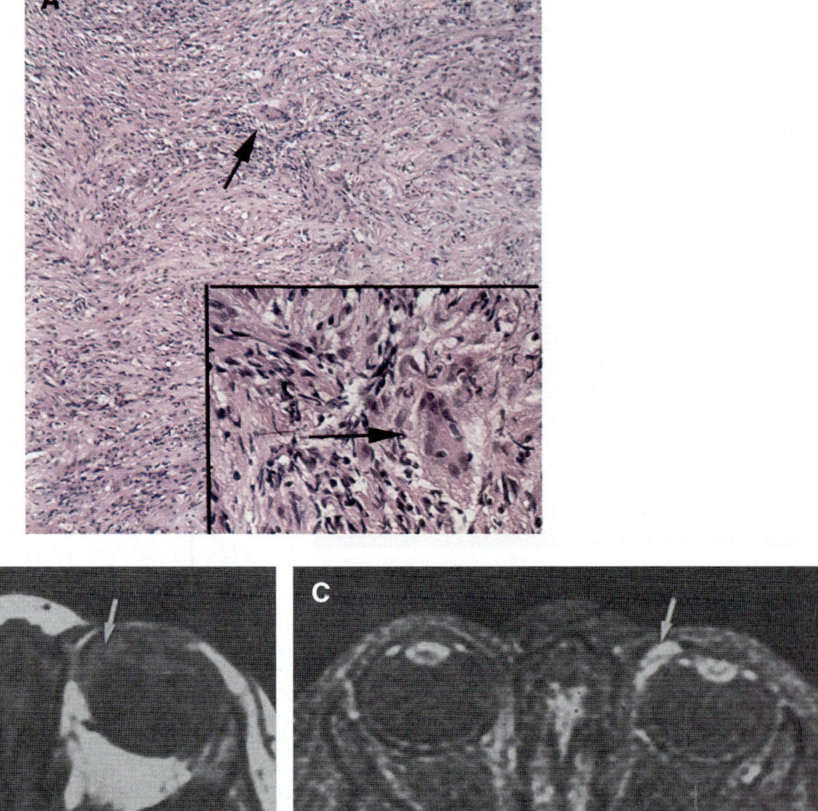


Fig. 6. Xanthogranuloma of the ciliary body. (*A*) Histopathologic examination (H & E stain) shows granulomatous inflammation with spindle-shaped histiocytic cells. Note the characteristic Touton giant cell (*arrow*). Precontrast T1-weighted (*B*) and postcontrast T1-weighted (*C*) MR imaging scans show an infiltrative enhancing mass involving the left eye (*arrows*). (*B* and *C* courtesy of A. Hidayat, MD, Washington, DC.)

topathologic findings and imaging studies of ciliary body melanoma. In contrast to medulloepitheliomas, melanomas of the ciliary body are acquired neoplasms. Unlike medulloepitheliomas, the surface of melanomas is smooth [4]. The classic tumor may be mushroom shaped [4]. For imaging studies, ultrasonographic findings may be useful, because medulloepitheliomas may demonstrate higher internal reflectivity when compared with ocular melanomas. In addition, cystic spaces and calcification, if seen, are suggestive of medulloepithelioma. In such cases, CT may be helpful in detecting calcification if it is not detected on ultrasonography.

In adults, other differential diagnoses of masses in the ciliary body region include adenoma or adenocarcinoma of the nonpigmented and pigmented ciliary epithelium, mesoectodermal leiomyoma, neurilemoma, metastatic carcinoma (Fig. 12), and granuloma (Fig. 13) [3,14,16]. Adenoma or adenocarcinoma of the ciliary epithelium is rare. The final diagnosis is often made by histopathologic examination of eyes enucleated for a clinical diagnosis of melanoma [4].

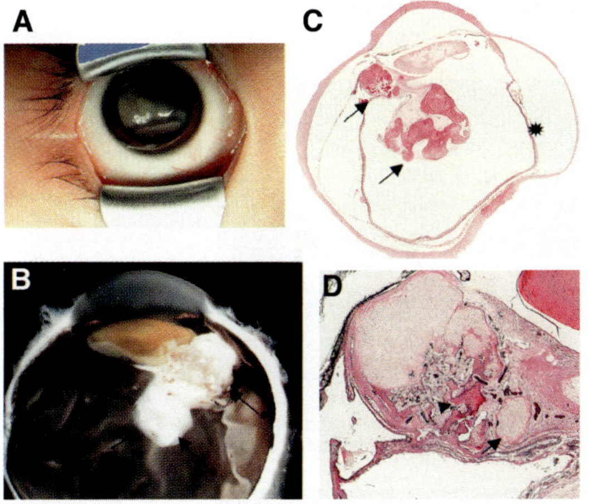


Fig. 7. Benign teratoid medulloepithelioma of the ciliary body. (*A*) Leukocoria with a tan-colored ciliary body mass behind the iris on clinical examination. (*B*) Gross examination shows a large lobulated tumor arising from the inferior ciliary body (*arrows*). Note the cut surface of the tumor, which shows whitish gelatinous areas with calcification. (*C*) At low magnification (H & E stain), a large lobulated mass (*arrows*) filled with cartilage and bone tissue is shown. Partial retinal detachment also seen (*). (*D*) At higher magnification, note a large island of well-developed cartilage (*arrow*) and bone (*arrowhead*) surrounded by vascularized spindle-shaped mesenchymal structures.

The tumors have MR imaging signal characteristics similar to those of melanoma and medulloepithelioma [13]. In addition to intraocular neoplasms, intraocular inflammation, such as granulomatous uveitis or tuberculosis (TB) granuloma, can mimic medulloepitheliomas if it presents with a mass in the ciliary body [4]. Fig. 14 shows the histopathologic findings and imaging of TB endophthalmitis.

### *Intracranial lesions associated with medulloepithelioma*

Ciliary body medulloepitheliomas have been associated with intracranial neoplasms other than central nervous system (CNS) medulloepitheliomas. Mamalis [18] first reported concurrent pinealoblastoma with benign teratoid medulloepithelioma of the ciliary body. Later, more complex intracranial abnormalities were demonstrated in a case of congenital malignant teratoid neoplasm of the eye and orbit, which is an unusual presentation of medulloepithelioma [19]. The abnormalities included agenesis of the corpus callosum, schizencephaly, and mass-like soft tissue prominence of the quadrigeminal plate. The authors suggested that clinicians be aware of associated intracranial neoplasms and CNS malformations in intraocular or orbital medulloepitheliomas [19]. In such cases, MR imaging should be the imaging modality of choice.

## Medulloepithelioma of the optic nerve

Medulloepitheliomas of the optic nerve are extremely rare congenital tumors. There are six case reports in the literature, with the age of these patients ranging from 20 months to 4.5 years [5]. Affected patients present with varied nonspecific complaints, such as ocular pain, strabismus, and proptosis [5].

On examination, patients usually have poor vision with abnormal pupillary responses. Fundus examination may demonstrate a mass in the region of the optic nerve, a swollen optic nerve, or disc pallor [5]. The tumor may extend anteriorly, appearing as exophytic masses from the optic nerve, or posteriorly with intracranial extension [5].

Management includes resection of the optic nerve via anterior enucleation combined with a craniotomy approach. A trial of adjuvant therapy, such as radiation and chemotherapy, has been used with varied success [5]. The prognosis is complicated by impairment secondary to extensive brain surgery and CNS system radiation. Similar to medulloepithelioma of the ciliary body, the prognosis is more favorable in cases that do not have intracranial extension [1–3,5]. It should be noted that optic nerve medulloepitheliomas may have a better prognosis when compared with medulloepitheliomas elsewhere in the CNS.

The diagnosis of medulloepitheliomas of the optic nerve is challenging. The final diagnosis often requires histopathologic examination [5]. The histopathologic classification and imaging features resemble those of medulloepitheliomas of the ciliary body [1,5]. Fig. 15 shows the histopathologic features of a malignant teratoid medulloepithelioma of the optic nerve. Fig. 16 shows MR imaging characteristics of the same patient as in Fig. 15.

The differential diagnosis of a mass in the region of the optic nerve head and optic nerve consists of optic nerve drusen, xanthogranuloma, papillitis, and optic nerve tumors like optic nerve gliomas, optic nerve sheath meningiomas, and optic nerve granuloma. Optic nerve drusen are benign, calcified, acellular lesions that are usually seen bilaterally [12,16]. On CT, they appear as discrete spherical high-density masses at the surface of the optic nerve [12,16]. In

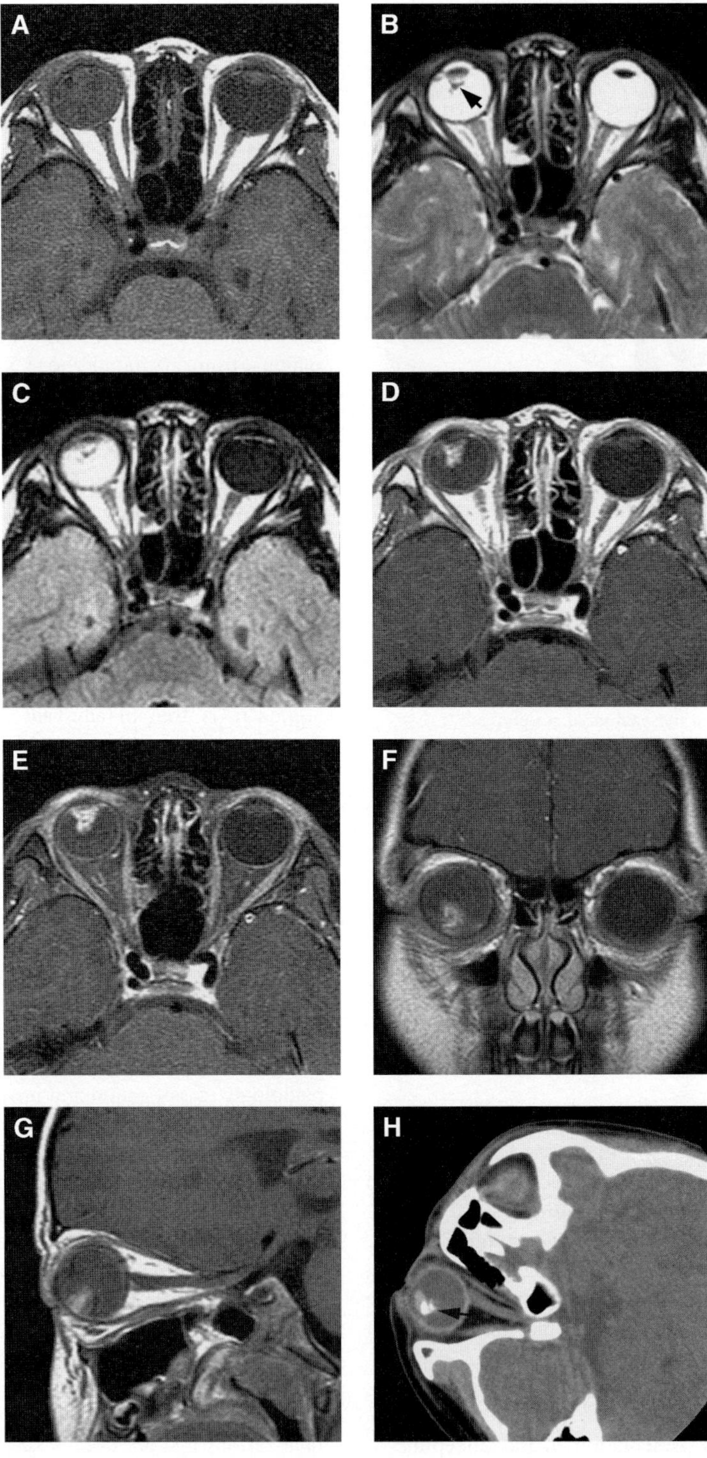
A
B
C
D
E
F
G
H

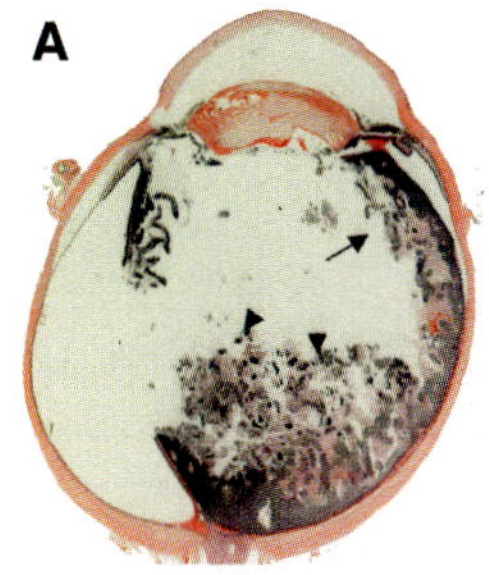


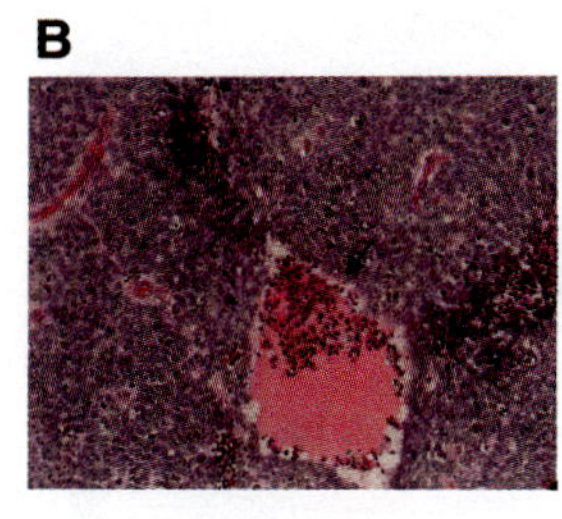


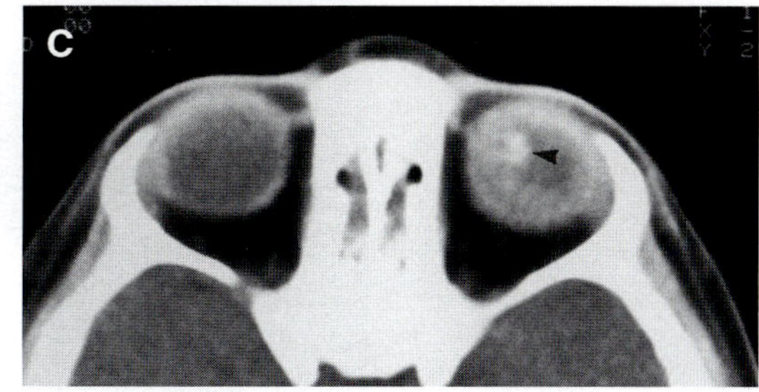


Fig. 9. Calcified retinoblastoma invading the ciliary body. (*A*) Low-magnification photograph shows exophytic retinoblastoma invading the ciliary body (*arrow*). Note an area of calcification (*arrowheads*). (*B*) Undifferentiated tumor cells with hyperchromatic nuclei and scant cytoplasm with necrosis (*arrow*) (H & E stain). (*C*) CT scan shows a retinoblastoma invading the ciliary body. Note calcification (*arrowhead*).

children, the lesions are more difficult to observe and calcification is rarely detectable on CT [12]. MR imaging is less sensitive in detecting optic nerve head drusen. Fig. 17 shows histopathologic findings and imaging of optic nerve drusen. For glioma, the most common location is the optic nerves [20]. A CT scan shows fusiform enlargement of the optic nerve with well-defined margins. A kinking or buckling appearance of the nerve is typical, whereas calcification is rare [12,20]. On MR imaging, the tumors appear hypointense to isointense with respect to the vitreous on T1-weighted series and hyperintense on T2-weighted series [20]. In contrast, optic nerve sheath meningiomas occur typically in adults, most commonly in middle-aged women [21]. On CT scans, meningiomas have a fusiform or tubular shape with a straightening appearance [20]. The tumors show marked enhancement; hence, the typical tram track sign may be observed [20]. Calcification may occur in 31% of cases [21] On MR imaging, the tumors show hypointensity on T1- and T2-weighted images with respect to the vitreous [20]. Of note, intracranial extension may present in optic nerve meningiomas, especially in younger patients [21]. CT and MR imaging of optic nerve gliomas and meningiomas are discussed elsewhere in this issue by Weber and his colleagues. Lastly, in cases in which optic nerve head or optic nerve medulloepitheliomas extend into the vitreous cavity or invade the surrounding structures, retinoblastomas involving the retina surrounding the optic nerve cannot be excluded.

## Medulloepithelioma of the central nervous system

Medulloepitheliomas of the CNS are rare embryonic intraepithelial tumors that originate from the primitive medullary plate and neural tube [22]. The tumor affects children between the ages of 6 months and 5 years [22]. Unlike medulloepitheliomas of the ciliary body and the optic nerve, the CNS tumors have a poor prognosis. The most common location is the cerebral hemisphere in the periventricular regions involving temporal, parietal, occipital, and frontal regions [22]. One series of eight cases showed an equal distribution between the supratentorial and infratentorial regions, however [23].

Medulloepitheliomas may be isodense or hypodense to brain, with variable heterogenicity [22]. Similar to ocular type tumors, CNS tumors are often associated with calcification and cystic changes. In addition, the brain may show necrosis and edema within the lesions [22,24]. With mixed tissue features, the contrast CT scan shows heterogeneous enhancement. Unlike ocular medulloepitheliomas, the CNS type is more aggressive. They may be disseminated or invade the adjacent skull in advanced cases [22,23]. MR imaging of cranial medulloepithelioma is variable. The tumors may demonstrate hypointensity or mixed signal intensity on T1-weighted images associated with marked enhancement compared with the brain signals. On T2-weighted images, heterogeneous isointensity to hyperintensity is observed [22].

Fig. 8. Teratoid medulloepithelioma of the ciliary body. Axial T1-weighted (*A*), T2-weighted (*B*), fluid-attenuated inversion recovery (*C*), enhanced T1-weighted (*D*), enhanced fat suppression T1-weighted (*E*), coronal enhanced T1-weighted (*F*), and sagittal enhanced T1-weighted (*G*) MR imaging scans and a CT scan (*H*) show a ciliary body medulloepithelioma (*arrow* in *B*) and calcification (*arrow* in *H*). (*A, B, E*, and *H from* Mafee MF, Valvassori GE, Becker M, editors. Imaging of the head and neck. 2nd edition. Stuttgart (Germany): Thieme; 2004. p. 189; with permission.)

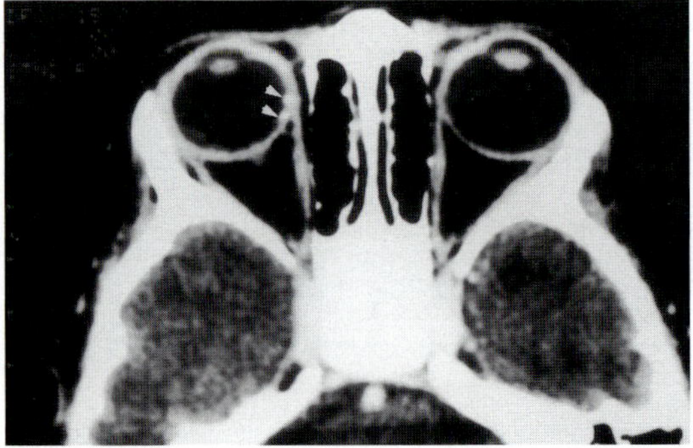

Fig. 10. Cytomegalovirus retinitis. CT scan in a child with AIDS complicated by CMV retinitis shows dystrophic calcifications (*arrowheads*).

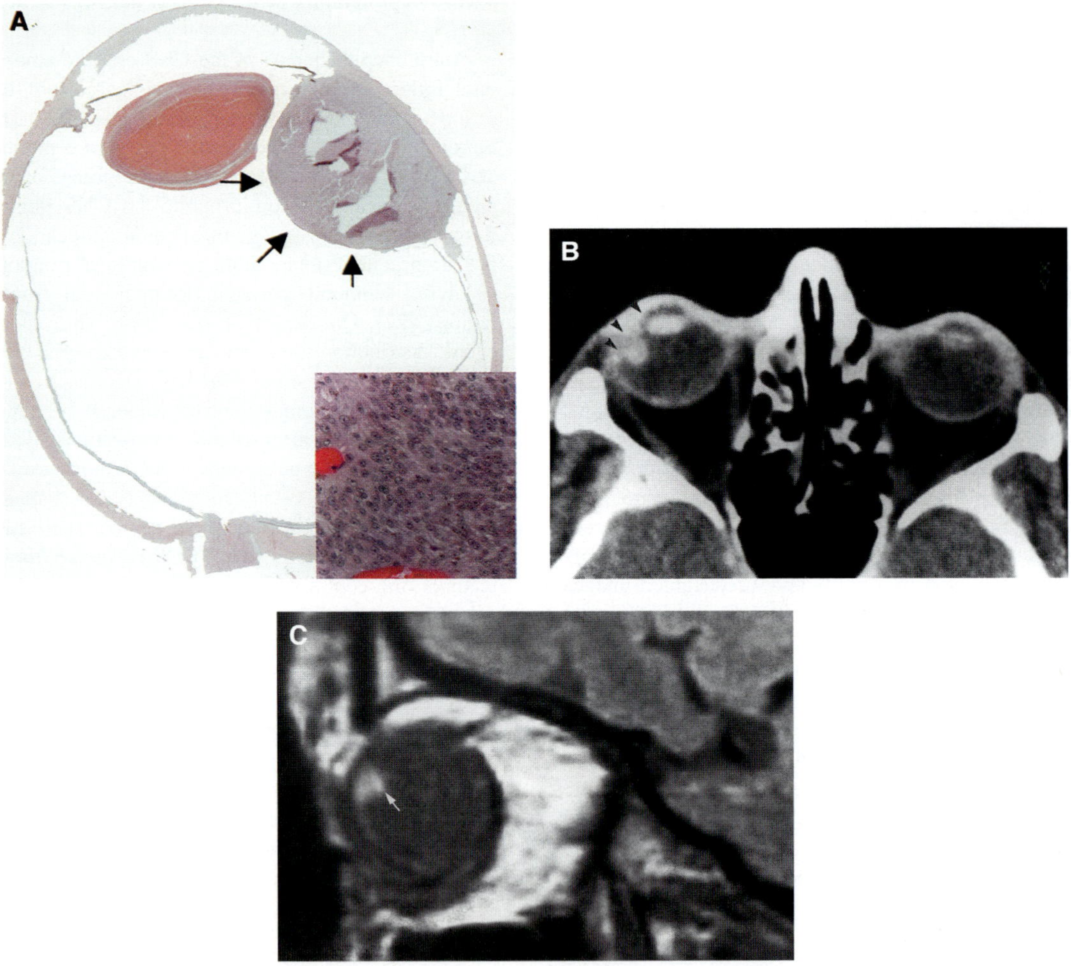

Fig. 11. Melanoma of the ciliary body. (*A*) Histopathologic findings of melanoma arising from the ciliary body region. Note a large localized mass with a smooth surface and densely packed basophilic cells (*arrows*). Higher magnification shows spindled B cells with variable pigmentation (*inset*, H & E stain). (*B*) CT scan shows a hyperdense mass (*arrowheads*) compatible with a large ciliary melanoma. (*C*) Proton-weighted MR imaging scan in another patient shows a ciliary body malignant melanoma (*arrow*).

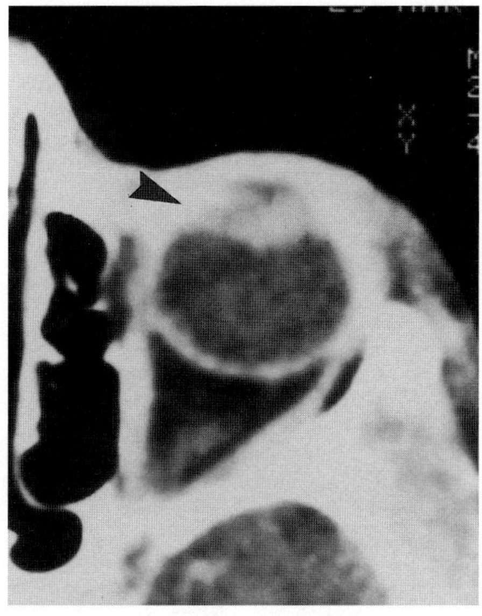

Fig. 12. Ciliary body metastasis from primary lung cancer. Axial enhanced CT scan shows a ciliary body metastasis (*arrowhead*).

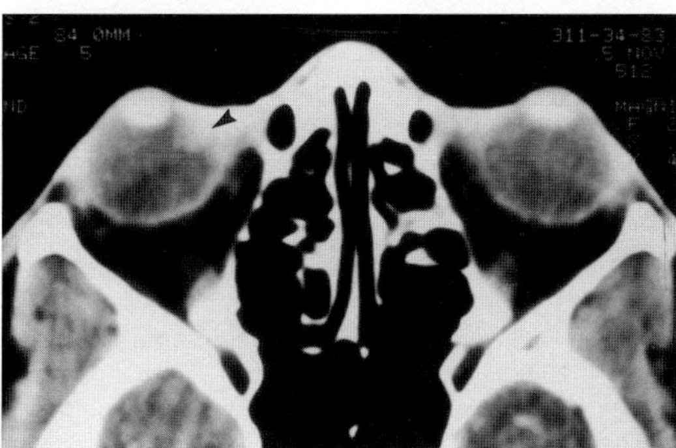

Fig. 13. Ocular granuloma in a middle-aged woman. Axial CT scan shows a mass in the anterior nasal aspect of the right eye. There is small calcification present (*arrowhead*). Because ciliary malignant melanoma could not be excluded, the eye was enucleated. The histopathological findings were consistent with chronic granuloma. (*From* Mafee MF, Valvassori GE, Becker M, editors. Imaging of the head and neck. 2nd edition. Stuttgart (Germany): Thieme; 2004. p. 174; with permission.)

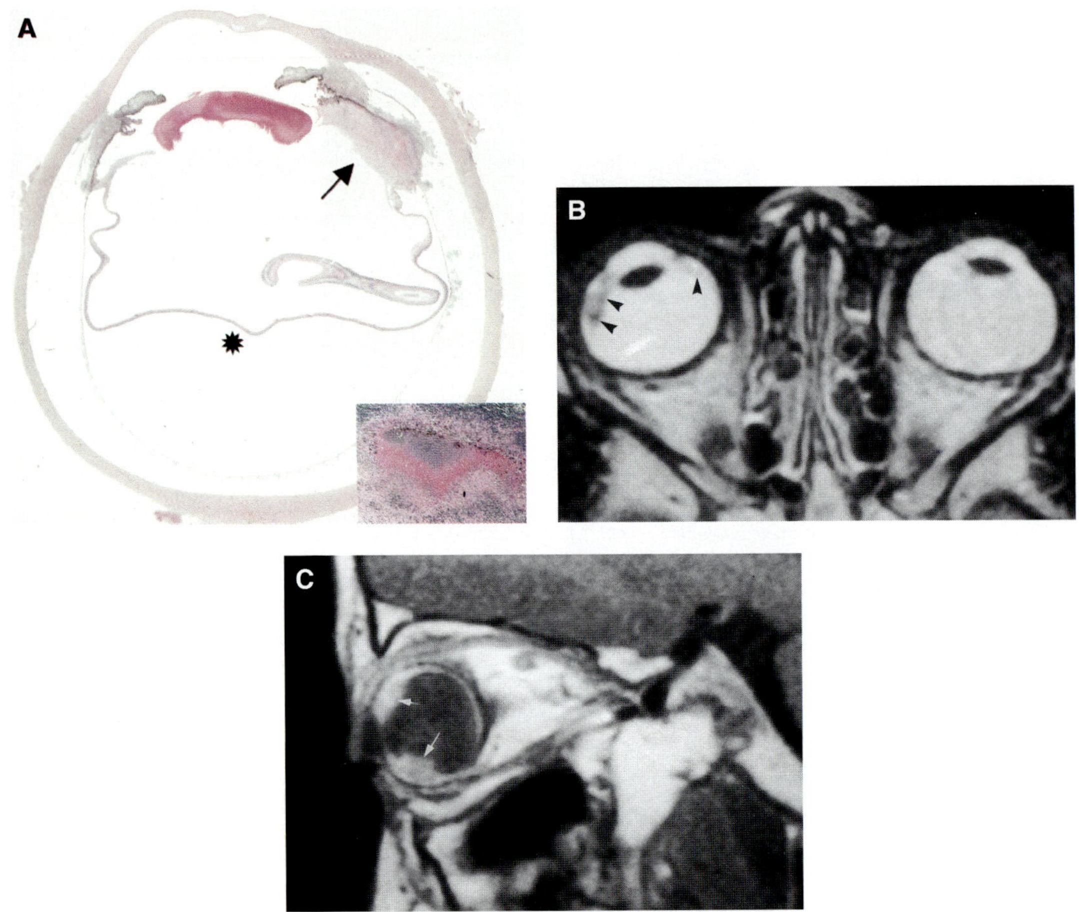

Fig. 14. Tuberculosis. (*A*) Low-magnification photograph shows a localized mass in the ciliary body region (*arrow*). Note the area of artifactual retinal detachment (*). Higher magnification shows a suppurative granuloma consistent with tuberculosis (*inset*, H & E stain). Axial T2-weighted (*B*) and enhanced sagittal T1-weighted (*C*) MR imaging scans show an infiltrative process involving the ciliary body of the right eye. The lesion is hypointense on T2-weighted MR imaging (*arrowheads* in *B*) and demonstrates marked diffuse enhancement (*arrows* in *C*). These MR imaging findings cannot be differentiated from those of ciliary body medulloepithelioma.

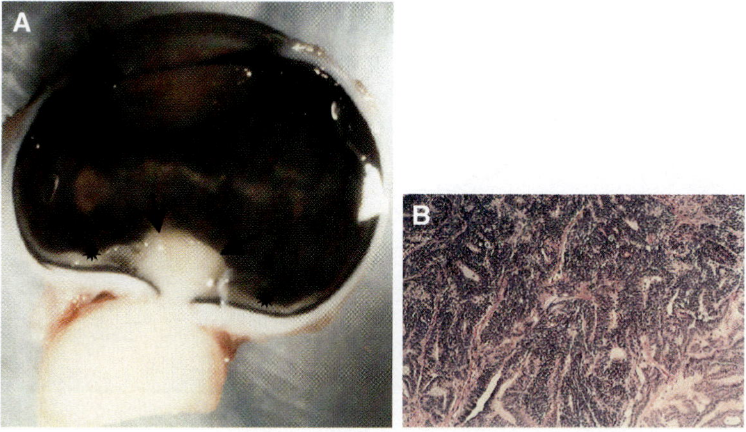


Fig. 15. Malignant teratoid medulloepithelioma of the optic nerve. (*A*) Tumor mass causes massive thickening of the optic nerve with tumor infiltration into the optic nerve head (*arrows*) and the surrounding retina (*). (*B*) Note the basophilic hyperchromatic cells with scant cytoplasm arranged in tubes and cords typical of medulloepithelioma (H & E stain).

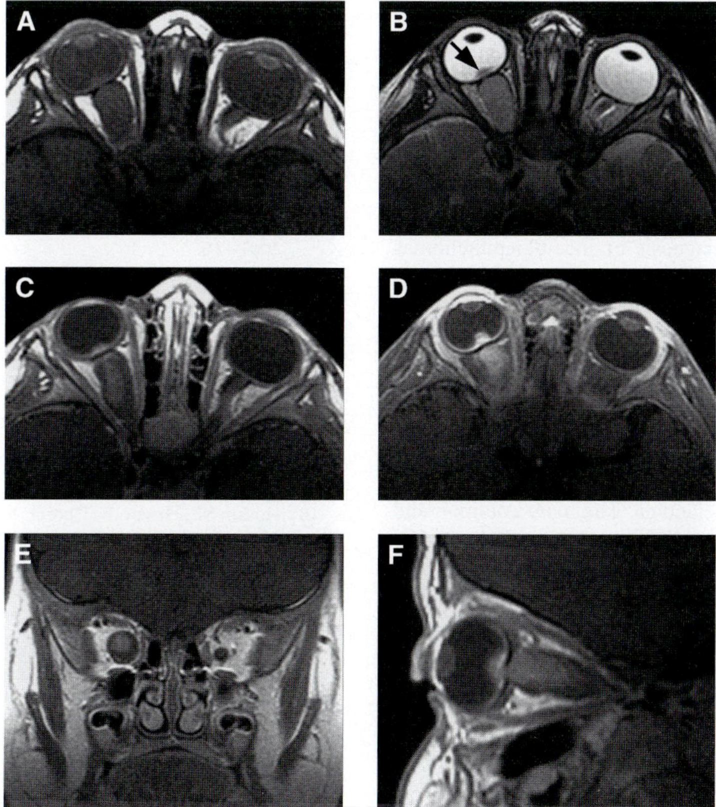


Fig. 16. Malignant teratoid medulloepithelioma of the optic nerve. Axial T1-weighted (*A*), T2-weighted (*B*), enhanced axial T1-weighted (*C*), enhanced axial T1-weighted with fat suppression (*D*), coronal enhanced T1-weighted (*E*), and sagittal enhanced T1-weighted (*F*) MR imaging scans show a medulloepithelioma involving the right optic disc (*arrow* in *B*). Note the marked involvement with increased contrast enhancement of the right optic nerve. (A–C *from* Mafee MF, Valvassori GE, Becker M, editors. Imaging of the head and neck. 2nd edition. Stuttgart (Germany): Thieme; 2004. p. 189; with permission).

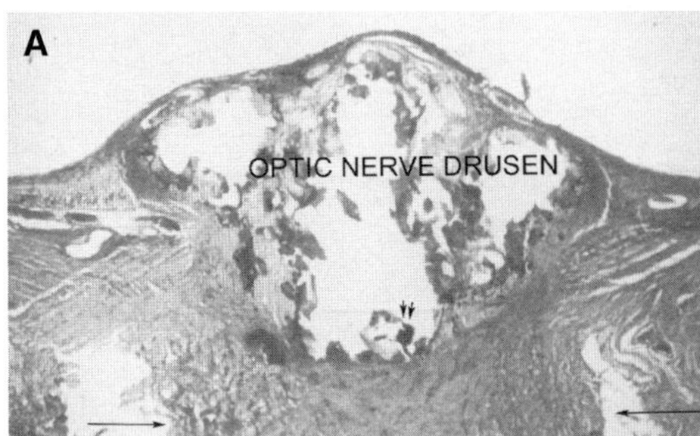


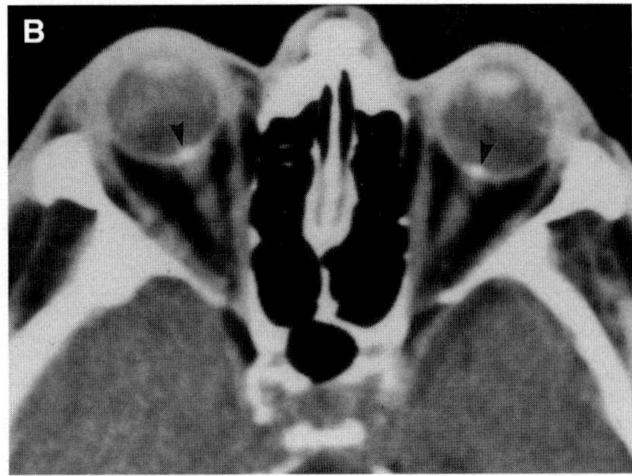


Fig. 17. Drusen of the optic nerve head. (*A*) Histopathologic findings of localized drusen of the optic nerve head (H & E stain). High magnification shows optic nerve (*arrowheads*) with calcification (*arrow*). (*B*) CT scan shows calcified deposits (*arrows*) at the center of the optic nerve heads (*arrowheads*).

In addition, similar findings of CT and MR imaging are seen in other primitive neuroectodermal tumors (PNETs), such as cerebral neuroblastoma, medulloblastoma, and pinealoblastoma [24]. The final diagnosis, similar to optic nerve medulloepitheliomas, requires histopathologic examination.

## Summary

The definitive diagnosis of medulloepitheliomas of the ciliary body and optic nerve is made by histopathologic examination. Familiarity with rare tumors aids clinicians in accurately diagnosing this rare neoplasm. CT and MR imaging findings can be helpful, especially if the mass is confined in an area of the ciliary body without involvement of the retina. The characteristic findings of cystic changes and possible calcification are suggestive of medulloepithelioma rather than melanoma. The more common and ominous retinoblastoma shares some radiologic features with medulloepithelioma, however, and is thus often a consideration. Clinical diagnosis of medulloepitheliomas of the optic nerve and CNS is more challenging. The diagnosis is often made by histopathologic examination. Lastly, coexisting CNS tumors and CNS anomalies have been reported in association with intraocular medulloepitheliomas and should be recognized.

## References

[1] Broughton WL, Zimmerman LE. A clinicopathologic study of 56 cases of intraocular medulloepitheliomas. Am J Ophthalmol 1978;85:407–18.

[2] Shields JA, Shields CL. Miscellaneous intraocular tumors. In: Shields JA, Shields CL, editors. Atlas of intraocular tumors. Philadelphia: Lippincott, Williams & Wilkins; 1999. p. 310–5.

[3] Shields JA, Eagle RC, Shields CL, et al. Congenital neoplasms of the nonpigmented ciliary epithelium (medulloepithelioma). Ophthalmology 1996;103(12): 1998–2006.

[4] Shields JA, Eagle RC, Shields CL, et al. Acquired neoplasms of the nonpigmented epithelium (adenoma and adenocarcinoma). Ophthalmology 1996;103(12): 2007–16.

[5] Chavez M, Mafee MF, Castillo B, et al. Medulloepithelioma of the optic nerve. J Pediatr Ophthalmol Strabismus 2004;41(1):48–52.

[6] Mullaney J. Primary malignant medulloepithelioma of the retinal stalk. Am J Ophthalmol 1974;77: 499–504.

[7] Carrillo R, Streeten BW. Malignant teratoid medulloepithelioma in an adult. Arch Ophthalmol 1979;97: 695–9.

[8] Husain SE, Husain N, Boniuk M, et al. Malignant nonteratoid medulloepithelioma of the ciliary body in adult. Ophthalmology 1998;105(4):596–9.

[9] Shields JA, Shields CL, Schwartz RL. Malignant teratoid medulloepithelioma of the ciliary body simulating persistent hyperplastic primary vitreous. Am J Ophthalmol 1989;107:296–8.

[10] Foster RE, Murray TG, Byrne SF, et al. Echographic features of medulloepithelioma. Am J Ophthalmol 2000;130(3):364–6.

[11] Karcioglu ZA, Abboud EB, Al-Mesfer SA, et al. Retinoblastoma in older children. J AAPOS 2002;6(1): 26–32.

[12] Mafee MF, Mafee RF, Malik M, et al. Medical imaging in pediatric ophthalmology. Pediatr Clin N Am 2003; 50(1):259–86.

[13] De Potter P, Shields CL, Shields JA, et al. The role of magnetic resonance imaging in children with intra-

ocular tumors and simulating lesions. Ophthalmology 1996;103:1774–83.

[14] Mafee MF, Ainbinder D, Afsani E, et al. The eye. Neuroimaging Clin N Am 1996;6(1):29–59.

[15] Peyman GA, Mafee MF. Uveal melanoma and similar lesions: the role of magnetic resonance imaging and computed tomography. Radiol Clin N Am 1987;25(3): 471–86.

[16] Wycliffe ND, Mafee MF. The magnetic imaging in ocular pathology. Top Magn Imaging 1999;10(6):384–400.

[17] Kaufman LM, Mafee MF, Song CD. Retinoblastoma and simulating lesions: role of CT, MR imaging and use of Gd-DTPA contrast enhancement. Radiol Clin N Am 1998;36(6):1101–17.

[18] Mamalis N, Font RL, Anderson CW, et al. Concurrent benign teratoid medulloepithelioma and pineoblastoma. Ophthalmic Surg 1992;23(6):403–8.

[19] Steinkuller PG, Font RL. Congenital malignant teratoid neoplasm of the eye and orbit: a case report and review of the literature. Ophthalmology 1997;104(1): 38–42.

[20] Liaw L, Vielvoye GJ, de Keizer RJW, et al. Optic nerve glioma mimicking an optic nerve meningioma. Clin Neurol Neurosurg 1996;98:258–61.

[21] Saeed P, Rootman J, Nugent RA, et al. Optic nerve sheath meningiomas. Ophthalmology 2003;110(10): 2019–30.

[22] Sundaram C, Vydehi BV, Reddy JJ, et al. Medulloepithelioma: a case report. Neurol India 2003;51(4): 546–7.

[23] Molloy PT, Yachnis AT, Rorke LB, et al. Central nervous system medulloepithelioma: a series of eight cases including two arising in the pons. J Neurosurg 1996;84(3):430–6.

[24] Dai AI, Backstrom JW, Burger PC, et al. Supratentorial primitive neuroectodermal tumors of infancy: clinical and radiologic findings. Pediatr Neurol 2003; 29(5):430–4.

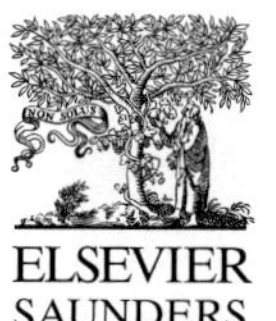
ELSEVIER
SAUNDERS

Neuroimag Clin N Am 15 (2005) 85 – 105

NEUROIMAGING
CLINICS OF
NORTH AMERICA

# Medical Imaging in Pediatric Neuro-Ophthalmology

Vito LaRocca, MD, MPH[a], Gleb Gorelick, MD[b], Lawrence M. Kaufman, MD, PhD[a,*]

[a]*Department of Ophthalmology and Visual Sciences, University of Illinois at Chicago, 1855 West Taylor Street, MC 648, Chicago, IL 60612, USA*
[b]*Department of Radiology, University of Illinois at Chicago, 1801 West Taylor Street, MC 711, Chicago, IL 60612, USA*

Recent advances in CT and MR imaging of the brain and orbit have contributed significantly to the practice of pediatric neuro-ophthalmology. In keeping with the purpose of this issue, our goal is to discuss clinical and imaging characteristics of certain congenital and acquired conditions of the eye, orbit, and visual pathway system as encountered in the practice of pediatric neuro-ophthalmology and neuroradiology.

## Congenital optic nerve anomalies

A variety of congenital anomalies of the optic nerve and optic disc (optic nerve head) may come to the attention of radiologists. These types of disorders range from a complete failure of development, optic nerve aplasia (Fig. 1), to a duplication of the nerve. Box 1 shows a list of those anomalies that may warrant medical imaging, some of which are discussed below [1,2].

### *Optic nerve hypoplasia*

Optic nerve hypoplasia, a specific clinical entity, is an increasingly common cause of infantile blindness in the United States. It is characterized by a small optic disc surface area and thin optic nerve caused by a congenital nonprogressive decrease in the number of optic nerve axons. Unilateral and bilateral optic nerve hypoplasia occurs with roughly equal frequency. Various pathophysiologic theories have been proposed, including failure of axons to normally develop; a destructive developmental event, such as a vascular insult; exaggerated apoptosis; or a genetic disorder.

All patients with optic nerve hypoplasia show visual field defects; localized defects as well as generalized constriction are seen. The loss of visual acuity is variable depending on the degree of involvement with axons from the macula, the center of sight.

Optic nerve hypoplasia is recognized as part of a spectrum of optic nerve, central nervous system (CNS), and hypothalamic-pituitary axis congenital anomalies [3]. From the ophthalmologist's perspective, optic nerve hypoplasia can be assigned into five sometimes overlapping groups: isolated unilateral or bilateral optic nerve hypoplasia (Fig. 2), with absence of the septum pellucidum (septo-optic dysplasia) (Fig. 3), with posterior pituitary ectopia or absence of the pituitary stalk, with hemispheric migration anomalies, or with intrauterine and/or perinatal hemispheric injuries [4]. Optic nerve hypoplasia is also associated with a variety of ocular and systemic disorders, including aniridia, albinism, maternal diabetes, fetal alcohol syndrome, and other maternal ingestions [5–7].

Neuroimaging is recommended in all cases of optic nerve hypoplasia. Attention should be directed to the width of the optic nerves and chiasm as well as

This study was supported in part by core grant EY1792 from the National Eye Institute, Bethesda, Maryland; by an unrestricted research grant from Research to Prevent Blindness, Inc., New York, New York; and by the Lions of Illinois Foundation, Maywood, Illinois.

* Corresponding author.
*E-mail address:* idoc00@sbcglobal.net (L.M. Kaufman).

1052-5149/05/$ – see front matter 
doi:10.1016/j.nic.2005.02.002

*neuroimaging.theclinics.com*

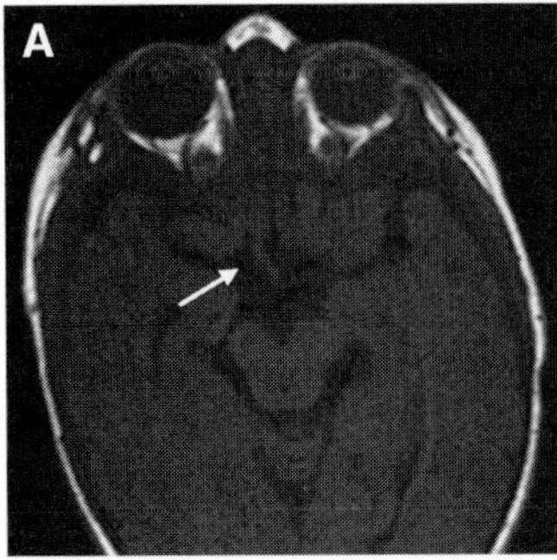

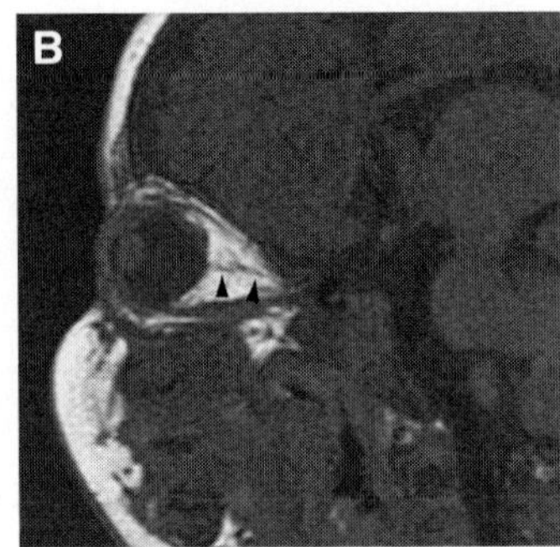

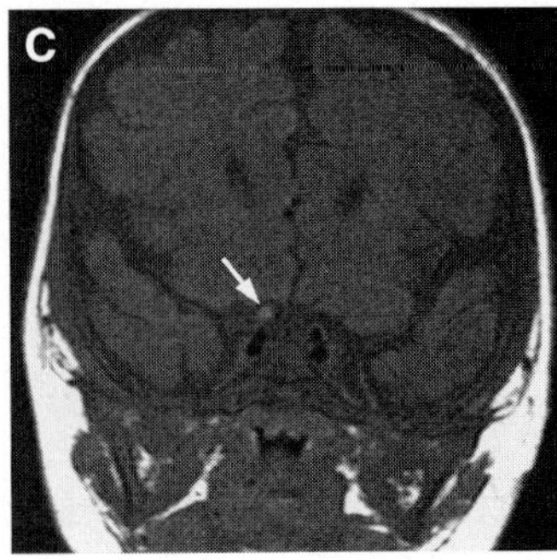


Fig. 1. Left optic nerve aplasia. This 2-month-old boy presented with microphthalmos at birth. Axial (*A*), sagittal (*B*), and coronal (*C*) T1-weighted MR images show left microphthalmos and an absent left optic nerve. Note the normal intracranial segment of the right optic nerve (*white arrow*). The thin line of low signal intensity in the expected location of the left optic nerve is likely compatible with a fibrous band of the optic nerve sheath (*arrowheads*).

to the hypothalamus–infundibulum–pituitary axis. With posterior pituitary ectopia, MR imaging shows hypoplasia or absence of the infundibulum, and in the case of absence of the infundibulum, precontrast T1-weighted images show a shift of the normal posterior pituitary bright spot to the origin of the pituitary stalk at the tuber cinereum.

### *Optic disc coloboma*

An ocular coloboma (Greek for mutilated) is a congenital anomaly that results from incomplete closure of the embryonic fissure, the cleft formed during infolding of the optic vesicle. The coloboma may be anterior, affecting only the iris, or posterior, affecting the optic disc, retina, or choroid. A coloboma limited to the optic disc presents as a deep white excavation enveloping the optic disc. Large optic nerve or chorioretinal coloboma may also be evident on medical imaging, seen as an aneurism-like outpouching of the sclera (Fig. 4). Medical imaging of the brain and orbit is often ordered in these cases in consideration of associated ocular and CNS anomalies, such as microphthalmia with a cyst (Figs. 5 and 6), CHARGE (coloboma, heart defects, atresia of the choanae, retardation of growth and development, genital and urinary abnormalities, ear abnormalities and/or hearing loss) syndrome, Walker-Warburg syndrome, and Aicardi syndrome [8].

**Box 1. Congenital optic disc anomalies**

- Optic nerve aplasia
- Optic nerve hypoplasia
- Optic nerve coloboma
- Morning glory disc
- Pseudopapilledema
- Optic pit
- Optic disc dysplasia
- Doubling of optic disc

### *Morning glory disc*

The morning glory disc is a congenital, non-progressive, coloboma-like anomaly of the optic nerve. The optic disc appears enlarged but within a larger excavation and with overlying glial tissue obscuring the disc. Medical imaging may show an aneurysm-like outpouching of the sclera at the optic nerve insertion to the globe [9]. Brain MR imaging and internal carotid artery MR angiography may also be ordered because of an association with transsphenoidal basal encephalocele and congenital constriction of the internal carotids (moyamoya disease) [10].

## Elevated optic disc in childhood

The normal optic disc lies flat in the plane of the retina. Any appearance of the optic disc protruding into the vitreous cavity represents an elevated disc. A variety of processes may result in an elevated disc, with benign and malignant causes. A selected list of those diagnoses of interest to the radiologist is shown in Box 2.

### *Pseudopapilledema*

In pseudopapilledema and true papilledema, the optic disc appears similarly elevated. Pseudopapille-

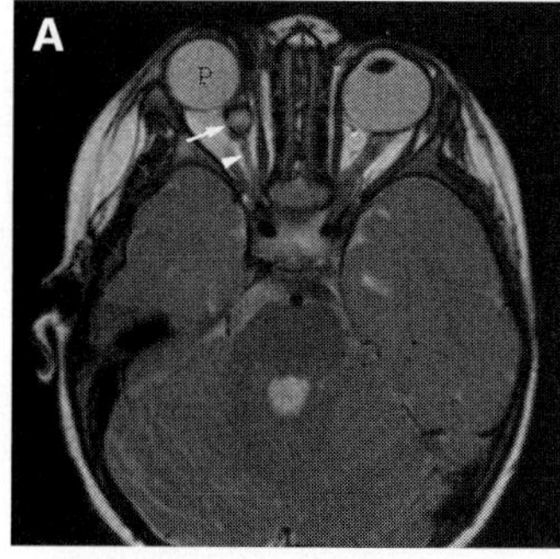


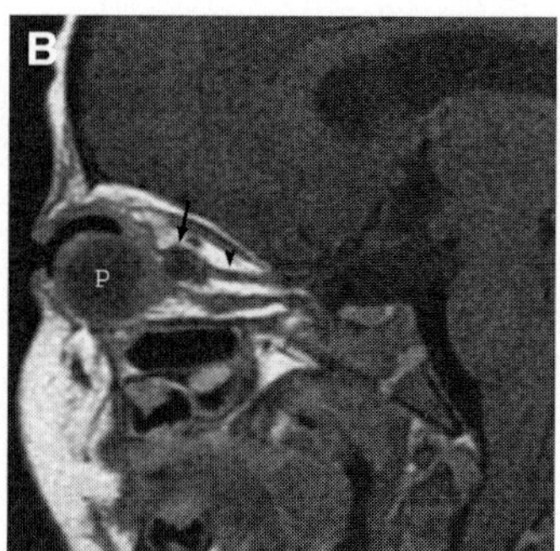


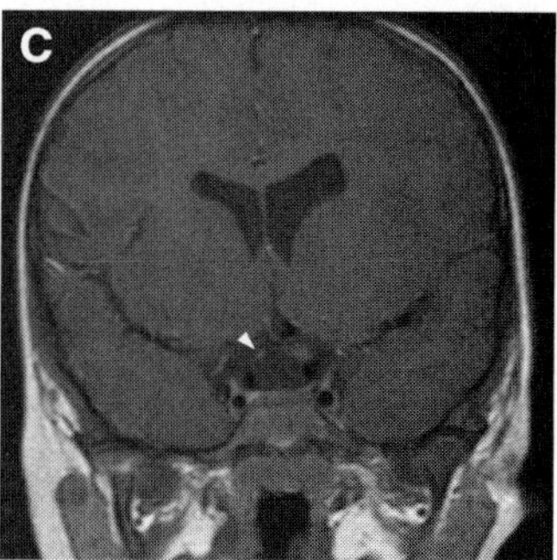


Fig. 2. Right anophthalmos with optic nerve hypoplasia. This 2-year-old girl, a twin, was born to a mother who took levothyroxine sodium (Synthroid) throughout pregnancy. The other twin appeared normal. Both children demonstrated normal development by the age of 3 years. Axial T2-weighted (*A*), sagittal (*B*), and coronal (*C*) T1-weighted MR images show a right eye prosthesis (P), small remnant of the of the optic vesicle (*arrow*), and marked hypoplasia of the right optic nerve (*arrowhead*).

dema is not a pathologic condition, however, but a normal congenital variant in the appearance of a healthy optic disc. There are several subtle clinical features that may allow the clinician to distinguish between the two. In certain cases, even an experienced ophthalmologist can find this distinction difficult, and this may result in the patient having medical imaging to aid in differentiation.

Pseudopapilledema has a few ocular and systemic associations, as seen in Box 2. Disc drusen, present in some patients with pseudopapilledema, are extracellular concretions of degenerate mitochondria, and they reside within the prelaminar portion of the optic nerve head. These drusen accumulate calcium that may be apparent on ultrasound or CT (Fig. 7) [11].

### *Papilledema in children*

Papilledema is defined as disc elevation caused by raised intracranial pressure, a feature of hydrocephalous and pseudotumor cerebri. Papilledema is a bilateral condition, although asymmetry may be seen on clinical examination. All children with newly identified papilledema should undergo medical imaging of the brain to evaluate for an intracranial mass or to distinguish between hydrocephalous and pseudotumor cerebri. The most common intracranial tumors in children include glioma, medulloblastoma, ependymoma, primitive neuroectodermal tumor, craniopharyngioma, choroid plexus papilloma, and ganglioneuroblastoma.

Rather than remembering a long list of specific lesions that can result in hydrocephalous, it may be more helpful to consider the various mechanisms that can lead to hydrocephalous, as shown in Box 2 [12–14]. Brain tumors can raise intracranial pressure not only through a mass effect but by leading to cerebral edema, cerebrospinal fluid (CSF) blockage, venous sinus blockage, and increased CSF production in the case of choroid plexus papilloma.

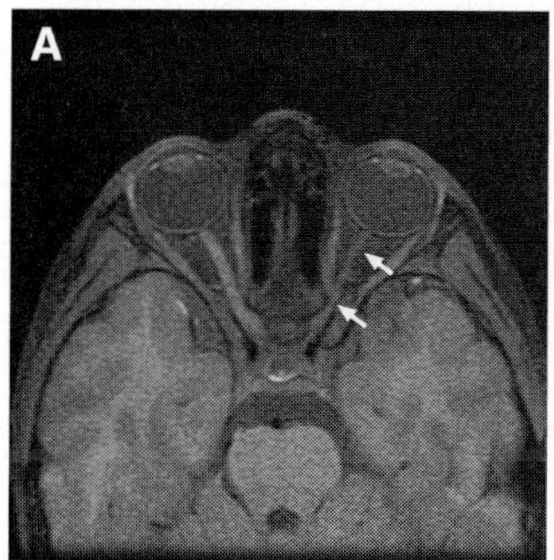


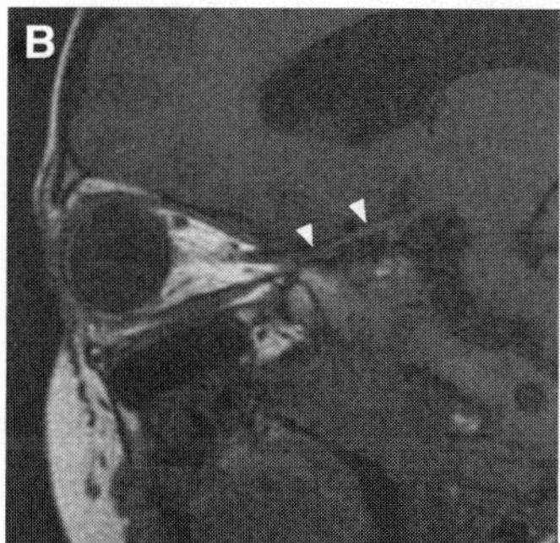


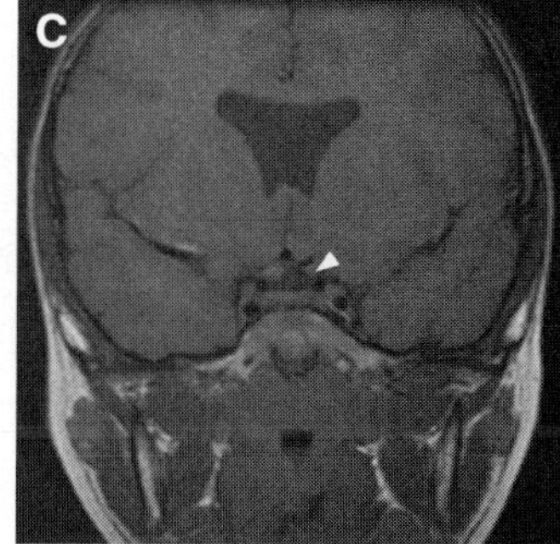


Fig. 3. Septo-optic dysplasia. This 5-year-old boy presented with poor vision and strabismus of the left eye since birth. Axial (*A*), sagittal (*B*), and coronal (*C*) T1-weighted MR images show hypoplasia of the intraorbital left optic nerve (*arrows*) and an absent septum pellucidum. Note the hypoplasia of the intracranial portion of the left optic nerve (*arrowheads*) and the relatively small size of the pituitary stalk.

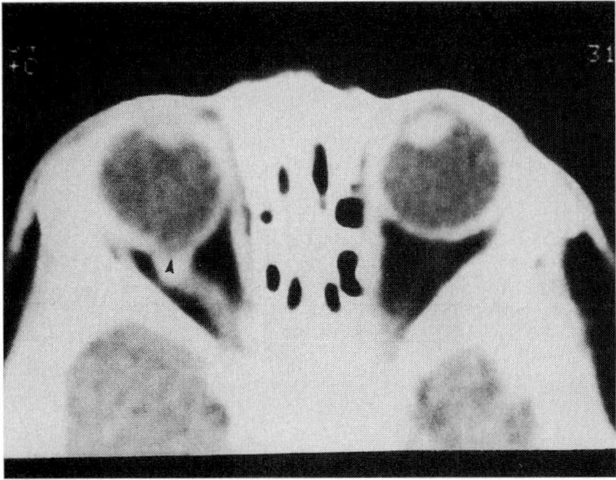

Fig. 4. Coloboma of the optic disc. A CT scan shows a focal cone-shaped deformity of the left optic nerve (*arrowhead*), characteristic of optic disc coloboma.

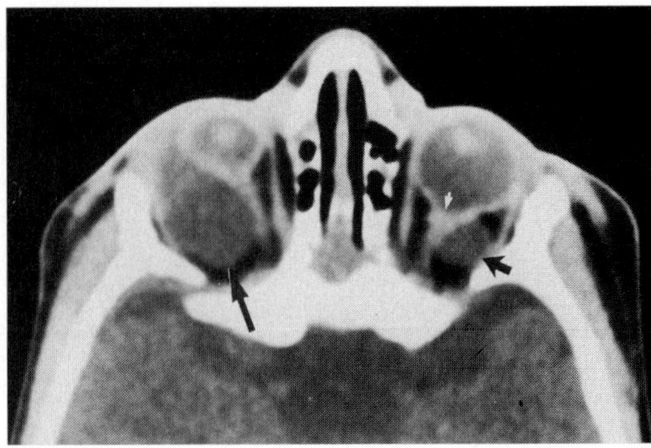

Fig. 6. Coloboma of the left optic nerve with bilateral colobomatous cysts. An axial CT scan shows deformity of the left optic disc related to the colobomatous defect (*white arrow*). Note the bilateral colobomatous cysts (*black arrows*).

### *Pseudotumor cerebri in children*

Pseudotumor cerebri (Fig. 8) is a syndrome defined as an elevation in intracranial pressure, with radiographic imaging showing an absence of an intracranial mass or hydrocephalus and CSF with normal composition. Unlike the case in adults, pseudotumor cerebri in children occurs in male and female patients with equal frequency, is not associated with obesity, and may spontaneously resolve [15]. The child typically presents with a stiff neck, headaches, nausea, vomiting, irritability, and diplopia and may have false localizing lateral rectus palsy. In approximately one third of pediatric pseudotumor cerebri cases, no identifiable cause is found, so-called "primary disease." Pseudotumor cerebri in children can be secondary to a broad range of conditions, including neurologic disease (eg, dural venous thrombosis, meningitis), intracranial otologic complications, systemic disease (eg, systemic lupus erythematosus, Addison disease, anemia), or the use or discontinuation of medications (eg, steroid withdrawal, tetracycline, vitamin A, growth hormone, thyroxin, nalidixic acid).

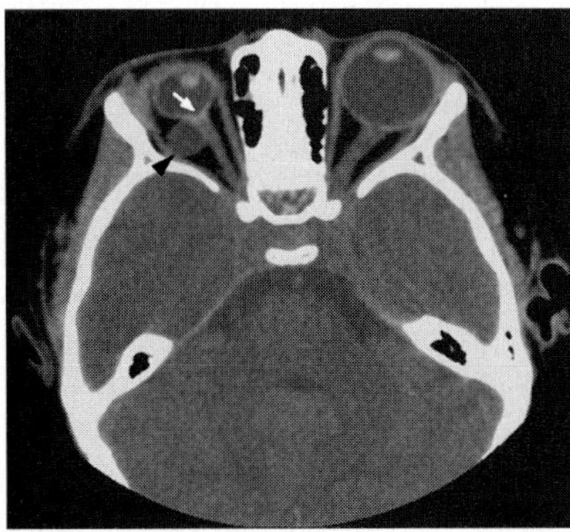

Fig. 5. Coloboma of the right optic nerve, colobomatous cyst, microphthalmia, and hypoplastic optic nerve. This 3-year-old girl was born with microphthalmia on the right side. An axial CT scan shows a colobomatous defect involving the right optic nerve (*arrow*), microphthalmia, a hypoplastic right optic nerve, and a colobomatous cyst (*arrowhead*).

### *Optic nerve compression*

Optic nerve compression occurs in children as a result of trauma, orbital tumors (Box 3 and Fig. 9), intracranial tumors, orbital cellulitis (Fig. 10), and stenosis of the optic canal, as seen in the craniosynostoses syndromes, osteopetrosis, and fibrous dysplasia [16]. The compression yields a clinical appearance similar to papilledema and progresses to irreversible optic atrophy unless corrected. Subtle cases of optic canal stenosis may be diagnosed on MR imaging by showing an absence of CSF surrounding the intracanalicular portion of the optic nerve.

## Optic neuritis in childhood

In comparison to adults, optic neuritis in children has no gender preference, is typically bilateral and anterior, and is only rarely caused by ischemia. In children, the demyelinization process of optic neuritis is most commonly related to active or resolved viral illness or occurs after immunization. Unlike adults,

**Box 2. Elevated optic disc in childhood**

*Congenital anomalies*
*Pseudopapilledema*
  Familial
  Disc drusen
  High hyperopia
  Down syndrome
  Kenny syndrome
  Alagille syndrome
  Linear sebaceous nevus syndrome
*Papilledema*
  *Hydrocephalus*
    Primary
    Space-occupying intracranial lesions
    Cerebral edema
    Reduction in size of cranial vault
    Blockage of cerebrospinal fluid (CSF) flow
    Blockage of CSF resorption
    Increased CSF production
  *Pseudotumor cerebri*
    Primary
    Secondary
*Optic nerve compression*
*Inflammatory disease*
  Papillitis and/or optic neuritis
  Uveitis
*Ischemia*
*Infiltrative disease*
  Leukemia
*Toxic optic neuropathies*
*Hereditary optic neuropathies*
  Leber heredity optic neuropathy
*Tumor*
  Optic glioma (juvenile astrocytoma)
  Optic disc hemangioma
  Retinal hamartoma
  Combined hamartoma of the retinal pigment epithelium (RPE) and retina
  Choroidal osteoma
  Retinoblastoma
  Retinoma
  Medulloepithelioma
*Vascular disease*
  Carotid-cavernous sinus fistula
*Systemic diseases*
  Malignant hypertension
  Diabetic papillopathy
  Mucopolysaccharidoses
*Shaken baby syndrome*

there is not a strong association between childhood optic neuritis and multiple sclerosis [17].

The workup of children with suspected optic neuritis requires medical imaging and lumbar puncture to confirm a demyelinization process and to rule out an intracranial neoplasm, encephalomyelitis, or meningitis. MR imaging of optic neuritis shows enhancement and enlargement of the affected portion of the optic nerve, which is best seen on postcontrast, fat-suppressed, T1-weighted images (Fig. 11).

## Optic atrophy in childhood

Damage to retinal ganglion cells anywhere along their course from their cell bodies in the inner retinas to their axons in the optic nerves, chiasm, and/or optic tracts or to their synapses in the lateral geniculate bodies can produce optic nerve atrophy [18,19]. Patients with optic atrophy present with loss of visual acuity, visual field, and color vision. The chalky-white appearance of the optic disc in optic

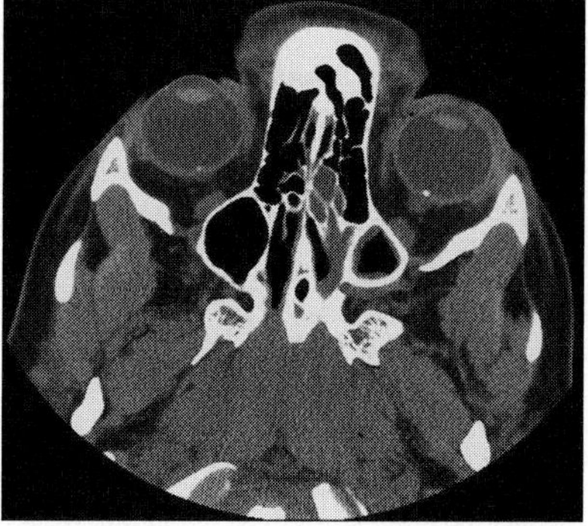

Fig. 7. Optic nerve head drusen in pseudopapilledema. This 8-year-old boy presented with visual hallucinations of shapes, forms, and color. He also had changes in depth perception. Funduscopic examination revealed elevated optic discs. The patient underwent cranial MR imaging, the results of which were normal. Opening CSF pressure was normal. An axial unenhanced CT scan shows bilateral calcifications at the center of the optic disc compatible with optic nerve head drusen buried within the disc.

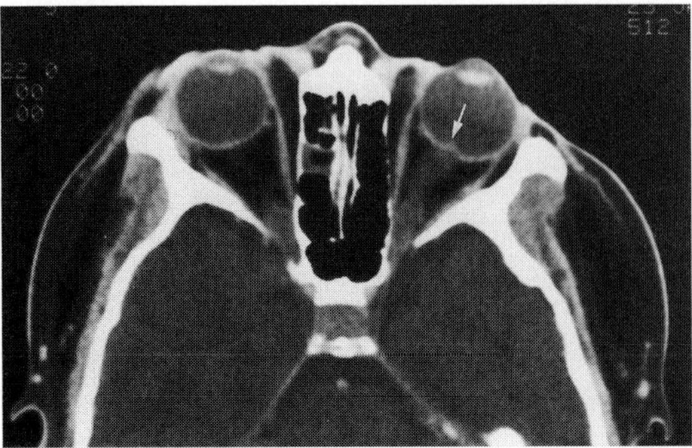

Fig. 8. Papilledema. An axial CT scan shows prominent optic discs (*white arrow*) in a child with pseudotumor cerebri.

atrophy does not become apparent immediately after injury to these cells but develops over 4 to 6 weeks after the insult. These vision and optic disc changes are nonspecific findings and belie the diverse causes of optic atrophy [20]. Patients with optic nerve atrophy who lack a clear-cut etiology require an evaluation, including medical imaging of the brain and orbit, in consideration of the etiologies listed in Box 4 [21].

## Blind child

The term "blindness" rarely refers to actual complete loss of vision. In the United States, educational and governmental agencies often use a legal definition of blindness as visual acuity of 20/200 or worse in the better eye or a constricted visual field that subtends an angle of less than 20°. In the authors' experience, it is useful to classify blind children into two broad categories, each with distinct etiologies: infantile blindness and acquired blindness. Infantile blindness can be further subdivided into patients with lesions anterior or posterior to the lateral geniculate nucleus.

### *Infantile cortical visual impairment*

Blind infants with disorders posterior to the lateral geniculate nucleus present by 2 to 3 months of age with blank stares or slow roving eye movements termed "searching nystagmus" and apparently healthy globes and optic discs on clinical examination [22]. These infants have normal pupil responses—pupil constriction in response to light involves pupillary fibers that leave the optic tracts just proximal to the lateral geniculate nucleus. "Cortical (or central) visual impairment" is now the preferred

**Box 3. Pediatric orbital tumors**

*Developmental orbital cysts*

- Choristoma: dermoid
- Teratoma
- Microphthalmos with cyst
- Congenital cystic eye

*Acquired orbital cysts*

- Cystic vascular lesion
- Hemangioma
- Lymphangioma
- Orbital varix
- Chocolate cyst
- Skin appendage cyst
- Epithelial implantation cyst
- Lacrimal duct cyst
- Optic nerve sheath cyst
- Hematic cyst
- Aneurysmal bone cyst
- Cystic myositis
- Orbital abscess
- Parasitic cysts
  - *Echinococcus granulosus*
  - *Cysticercus cellulosae*

*Adjacent structure cysts*

- Mucocele
- Dacryocele
- Mucopyocele
- Cephalocele
- Meningocele
- Encephalocele
- Meningoencephalocele
- Porencephalic cyst
- Dentigenous cysts

*Vascular lesions*

- Capillary hemangioma
- Cavernous hemangioma
- Lymphangioma (lymphohemangioma)
- Orbital varix
- Arteriovenous malformation
- Hemangiopericytoma
- Malignant hemangioepithelioma

Organizing hematoma (eg, hematic cyst, cholesterol granuloma)
Sturge-Weber syndrome
Klippel-Trenaunay-Weber syndrome

*Inflammatory masses*

Preseptal and orbital cellulitis
Nonspecific orbital inflammatory syndromes (NSOIS) and/or orbital pseudotumor
Specific orbital inflammatory disease
- Thyroid ophthalmopathy
- Sarcoidosis
- Wegener granulomatosis
- Idiopathic midline destructive disease
- Polyarteritis nodosa
- Systemic lupus erythematosus
- Painful external ophthalmoplegia (Tolosa-Hunt syndrome)
- Angiolymphoid hyperplasia with eosinophilia (Kimura disease)
- Multifocal fibrosclerosis
- Amyloidosis

*Histiocytic, hematopoietic, and lymphoproliferative masses*

Langerhans cell histiocytosis
- Histiocytosis X, Hand-Schuller-Christian disease, Letterer-Siwe disease

Non-Langerhans cell histiocytosis
- Juvenile xanthogranuloma

Sinus histiocytosis
Leukemia
- Granulocytoma sarcoma

Lymphoma

*Mesodermal tumors*

Fibroma
Myofibromatosis
Lipoma
Leiomyoma
Fibrous dysplasia
Juvenile ossifying fibroma
Giant cell (reparative) granuloma of bone
Aneurysmal bone cyst
Cartilaginous hamartoma
Sarcoma: osteogenic sarcoma, leiomyosarcoma, fibrosarcoma, malignant fibrous histiocytoma, alveolar soft part sarcoma
Rhabdomyosarcoma

*Neurogenic tumors*

Glioma
Meningioma
Neurofibroma
Schwannoma
Esthesioneuroblastoma
Paraganglioma
Melanotic neuroectodermal tumor

*Lacrimal gland tumors*

Pleomorphic adenoma (benign mixed tumor)
Adenocarcinoma (malignant mixed tumor)

*Metastatic tumors*

Neuroblastoma
Ewing sarcoma
Wilms tumor

terminology to describe these patients in recognition of the spectrum of vision loss as a result of cortical lesions. Medical imaging is often pursued in these patients in consideration of the etiologies listed in Box 5 [23,24].

### *Infantile globe and optic nerve blindness*

Infants with blinding disorders of the visual system anterior to the lateral geniculate nucleus present by 2 to 3 months of age with impaired vision and true nystagmus—rapid involuntary oscillations of the eyes. In most cases, the etiology of loss of vision is apparent to the ophthalmologist during the clinical examination (Box 6). Some of these patients may warrant medical imaging, for instance, infants with intraocular masses, congenital ocular anomalies, or an optic nerve disorder (see article on imaging of retinoblastoma by Apushkin et al and article by Weber et al elsewhere in this issue).

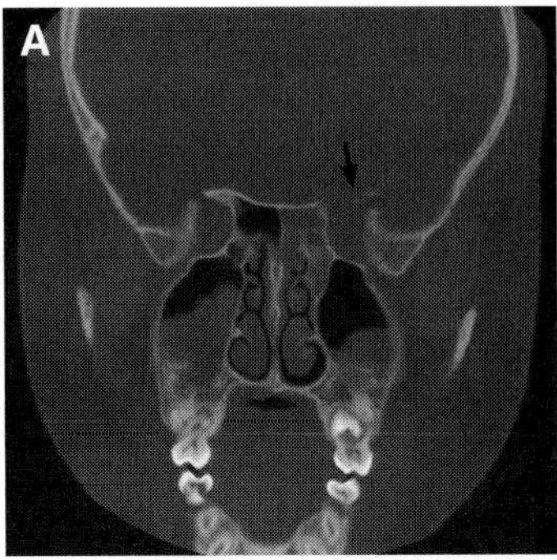


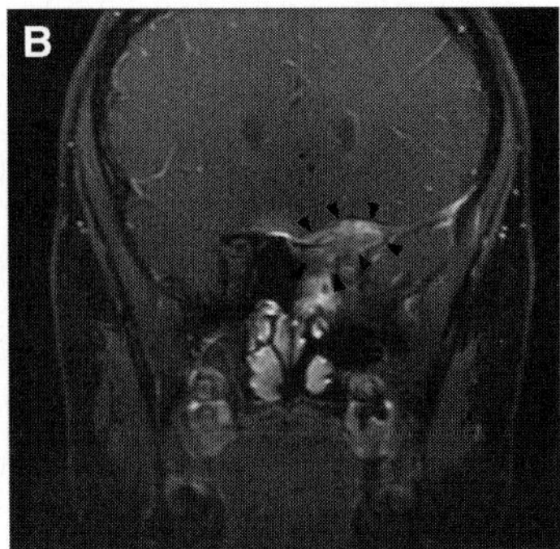


Fig. 9. Langerhans cell histiocytosis. This 10-year-old boy presented with rapid loss of visual acuity in the left eye associated with optic nerve compression. (*A*) Coronal CT scan shows a lytic lesion involving the left anterior clinoid (*arrow*). Notice widening of the superior orbital fissure at this level, and involvement of the left sphenoid sinus. (*B*) Coronal enhanced, fat-suppressed, T1-weighted MR image shows marked enhancement of an infiltrative process involving the left optic nerve, paraclinoid region, and sphenoid sinus (*arrowheads*). Vision recovered following short course radiation therapy.

*Acquired blindness in childhood*

In many respects, the evaluation and differential diagnosis of a child with acquired blindness is similar to that of an adult. However, the most common causes of acquired visual impairment in children are uncorrected refractive error and amblyopia. After these causes have been excluded, the ophthalmologist must consider organic ocular or CNS disease; some of these diagnoses are shown in Box 7. A diagnostic workup with medical imaging may be indicated in certain of these cases.

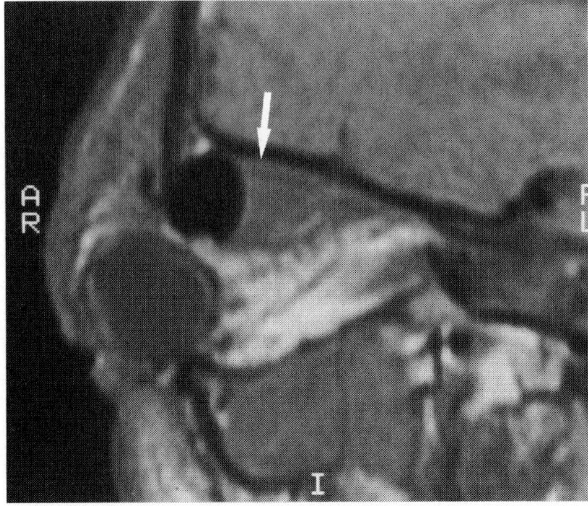


Fig. 10. Subperiosteal abscess. A sagittal T1-weighted MR image shows a large subperiosteal abscess with an air-fluid level (*arrow*). Note the proptosis and deformity of the globe.

## Nystagmus in childhood

Nystagmus, a clinical sign rather than a diagnostic entity, is an involuntary rhythmic eye oscillation. The eye movements may be primarily horizontal, vertical, or rotational and may show a variety of wave forms, such as pendular or jerk. Nystagmus is most often bilateral but can be unilateral. Specific types of nystagmus have been named according to the wave form of the oscillations, the direction of the predominant component, the timing of onset, or the underlying etiology (Box 8).

*Congenital nystagmus*

Congenital nystagmus typically presents in infants between 1 and 4 months of age [25]. This type of nystagmus may be further classified as having an afferent (sensory) or efferent (motor) etiology. Sensory nystagmus is a secondary process and occurs in infants with a congenital or early-onset primary loss of vision caused by lesions anterior to the lateral geniculate nucleus (see Box 6). Children who acquire blindness after 1 year of age do not develop sensory nystagmus.

Congenital motor nystagmus results from a primary disorder of the ocular motor control pathways. Infants with motor nystagmus have healthy globes and optic nerves as well as relatively preserved vision. Motor nystagmus can be idiopathic (essential) or familial, with both showing normal CNS imaging. Alternatively, congenital motor nystagmus can be due to a variety of CNS congenital abnormalities or early-onset insults, with positive CNS imaging.

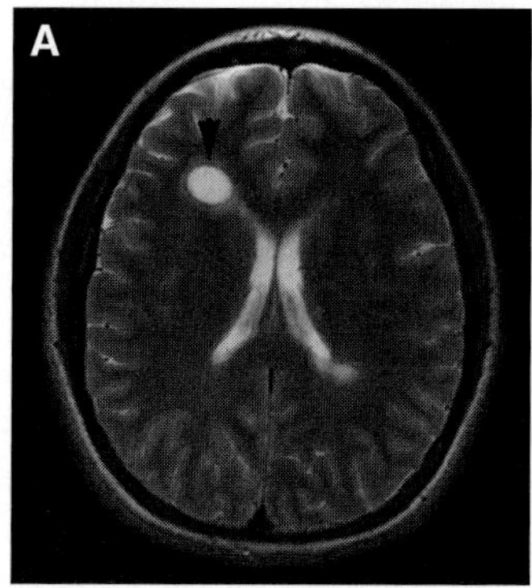


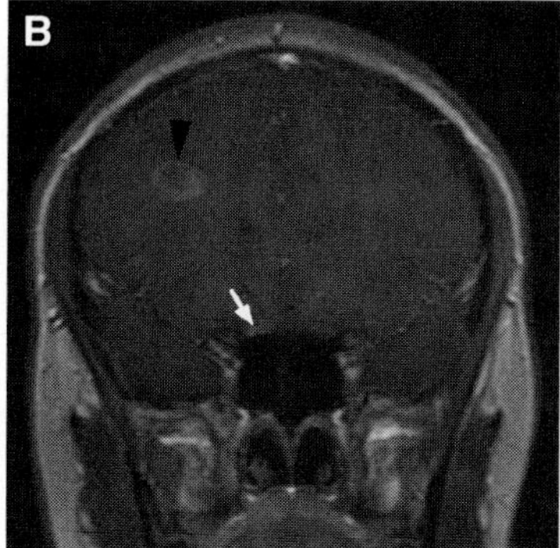


Fig. 11. Multiple sclerosis (MS) and right optic neuritis in a 15-year-old girl. (*A*) Axial T2-weighted MR image shows a large characteristic MS plaque involving the forceps minor of the corpus callosum on the right side. (*B*) Coronal enhanced T1-weighted MR image shows enhancement of the intracranial segment of the right optic nerve (*arrow*) as well as an active frontal MS plaque (*arrowhead*).

*Acquired nystagmus*

Nystagmus presenting after 6 months is considered acquired. Children with acquired nystagmus often undergo medical imaging of the brain and orbits to exclude a neoplastic or anatomic etiology.

**Box 4. Optic atrophy in childhood**

- Compressive intracranial lesions
- Compressive optic canal lesions
- Compressive orbital lesions
- Chronic papilledema
  - Hydrocephalus
  - Pseudotumor cerebri
- Postoptic neuritis
- Optic nerve hypoplasia
- Hereditary optic neuropathy
- Toxic and/or nutritional optic neuropathy
- Neurodegenerative disorders with optic atrophy
- Hypoxia and/or ischemia
- Trauma
- Radiation optic neuropathy
- Paraneoplastic syndromes
- Ocular disorders
  - Retinopathy of prematurity
  - Pigmentary retinopathy
  - Glaucoma
  - Retinal detachment
  - Uveitis

Ocular motor control pathways are extensive and complex. Acquired lesions anywhere along these pathways may result in nystagmus, but in many of these cases, the clinician cannot determine the site of the lesion based on the clinical features of the nystagmus. In these cases, medical imaging of the brain and orbits is undirected. A few specific types of acquired nystagmus result from localized CNS lesions. In these cases, medical imaging can be directed to areas of interest, such as the cervical-medullary junction for downbeat nystagmus, dorsal midbrain for convergence-retraction nystagmus, or suprasellar region for see-saw nystagmus.

Spasmus nutans is a syndrome of asymmetric shimmering, low-amplitude, and high-frequency nystagmus; head bobbing; and torticollis. It occurs in children between the ages of 6 and 18 months [26]. The process is self-limiting and resolves over months to a few years without sequelae. Brain and orbit

**Box 5. Causes of cortical visual impairment**

- Perinatal hypoxia
- Postnatal hypoxia
- Peri- and intraventricular hemorrhage
- Cerebral malformations
- Head trauma
- Metabolic and neurodegenerative conditions
- Meningitis, encephalitis, and sepsis
- Hydrocephalus, ventricular shunt failure
- Preictal, ictal, or postictal phenomenon

**Box 6. Causes of infantile blindness as a result of globe and optic nerve disorders**

*Anterior segment abnormalities*

- Cataract
- Corneal opacities and anomalies: anterior segment dysgenesis
- Glaucoma
- Microphthalmia

*Posterior segment abnormalities*

- Macular hypoplasia: albinism, aniridia
- Optic nerve and chorioretinal coloboma
- Optic nerve atrophy
- Optic nerve hypoplasia
- Persistent hyperplasia of the primary vitreous
- Hereditary retinal dystrophy
- Retinoblastoma
- Retinopathy of prematurity
- TORCH (toxoplasma, other viruses, rubella, cytomegalovirus, herpesvirus) syndromes

imaging is normal. However, children with visual pathway tumors, typically glioma of the chiasm (Figs. 12 and 13), may present with symptoms that mimic those of spasmus nutans, resulting in a so-called "masquerade" syndrome [27].

## Ocular motor disorders

"Strabismus" is the general term used to describe any type of eye misalignment or eye movement disorder. Various other terms and subgroupings, as summarized in Table 1, are used to indicate the nature and direction of the misalignment, timing of onset, relation to refractive error, and visual disturbance. Of paramount importance to the clinician when encountering a patient with strabismus is the etiology of the condition. In most cases, the ophthalmologist can assign a strabismic patient into one of six etiologic groups based on the clinical features of the strabismus.

### *Benign childhood strabismus*

This is the most common type of strabismus; the etiology is actually idiopathic, and it occurs in children less than 6 years of age who are usually otherwise healthy. Onset may be infantile or acquired and includes comitant esotropia, accommodative esotropia, and comitant exotropia. Infrequently, these patients require a workup or medical imaging for those cases with unusual features.

### *Sensory strabismus*

The maintenance of well-aligned eyes is an active process and requires adequate vision in both eyes. If there is a significant loss of vision in one or both eyes

**Box 7. Causes of acquired blindness in childhood**

- Amblyopia
- Uncorrected refractive errors
- Cataracts, acquired
- Glaucoma
- Retinal detachment
- Optic atrophy
- Optic neuritis
- Pigmentary retinopathy
- Uveitis
- Tumors
  - Retinoblastoma
  - Optic glioma
  - Medulloepithelioma
  - Craniopharyngioma
  - Chiasmal glioma
- Neurodegenerative diseases
  - Gangliosidoses
  - Lipidoses
  - Mucopolysaccharidoses
  - Leukodystrophies
- Infectious or inflammatory diseases
  - Encephalitis
  - Meningitis
  - Corneal ulcer
- Hematologic disorders: leukemia
- Vascular disorders
- Collagen vascular diseases
- Trauma
  - Contusion and/or avulsion of optic nerve or chiasm
  - Vitreous and/or retinal hemorrhage
  - Intraocular foreign body
  - Globe laceration
  - Hyphema
- Drugs and toxins

**Box 8. Nystagmus in childhood**

- Congenital
  - Motor
  - Sensory
- Spasmus nutans
- Diencephalic syndrome
- Associated with infantile strabismus
- Periodic alternating nystagmus
- See-saw nystagmus
- Convergence retraction nystagmus
- Downbeat nystagmus
- Opsoclonus
- Neurodegenerative disorders nystagmus
- Systemic disorders associated with nystagmus
  - Down syndrome
  - Hypothyroidism
- Nutritional
- Toxic and/or metabolic

from any etiology, a secondary eye misalignment may develop. These deviations are usually comitant and in an esotropic or exotropic direction. Medical imaging may be pursued in these patients to evaluate the loss of vision, but the strabismus itself does not require a workup.

*Restrictive strabismus*

This type of strabismus results from orbital disorders that limit the free movement of the extraocular muscles and globes. The process may be unilateral or bilateral and includes diagnoses like orbital tumors, blow-out fractures, thyroid ophthalmopathy, and orbital pseudotumor. The strabismus in usually incomitant with horizontal and vertical misalignment, and the affected eye(s) shows a limitation of ocular rotations. An orbital CT scan or MR imaging is often ordered as part of the workup.

*Paralytic strabismus*

This group includes patients with lesions of the nucleus or pathways of cranial nerves (CNs) III, IV, or VI. Figs. 14–17 illustrate these areas of concern. The strabismus is incomitant, and the affected eye(s) shows a limitation of rotation in the direction of the paralytic muscle(s). When ordered, medical imaging in patients with paralytic strabismus should include brain and orbit studies, without and with contrast, with attention to the entire course of the affected nerve.

For children with isolated unilateral CN IV palsy, the specific etiology is most often congenital or traumatic; thus, medical imaging may be limited in these cases [28].

Isolated CN VI palsy in children usually occurs on a viral, postviral, postimmunization, otogenic (petrous apicitis), traumatic, or congenital basis [29]. Up to 80% of the cases of acquired isolated CN VI palsy are self-limiting [30]. Ophthalmologists often expectantly observe these patients and only pursue a workup with medical imaging if the patient fails to show a spontaneous improvement 3 to 4 weeks after the onset.

Up to 50% of children with isolated CN III palsy have a congenital or idiopathic etiology. Other benign

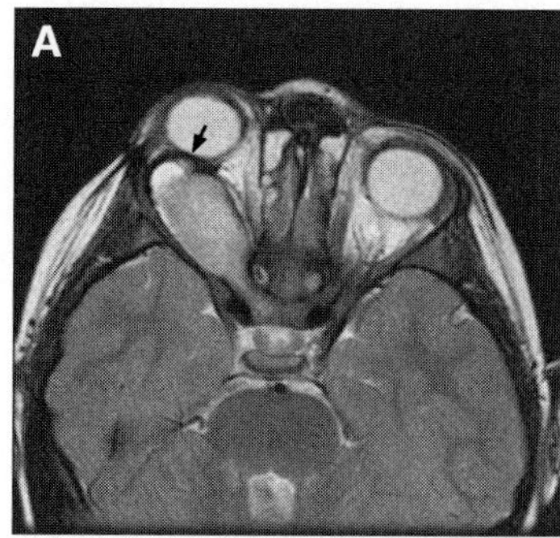


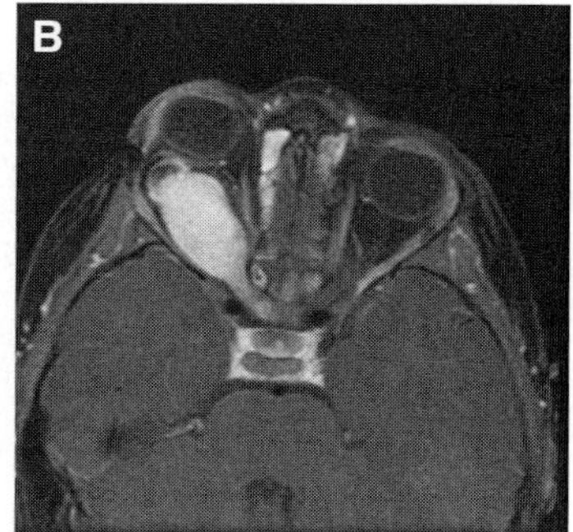


Fig. 12. Pilocytic astrocytoma (glioma) of the right optic nerve. This girl presented at the age of 1 year with a 3-month history of right-sided proptosis. The results of a biopsy were compatible with benign pilocytic glioma. She underwent eight cycles of chemotherapy without a reduction in tumor size. (*A*) Axial T2-weighted MR image shows a large right optic nerve mass indenting the globe (*arrow*) and extending intracranially to involve the optic chiasm (not shown here). (*B*) Axial enhanced, fat-suppressed, T1-weighted MR image at the same level shows marked enhancement of the tumor.

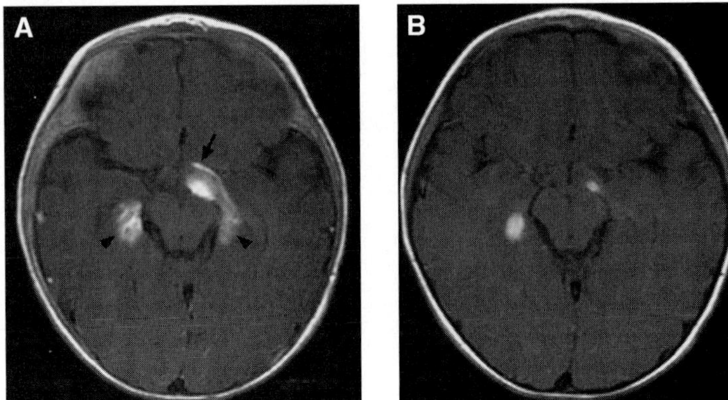


Fig. 13. Bilateral optic nerve gliomas in a patient with known neurofibromatosis type 1. (*A*) Enhanced T1-weighted MR image demonstrates marked thickening and enhancement of the optic chiasm (*arrow*) and radiations (*arrowheads*). (B) Enhanced T1-weighted MR image at the same level after chemotherapy shows a marked response.

etiologies include trauma, infection, inflammation, and ophthalmoplegic migraine. Regardless, most of these patients have medical imaging performed to rule out an intracranial tumor or, much less likely, an aneurysm (Figs. 18 and 19) [31].

In children with multiple cranial neuropathies or showing other neurologic deficits, more precise localization of a lesion can be inferred by knowledge of the neuroanatomy. Medical imaging can then be directed to an area of interest.

Table 1
Strabismus terminology

| Term | Definition |
|---|---|
| Infantile strabismus | Onset before 6 mo of age |
| Acquired strabismus | Onset after 6 mo of age |
| Comitant strabismus | Amplitude of ocular misalignment remains the same as patient looks in different directions, includes benign childhood and sensory strabismus |
| Incomitant strabismus | Amplitude of ocular misalignment changes as patient looks in different directions, includes paretic, restrictive and syndromic strabismus, and complex ocular motor disorders |
| Tropia | Manifest ocular misalignment, may be constant or intermittent |
| Phoria | Latent ocular misalignment, requires interruption of fusion to allow detection |
| Esodeviation | Inward misalignment of one eye, may be manifest (esotropia) or latent (esophoria) |
| Exodeviation | Outward misalignment of one eye, may be manifest (exotropia) or latent (exophoria) |
| Hyperdeviation | Upward misalignment of one eye, may be manifest (hypertropia) or latent (hyperphoria) |
| Hypodeviation | Downward misalignment of one eye, may be manifest (hypotropia) or latent (hypophoria) |
| Intermittent strabismus | Ocular misalignment is intermittently manifest |
| Constant strabismus | Ocular misalignment is constantly manifest |
| Alternating strabismus | Misaligned eye switches from one eye to the other |
| Accommodative strabismus | Strabismus that improves with correction of patient's farsightedness |
| Diplopia | Double vision, occurs when eyes are misaligned and suppression is not available |
| Suppression | CNS process that eliminates diplopia by preventing image from misaligned eye from reaching consciousness, a sensory adaptation to strabismus in children less than 6 years old |
| Amblyopia | CNS process of degradation of visual acuity in response to constant suppression or blurred image from one or both eyes |
| Fusion | CNS process of bringing the images from right and left eye into a single visual perception |
| Stereopsis | Depth perception |

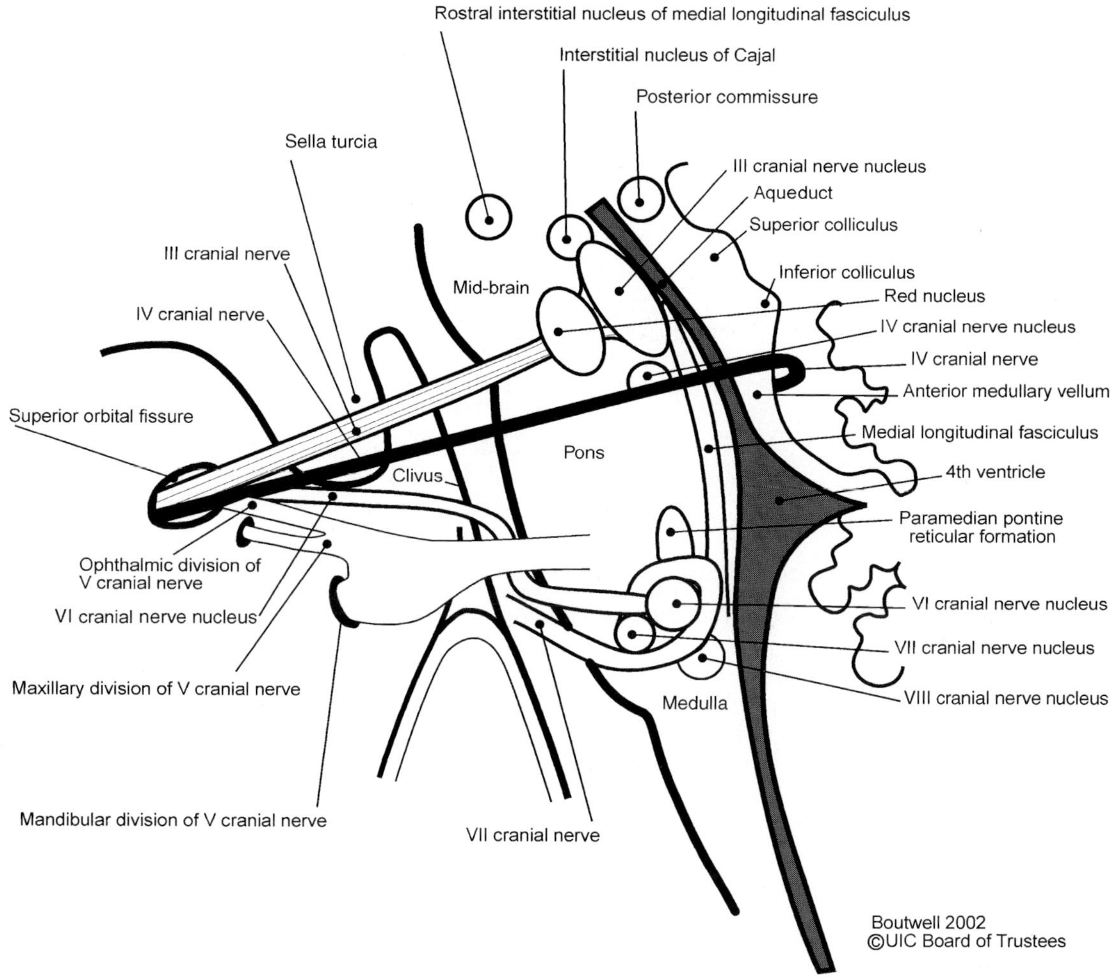


Fig. 14. Diagram of lateral view of the brain stem shows the nuclei and pathways of CN III, CN IV, and CN VI. (Illustration by Adrienne J. Boutwell and Lisa J. Birmingham © University of Illinois at Chicago Board of Trustees 2002; with permission.)

*Complex ocular motor disorders*

Maintaining well-aligned eyes and normal ocular rotations is a complex process and involves numerous CNS ocular motor control centers and pathways above the level of the CN nuclei. Congenital anomalies or acquired lesions of these centers or pathways can lead to predictable and unpredictable ocular motor deficits, a few of which are presented below.

Horizontal gaze palsy (the inability to move both eyes simultaneously into the right or left gaze) results from lesions of the contralateral frontal eye fields or the ipsilateral paramedian pontine reticular formation (PPRF) [32]. The PPRF is a paired midline structure adjacent to the CN VI nucleus and coordinates ipsilateral horizontal gaze via fibers to the ipsilateral CN VI nucleus and the contralateral medial rectus subnucleus of CN III.

Dorsal midbrain syndrome (Parinaud syndrome) results from a lesion of the rostral dorsal mesencephalon in the area of the posterior commissure [33]. Affected patients show impaired upgaze (inability to move both eyes simultaneously into upgaze); retracted upper eyelids (Collier sign); convergence-retraction nystagmus (rhythmic contraction of all the rectus muscles, resulting in jerky convergence and retraction movements of the eyes); and light-near dissociation (pupils respond poorly to light but constrict with near gaze). Infants may also tonically hold their eyes in downgaze, giving rise to the "setting sun" sign. The dorsal midbrain syndrome is a common feature in infants with hydrocephalus. Other diagnostic considerations include ventriculo-

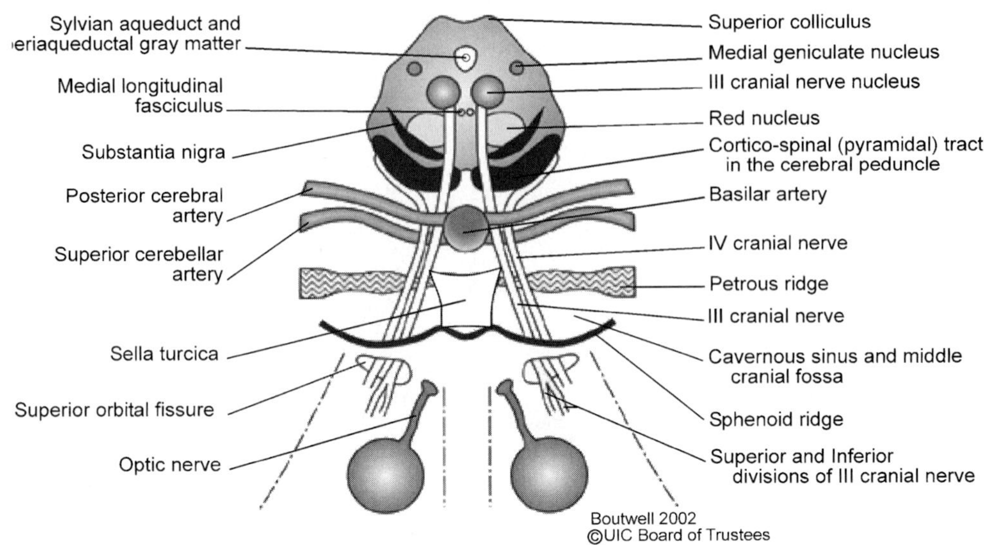


Fig. 15. Diagram of axial view of the midbrain at level of the superior colliculus highlights CN III. (Illustration by Adrienne J. Boutwell and Lisa J. Birmingham © University of Illinois at Chicago Board of Trustees 2002; with permission.)

peritoneal (VP) shunt failure, pineal tumor, arteriovenous malformation, and trauma.

Double elevator palsy refers to the inability to move an eye into upgaze because of a lesion of a purported supranuclear center that coordinates ocular elevation. The center probably resides near the dorsal midbrain and directs upgaze via fibers to the superior rectus subnucleus and inferior oblique subnucleus within the CN III nucleus. The inability to elevate an eye because of a supranuclear lesion must be distinguished from isolated palsy of the superior rectus muscle and from restrictive strabismus.

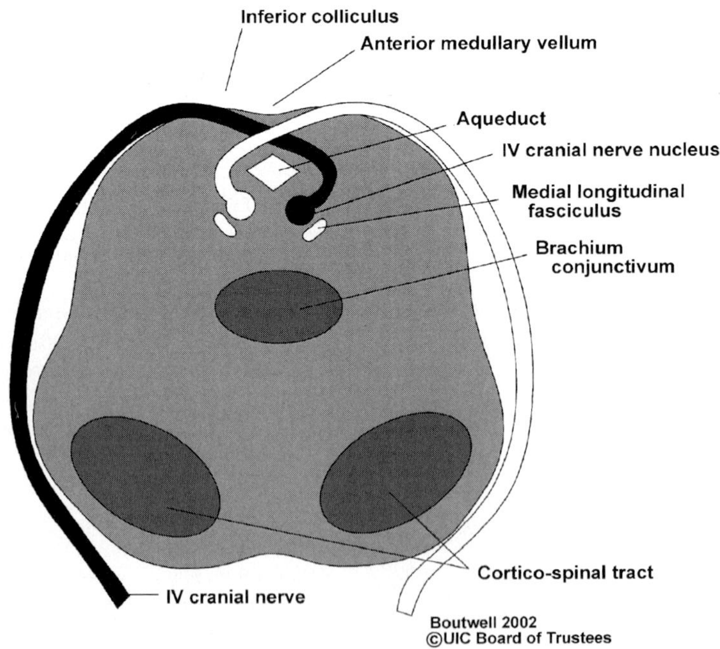


Fig. 16. Diagram of axial view of the midbrain at level of the inferior colliculus highlights CN IV. (Illustration by Adrienne J. Boutwell and Lisa J. Birmingham © University of Illinois at Chicago Board of Trustees 2002; with permission.)

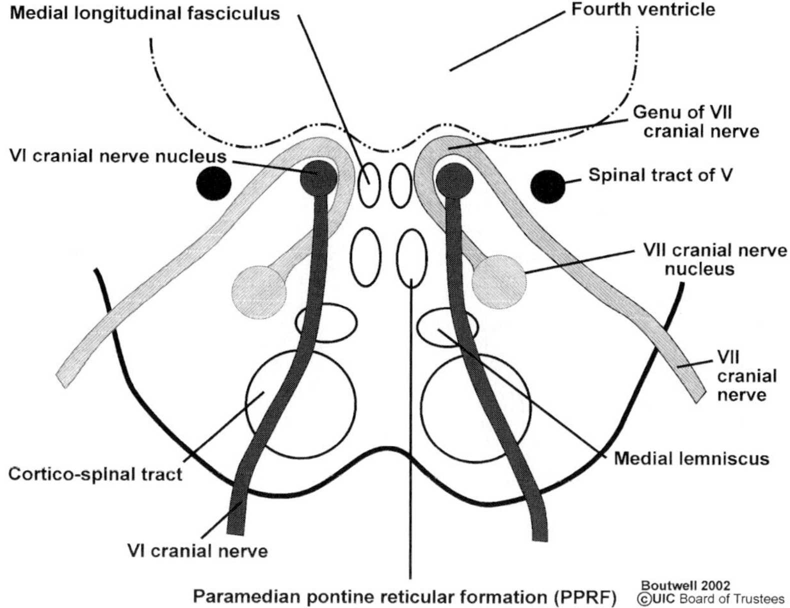


Fig. 17. Diagram of axial view at the level of the pontine-medullary junction highlights CN VI. (Illustration by Adrienne J. Boutwell and Lisa J. Birmingham © University of Illinois at Chicago Board of Trustees 2002; with permission.)

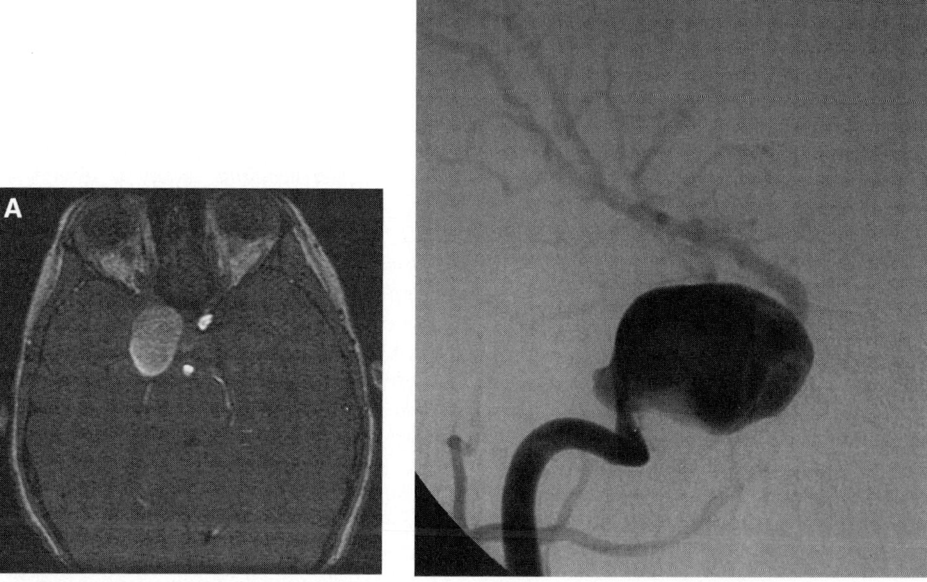


Fig. 18. Giant carotid artery aneurysm presenting with oculomotor nerve palsy. An axial gradient echo source image from an MR angiogram (*A*) and an oblique image from a standard angiogram (*B*) show a giant aneurysm of the cavernous portion of the right internal carotid artery in this 10-year-old boy. The patient underwent balloon occlusion sacrifice of the right internal carotid artery. The CN III function has recovered completely.

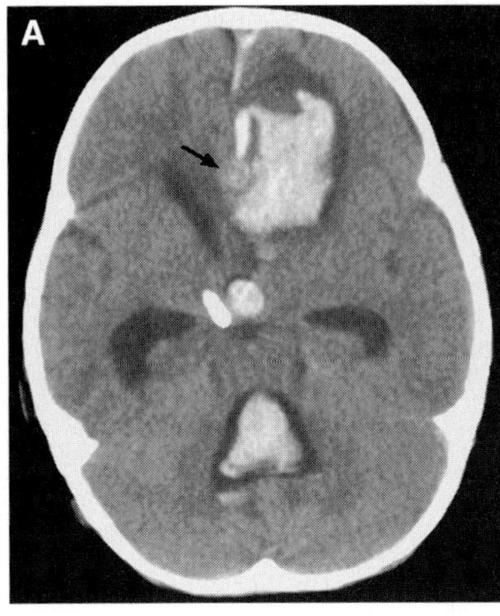

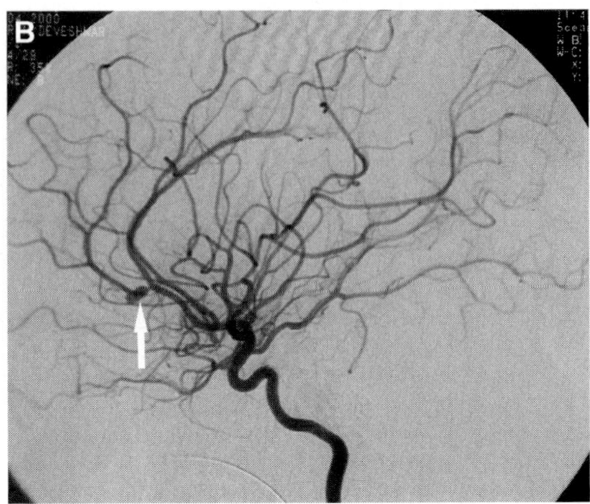

Fig. 19. Traumatic anterior cerebral artery aneurysm with intracranial hemorrhage. This 1-year-old girl was involved in a serious motor vehicle accident. An initial CT scan of the head was normal. She later presented with signs of hydrocephalus and a fully dilated left pupil. (*A*) Unenhanced CT scan demonstrates an extensive intraparenchymal hematoma in the left frontal lobe (*arrow*), intraventricular hemorrhage, and hydrocephalus. A round hyperdense focus at the interhemispheric fissure (*arrow*) represents a posttraumatic right anterior cerebral artery aneurysm at the origins of the pericallosal and callosomarginal arteries, as demonstrated on a lateral standard angiographic image (*B*).

Congenital ocular motor apraxia is characterized by an inability to initiate voluntary horizontal gaze movements to the right or left. Other pathways involving horizontal gaze remain intact, so that eye movements to the right and left can be initiated by convergence, the vestibulo-ocular reflex (doll's head maneuver), or optokinetic nystagmus [34]. Vertical eye movements are typically preserved in congenital ocular motor apraxia but not so in acquired cases. Children with congenital ocular motor apraxia use a characteristic head thrust movement to drive their eyes into side gaze, a maneuver that takes advantage of the vestibulo-ocular reflex.

### *Syndromic strabismus*

This is a heterogeneous group that includes a number of specific diagnoses, each with a stereotypical presentation and not belonging in the aforementioned etiologic categories.

Duane syndrome is a congenital disorder and results from developmental hypoplasia of the nucleus of CN VI and subsequent anomalous innervation of the ipsilateral lateral rectus muscle by fibers from CN III. The pathologic process is idiopathic yet benign and nonprogressive. Patients with Duane syndrome show decreased abduction and narrowing of the lid fissure on adduction of the affected eye(s). Duane syndrome may be confused clinically with CN VI palsy, and these patients may undergo medical imaging to help in this differentiation. Duane syndrome occurs most often in isolation but is also associated with a variety of systemic conditions, including hemifacial microsomia, Goldenhar syndrome, Wildervanck syndrome, and deafness among others [35].

Brown syndrome is a disorder of the superior oblique muscle tendon's inability to slide through its pulley (trochlea). Clinically, patients with Brown syndrome show an inability to elevate the affected eye(s) in adduction. Onset may be congenital or acquired. The acquired variety is usually caused by an acute inflammatory process (Fig. 20) that may respond to treatment with local or systemic anti-inflammatory medication. CT or MR imaging usually demonstrates thickening of the reflected portion of the superior oblique tendon [36].

Congenital fibrosis syndrome is a congenital dystrophy of the extraocular and levator muscles and is characterized by normal muscle fibers replaced with contracted inelastic fibrotic tissue [37]. A single muscle or multiple muscles may be involved but usually symmetrically. These patients have blepharoptosis, incomitant vertical and horizontal strabismus, and limitation of ocular rotations. Medical imaging shows thickening or atrophy of the affected extraocular muscles [38] and may also reveal associated CNS anomalies [39].

Other diagnostic entities that fall into this group of strabismus syndromes include Möbius syndrome,

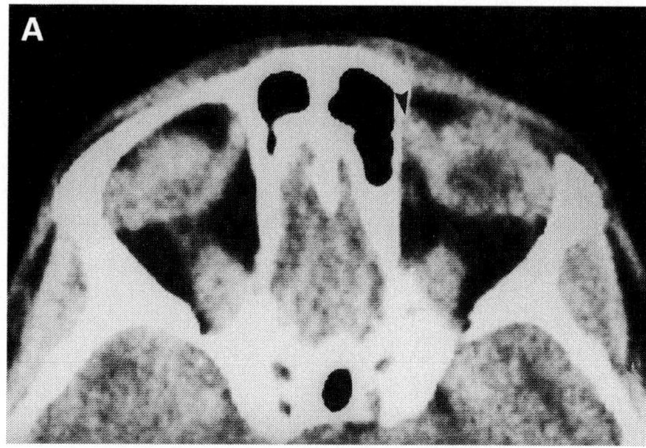


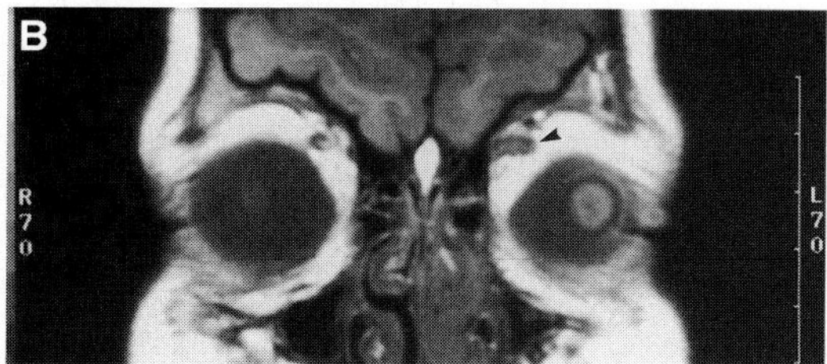


Fig. 20. Brown syndrome. Axial CT (*A*) and coronal T1-weighted MR (*B*) images show enlargement of the reflected portion of the left superior oblique muscle (*arrowheads*) in two different patients with Brown syndrome.

chronic progressive external ophthalmoplegia, Kearns-Sayre syndrome, various mitochondrial disorders, the Fisher variant of Guillain-Barré syndrome, and ocular myasthenia gravis.

## Ocular torticollis

Torticollis (or wry neck) refers to the maintenance of the head in an abnormal position rather than an upright posture. Torticollis results from a variety of disparate disorders, such as contractions of neck musculature, neck masses, cervical spine diseases, unilateral hearing deficit, or lesions of the peripheral or central posture maintenance pathways. Ocular torticollis is the adoption of an abnormal head posture in compensation for some deficit of the ocular sensory or motor system, so as to improve visual acuity, to preserve fusion and stereopsis, or to avoid diplopia (Box 9) [40,41]. Patients with incomitant strabismus may have some position of gaze where their eyes remain well aligned. These patients then turn their head so as to maintain their eyes in this position, thereby preserving fusion and avoiding diplopia. Patients with ptosis maintain a chin-up head posture to "look under" their droopy lids. In null-point nystagmus, the ocular oscillations dampen in one particular position of gaze (the null-point), which allows for improved visual acuity [42]. These patients may assume an abnormal head position to maintain their eyes in the null-point.

In some children with presumed ocular torticollis, the ophthalmologist may be uncertain as to the etiology of the torticollis because of conflicting clinical features or the quality of the eye examination. These patients may have medical imaging to rule out identifiable orbital or CNS lesions.

## Pupil abnormalities in childhood

Any abnormality in the innervation of the iris results in anisocoria, a round and central pupil but of unequal size between the two eyes. Anisocoria caused by an interruption of sympathetic innervation results in a smaller (miotic) ipsilateral pupil; disruption of parasympathetic innervation results in a dilated (mydriatic) ipsilateral pupil. Figs. 21 and 22 illustrate the neuroanatomic pathways of iris innervation. Disruption of iris anatomy (from trauma, inflammation, degeneration, or a congenital anomaly) can similarly result in anisocoria and can also alter the position and shape of the pupil.

Anisocoria in children is most often physiologic, that is, a variation of normal. The child with innervational anisocoria must be evaluated for a lesion of the sympathetic or parasympathetic pathway.

**Box 9. Ocular torticollis in childhood**

- Paralytic strabismus: superior oblique palsy
- Acquired "pattern" strabismus
- Restrictive strabismus
- Syndromic strabismus
- Complex ocular motor disorders
- Infantile strabismus
- Ptosis
- Unilateral blindness
- Large refractive errors
- Congenital "null-point" nystagmus
- Spasmus nutans
- Periodic alternating nystagmus
- Lens subluxation

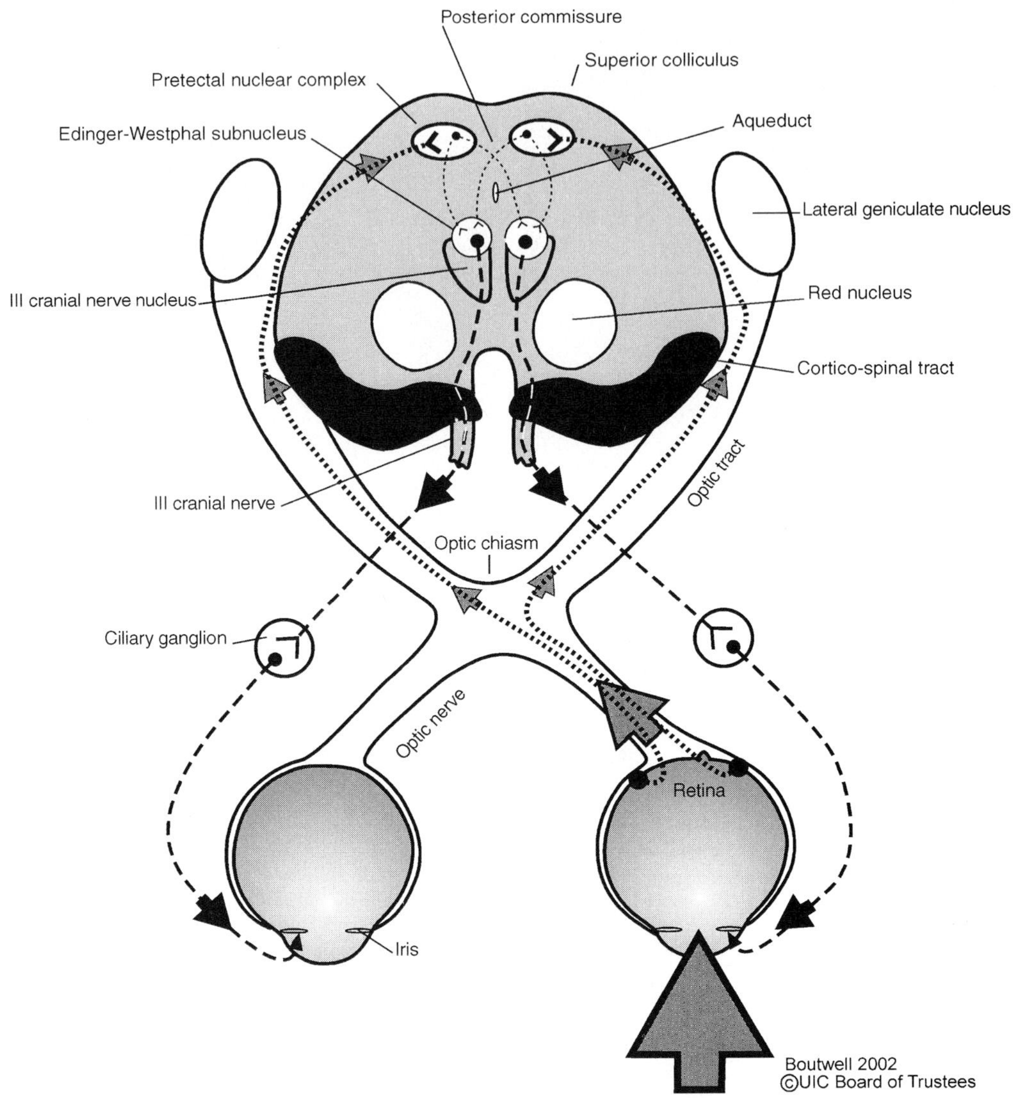


Fig. 21. Pupillary light reflex and parasympathetic pathways of pupil innervation. Light presented to an eye stimulates the retina. Pupillomotor afferent fibers enter the optic nerve and pass ipsilaterally and contralaterally through the optic chiasm into both optic tracts. Unlike the visual fibers, the pupillomotor fibers bypass the lateral geniculate nucleus and then terminate in the pretectal nuclear complex at the level of the superior colliculus. Crossed and uncrossed intercalated neurons travel from the pretectal nuclear complex to the Edinger-Westphal nuclei (the visceral component of CN III nucleus). Parasympathetic fibers to the iris originate in the Edinger-Westphal nucleus and travel to the iris sphincter muscle via the ipsilateral CN III after synapsing in the ciliary ganglion within the orbit. Note that unilateral stimulation of the retina results in bilateral symmetric pupil constriction. (Illustration by Adrienne J. Boutwell and Lisa J. Birmingham © University of Illinois at Chicago Board of Trustees 2002; with permission.)

*Sympathetic deinnervation of the iris*

A lesion at any point along the sympathetic pathway of iris innervation results in an ipsilateral Horner syndrome (see Fig. 22). A lesion proximal to the take-off of the sudomotor fibers to the face results in the classic triad of ptosis, miosis, and anhydrosis. More distal lesions may lack the anhydrosis or ptosis.

Pharmacologic testing of pupil function to localize a Horner syndrome lesion to the first, second, or third order is critically important but is challenging to interpret in children. Instead, the authors routinely order MR imaging, without and with contrast, of the

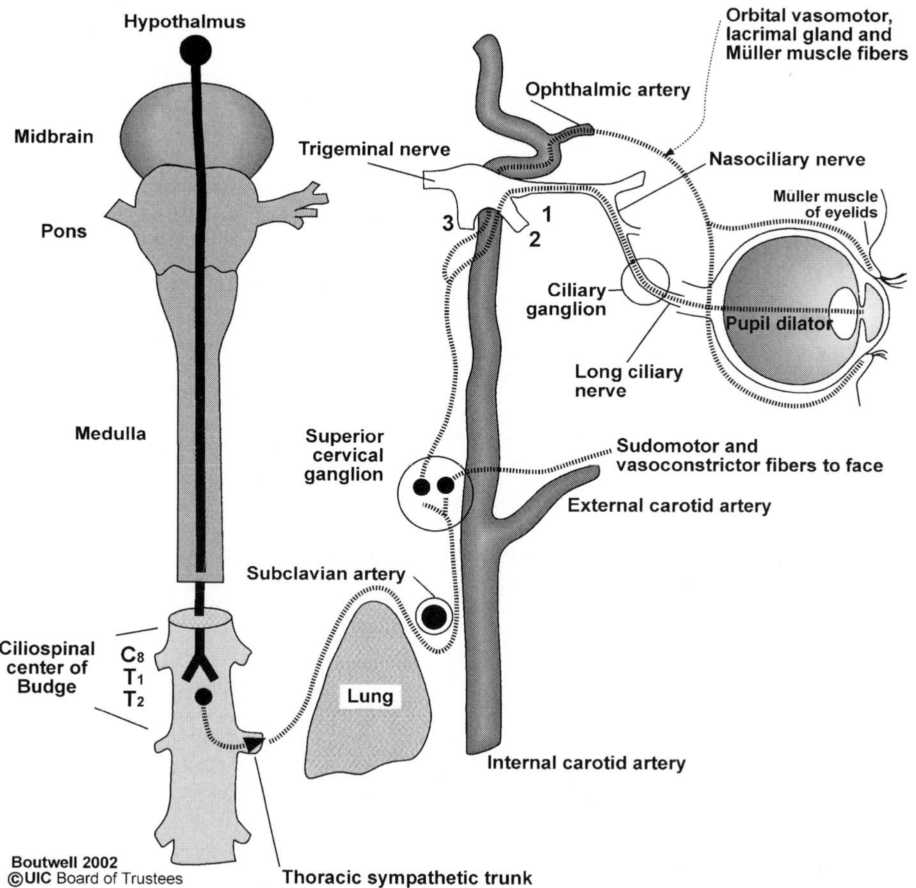


Fig. 22. Sympathetic pathways of pupil innervation. First-order neurons of sympathetic innervation to the iris dilator muscle originate in the posterior hypothalamus and travel down the brain stem to terminate in the spinal cord at the C8 to T2 level in the ciliospinal center of Budge. Second-order neurons leave the spinal cord and travel through the paravertebral sympathetic chain to terminate in the superior cervical ganglion, located alongside the internal carotid artery at the skull base. Third-order (and final) neurons ascend alongside the internal carotid artery to enter the orbit, pass through the ciliary ganglion without synapsing, and then innervate the iris dilator muscle. Sympathetic innervation for facial sweating and to the smooth Müller muscle of the eyelid also travels in these pathways. Unilateral interruption of these pathways results in ipsilateral Horner syndrome, with miosis, ptosis, and anhydrosis. (Illustration by Adrienne J. Boutwell and Lisa J. Birmingham © University of Illinois at Chicago Board of Trustees 2002; with permission.)

head, orbit, neck, and upper chest to image the entire sympathetic pathway. Isolated Horner syndrome in children most often has a benign etiology (congenital, traumatic, or familial) [43]. Medical imaging is pursued to exclude a mass lesion, most commonly neuroblastoma of the upper chest.

### *Parasympathetic deinnervation of the iris*

Parasympathetic innervation to the globe originates in the Edinger-Westphal subnucleus of CN III (see Fig. 21). The parasympathetic fibers then travel in the ipsilateral fascicle and nerve of CN III to reach the orbit. Lesions of CN III result in paralytic strabismus as well as parasympathetic deinnervation of the iris with an enlarged, unreactive pupil. Diagnostic possibilities were discussed previously (see section on paralytic strabismus).

Adie tonic pupil, a syndrome of parasympathetic deinnervation of the iris unrelated to a mass lesion and not involving the motor fibers of CN III, is rare in children.

## Summary

This article provides an outline of the congenital and acquired conditions encountered in the practice of pediatric neuro-ophthalmology. Although some entities can be effectively evaluated clinically, CT and MR imaging studies may prove instrumental in many instances for detailed evaluation, narrowing of the differential diagnosis, or exclusion of underlying CNS pathologic findings.

## Acknowledgments

The authors thank Jay Shah, BSc, for his invaluable help with image processing. This work was approved by the Institutional Review Board of the University of Illinois at Chicago.

## References

[1] Apple DJ, Rabb MF, Walsh PM. Congenital anomalies of the optic disc. Surv Ophthalmol 1982;27(1): 3–41.

[2] Golnik KC. Congenital optic nerve anomalies. Curr Opin Ophthalmol 1998;9(6):18–26.

[3] Campbell CL. Septo-optic dysplasia: a literature review. Optometry 2003;74(7):417–26.

[4] Brodsky MC, Glasier CM. Optic nerve hypoplasia. Clinical significance of associated central nervous system abnormalities on magnetic resonance imaging. Arch Ophthalmol 1993;111(1):66–74.

[5] Brown GC. Optic nerve hypoplasia and colobomatous defects. J Pediatr Ophthalmol Strabismus 1982;19(2): 90–3.

[6] Chan T, Bowell R, O'Keefe M, et al. Ocular manifestations in fetal alcohol syndrome. Br J Ophthalmol 1991;75(9):524–6.

[7] Mansour AM, Bitar FF, Traboulsi EI, et al. Ocular pathology in congenital heart disease. Eye 2004;19(1): 29–34.

[8] Berk AT, Yaman A, Saatci AO. Ocular and systemic findings associated with optic disc colobomas. J Pediatr Ophthalmol Strabismus 2003;40(5):272–8.

[9] Auber AE, O'Hara M. Morning glory syndrome. MR imaging. Clin Imaging 1999;23(3):152–8.

[10] Krishnan C, Roy A, Traboulsi E. Morning glory disk anomaly, choroidal coloboma, and congenital constrictive malformations of the internal carotid arteries (Moyamoya disease). Ophthalmic Genet 2000;2l(1): 21–4.

[11] Kurz-Levin MM, Landau K. A comparison of imaging techniques for diagnosing drusen of the optic nerve head. Arch Ophthahmol 1999;l17(8):1045–9.

[12] Chan DQ. Neurologic, ophthalmic, and neuropsychiatric manifestations of pediatric systemic lupus erythematosus. Optom Vis Sci 2000;77(8):388–94.

[13] Mottow LS, Jakobiec FA. I. Idiopathic inflammatory orbital pseudotumor in childhood. I. Clinical characteristics. Arch Ophthalmol 1978;96(8):1410–7.

[14] Vaphiades MS, Eggenberger E. Childhood sarcoidosis. J Neuroophthalmol 1998;18(2):99–101.

[15] Phillips PH, Repka MX, Lambert SR. Pseudotumor cerebri in children. J AAPOS 1998;2(1):33–8.

[16] Dollfus H, Vinikoff L, Renier D, et al. Insidious craniosynostosis and chronic papilledema in childhood. Am J Ophthalmol 1996;122(6):910–1.

[17] Boomer JA, Siatkowski RM. Optic neuritis in adults and children. Semin Ophthalmol 2003;18(4):174–80.

[18] Repka MX, Miller NR. Optic atrophy in children. Am J Ophthalmol 1988;106(2):191–3.

[19] Towbin R, Garcia-Revillo J, Fitz C. Orbital hydrocephalus: a proven cause for optic atrophy. Pediatr Radiol 1998;28(12):995–7.

[20] Mudgil AV, Repka MX. Childhood optic atrophy. Clin Exp Ophthalmol 2000;28(1):34–7.

[21] Sadun F, De Negri AM, Carelli V, et al. Ophthalmologic findings in a large pedigree of 11778/Haplogroup J Leber hereditary optic neuropathy. Am J Ophthalmol 2004;137(2):271–7.

[22] Dutton GN, Jacobson LK. Cerebral visual impairment in children. Semin Neonatol 2001;6(6):477–85.

[23] Repka MX. Ophthalmological problems of the premature infant. Ment Retard Dev Disabil Res Rev 2002; 8(4):249–57.

[24] Van Hof-van Duin J, Mohn G. Visual defects in children after cerebral hypoxia. Behav Brain Res 1984;14(2):147–55.

[25] Maybodi M. Infantile-onset nystagmus. Curr Opin Ophthalmol 2003;14(5):276–85.

[26] Gottlob I, Zubcov A, Catalano RA, et al. Signs distinguishing spasmus nutans (with and without central nervous system lesions) from infantile nystagmus. Ophthalmology 1990;97(9):1166–75.

[27] Arnoldi KA, Tychsen L. Prevalence of intracranial lesions in children initially diagnosed with disconjugate nystagmus (spasmus nutans). J Pediatr Ophthalmol Strabismus 1995;32(5):296–301.

[28] Tarczy-Hornoch K, Repka MX. Superior oblique palsy or paresis in pediatric patients. J AAPOS 2004;8(2): 133–40.

[29] Afifi AK, Bell WE, Menezes AH. Etiology of lateral rectus palsy in infancy and childhood. J Child Neurol 1992;7(3):295–9.

[30] Holmes JM, Droste PJ, Beck RW. The natural history of acute traumatic sixth nerve palsy or paresis. J AAPOS 1998;2(5):265–8.

[31] Tamhankar MA, Liu GT, Young TL, et al. Acquired, isolated third nerve palsies in infants with cerebrovascular malformations. Am J Ophthalmol 2004;138(3): 484–6.

[32] Yee RD, Duffin RM, Baloh RW, et al. Familial, congenital paralysis of horizontal gaze. Arch Ophthalmol 1982;100(9):1449–52.

[33] Cho BK, Wang KC, Nam DH, et al. Pineal tumors: experience with 48 cases over 10 years. Childs Nerv Syst 1998;14(1–2):53–8.

[34] Steinlin M, Thun-Hohenstein L, Boltshauser E. Congenital oculomotor apraxia. Presentation—develop-

mental problems—differential diagnosis. Klin Monatsbl Augenheilkd 1992;200(5):623–5.

[35] Shauly Y, Weissman A, Meyer E. Ocular and systemic characteristics of Duane syndrome. J Pediatr Ophthalmol Strabismus 1993;30(3):178–83.

[36] Tien RD, Duberg A, Chu PK, et al. Superior oblique tendon sheath syndrome (Brown syndrome): MR findings. AJNR Am J Neuroradiol 1990;11(6):1210.

[37] Mafee MF. The orbit. In: Mafee MF, Valvassori GE, Becker M, editors. Imaging of the head and neck. Stuttgart (Germany): Thieme; 2004. p. 196–294.

[38] Hertle RW, Katowitz JA, Young TL, et al. Congenital unilateral fibrosis, blepharoptosis, and enophthalmos syndrome. Ophthalmology 1992;99(3):347–55.

[39] Pieh C, Goebel HH, Engle EC, et al. Congenital fibrosis syndrome associated with central nervous system abnormalities. Graefes Arch Clin Exp Ophthalmol 2003;241(7):546–53.

[40] Rubin SE, Wagner RS. Ocular torticollis. Surv Ophthalmol 1986;30(6):366–76.

[41] Mitchell PR. Ocular torticollis. Trans Am Ophthalmol Soc 1999;97:697–769.

[42] Hertle RW, Zhu X. Oculographic and clinical characterization of thirty-seven children with anomalous head postures, nystagmus, and strabismus: the basis of a clinical algorithm. J AAPOS 2000;4(1):25–32.

[43] Jeffery AR, Ellis FJ, Repka MX, et al. Pediatric Horner syndrome. J AAPOS 1998;2(3):159–67.

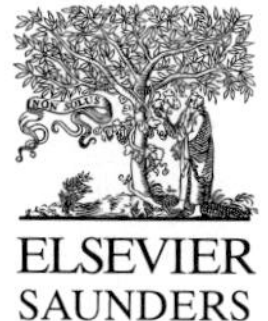

ELSEVIER
SAUNDERS

Neuroimag Clin N Am 15 (2005) 107 – 120

NEUROIMAGING
CLINICS OF
NORTH AMERICA

# Vascular Lesions of the Orbit in Children

Larissa T. Bilaniuk, MD[a,b,*]

[a]*University of Pennsylvania School of Medicine, Philadelphia, PA, USA*
[b]*Department of Radiology, Children's Hospital of Philadelphia, 34th Street and Civic Center Boulevard, Philadelphia, PA 19104, USA*

Vascular orbital lesions in the pediatric population represent an important group of lesions because they can present very early in life and may affect vision and ocular motility and can cause prominent proptosis and disfigurement. Prompt and accurate diagnosis and localization of these lesions are essential for proper management and avoiding serious complications. Failure to recognize the specific nature of the lesion could lead to inappropriate therapy. Although clinical characterization and diagnosis are important, the detection, delineation, and characterization of deep orbital lesions have always required some type of imaging. Over the years, tremendous progress has been made in the imaging of the orbit [1–4]. The results of modern imaging combined with sophisticated clinical, histopathologic, electron microscopic evaluations, and basic research, including genetic studies, have lead to a better understanding of this complex and still controversial group of orbital lesions [5–12]. Varied opinions remain as to the origin and nature of many of the orbital vascular lesions. It is important for the radiologist to be familiar with embryologic, clinical, hemodynamic, and pathophysiologic aspects of these lesions to reach correct conclusions based on the imaging characteristics.

In the pediatric population, when all types of orbital lesions are included, the reported incidence of vascular orbital lesions, as given in six different series, ranges from 5.5% to 22% [13–18]. This great variability in incidence is caused by a combination of factors: the referral pattern for a given physician and institution; the criteria for inclusion into the study series (ie, the inclusion of only cases in which a biopsy was performed versus clinically, radiologically, or histopathologically diagnosed cases); the special interests of a given physician or department; and the type of diagnostic studies that were used. For example, a series that covers a period of many years will consist of cases diagnosed with various imaging modalities, some much more sophisticated and precise than others, and therefore, not all diagnoses may be correct. Modern imaging has obviated the need for a diagnostic biopsy in many instances; therefore, a series from the pre-modern imaging era based only on histopathologic results will differ from a more recent series because the diagnosis of many lesions presently does not require that a biopsy be performed.

Over the years, there has been tremendous confusion and disagreement about the classification and nomenclature of vascular lesions, including those occurring in the orbit. New classifications and new nomenclature for vascular lesions have been proposed by various investigators based on pathogenesis, histopathology, and hemodynamic studies [19–24].

As proposed by Mulliken and Glowacki [19], the number one step in approaching a vascular lesion is to decide whether the lesion is a vascular tumor or a vascular malformation. A vascular tumor such as a hemangioma is related to an angiogenic growth factor affect and is composed of sinusoidal channels that have rapidly proliferating endothelial cells. A vascular malformation results from a localized error in angiogenic development, and its channels do not

* Department of Radiology, Children's Hospital of Philadelphia, 34th Street and Civic Center Boulevard, Philadelphia, PA 19104.

*E-mail address:* bilaniuk@email.chop.edu

1052-5149/05/$ – see front matter 
doi:10.1016/j.nic.2005.03.001

contain rapidly dividing endothelial cells. A vascular malformation enlarges slowly in proportion to the growth of a child, unless the lesion hemorrhages or is inflamed. Although most malformations occur sporadically, in some instances, genetic studies have revealed mutated genes, indicating that genes play an important role in regulation of angiogenesis [9,10].

The ongoing conflict concerning the classification and nomenclature of the orbital vascular lesions has had a negative affect on scientific progress in the study of these lesions and has led at times to the mismanagement of a patient, resulting in severe complications. The degree of difficulty in surgical resection and the incidence and severity of complications vary with the type of vascular lesion, whether it is a hemangioma, a malformation (the so-called "cavernous hemangioma") a venous lymphatic malformation, a varix, or an arteriovenous malformation. Because the influence of the conflict had extended beyond the academic debate into clinical practice, the Orbital Society was prompted to draft and reach a consensus on the classification of orbital vascular malformations [25]. The Society accepted a hemodynamic classification of orbital vascular malformations because this classification emphasized features most pertinent to the management of such lesions [25]. In this consensus, lesions are classified according to their hemodynamic relationships: no-flow (so-called "lymphangiomas"), venous flow (so-called "primary varices"), and arterial flow (arteriovenous malformation) [25]. The objective of the Orbital Society is to create universally accepted terminology that should allow a better comparison of therapeutic protocols, lead to better statistical results in reports dealing with various aspects of the lesions, and most importantly, to improve the management of these lesions.

## Hemangiomas

In one series [26] of orbital vascular lesions that included all age groups, hemangiomas were reported as the most frequent vascular tumor. When the statistics from six series [13–18] of pediatric orbital lesions are combined, the incidence of capillary hemangioma is 5.6%. Among the six series, the incidence ranges from 0% to 11.8%. Hemangiomas, which are vascular neoplasms resulting from vasoformative tissue proliferation, are the most common pediatric orbital tumors. Although they have been referred to as infantile hemangioma, juvenile hemangioma, hypertrophic hemangioma, and hemangioblastoma, the most common and most widely accepted term for these tumors is "capillary hemangioma." Mulliken and Glowacki [19], who revised and simplified the classification of birthmarks and vascular tumors based on the pathogenesis and behavior of these neoplasms, recommend using just the term "hemangioma." Because the term capillary hemangioma is so commonly used throughout the world and because the term hemangioma is used sometimes incorrectly to refer to vascular malformations (ie, cavernous hemangiomas), many practitioners still hold onto the term capillary hemangioma. This article uses the term hemangioma. Perhaps in time, as more physicians in various specialties become familiar with the correct and simplified terminology proposed by Mulliken and Glowacki [19] and become more aware of the distinction between vascular neoplasms and malformations, it will be possible to drop the adjective *capillary* from the term.

No definite hereditary or familial pattern has been noted in connection with hemangiomas, although they are reported to be more common in females, with an approximate female:male ratio of 3:2 [27,28]. There is no geographic predilection. In his experience, Mulliken [21] has found hemangiomas to be uncommon in African American children.

Hemangiomas typically present at birth or shortly thereafter. Approximately one third of hemangiomas are noted at birth. They characteristically go through a proliferative phase within 3 to 6 months after diagnosis [19,21,27]. During this time, there is generally a marked enlargement of the lesion, which can alarm both the parents and the pediatrician. After a period of stabilization and an intermediate stage, the tumor enters an involutional phase, which is usually complete by 5 to 7 years of age but may last longer. Generally, the faster the lesion enlarges, the faster it involutes [27]. Congenital hemangiomas, those that proliferate in utero, are fully grown at birth and begin to involute shortly thereafter, and their regression proceeds more rapidly than that of postnatal hemangiomas, within an average range of 6 to 14 months [29]. This behavior of congenital hemangiomas prompted a study [29] that led the investigators to postulate that intrauterine hemangiomas may result from a localized low concentration of trophoblastic interferon, which is known to inhibit angiogenesis by lowering the concentration of basic fibroblast growth factor, a known stimulator of angiogenesis. It is further postulated that the postnatal appearance of a hemangioma might result from a sudden decrease in trophoblastic interferon as the infant separates from placental circulation [29].

The histopathology of a hemangioma varies depending on its phase. During the proliferative phase, the tumor consists of clusters of endothelial cells with increased mitosis around some small irregular vascular spaces. Also, the number of mast cells is much greater than is seen in normal tissue [30]. Mast cells are believed to play a role in the development and early involution of the hemangioma. When the tumor enlarges, the vascular structures become better formed. As it begins to involute, which starts from the center, fibro-fatty tissue is deposited around the blood vessels and lobules of endothelial cells. There is a progressive diminution in the cellular component of both endothelial and mast cells, and the tumor eventually consists mostly of fatty and fibrous tissue without vessels. Finally, there is complete atrophy of the vasculature [28].

The clinical presentation of the orbital hemangioma depends on its location and its size. Very superficial hemangiomas with skin involvement result in fine lobulation of the skin that has a bright red color. Subcutaneous lesions appear dark blue or purple as viewed through the skin and have a spongy consistency on palpation. Deep lesions are not associated with skin discoloration and manifest by mass effect. However, there are also hemangiomas that consist of various combinations of superficial, subcutaneous, and deep components.

Proptosis, or displacement of the globe, is a frequent finding with hemangiomas. At times, the proptosis can be so severe that it results in corneal exposure and stretching of the optic nerve. With a Valsalva maneuver, the hemangiomas enlarge and change in color to deep blue [27]. This is believed to be caused by inflow of the less oxygenated blood into the lesion.

Of all of the complications related to adnexal hemangiomas, visual loss resulting from amblyopia is the most common and most serious. Amblyopia is reported to occur in 43% to 60% of patients [27,28, 31,32]. Amblyopia can be caused by the involvement and affect of the tumor on the lid, globe, extraocular muscles, and optic nerve. Visual loss caused by depravation amblyopia can result from obstruction of the visual access by a large hemangioma in the eyelid. If the tumor indents the globe and cornea and produces astigmatism, then an anisometropic amblyopia results. If the tumor involves the extraocular muscles or by its mass effect limits ocular motility, then strabismus can result, leading to amblyopia. Each of the affects of the tumor can act alone or in combination. Prolonged unilateral eyelid closure in infants can result in axial elongation of the globe and myopia. Finally, a rapid increase in retrobulbar hemangioma can stretch and injure the optic nerve. The longer the visual access is occluded the more severe the amblyopia. Patients who have a hemangioma that obstructs the visual access need to be carefully monitored.

The high incidence of amblyopia with periocular hemangioma is related to the fact that the tumor manifests itself within the first months of life. Animal studies [28] have revealed that even short periods of abnormal visual input during the first months of life may result in significant and permanent abnormalities of the visual pathways.

Patients who have orbital hemangiomas may have coexisting hemangiomas elsewhere in the body. Hemangiomas involving the airway (subglottal, peritracheal, and oral and nasal) are the most important to detect because they can cause respiratory difficulties and result in hypoxia-anoxia. Intubation can cause a hemangioma to hemorrhage, and compression of the esophagus by a hemangioma can result in aspiration. There have been few reports of the coexistence of central nervous system abnormalities with facial hemangiomas [33].

Although prompt identification and correct characterization and delineation of the lesion are important for proper management, no matter which part of the body is involved, these factors are critical in cases of orbital hemangiomas. A delay or mistake in the diagnosis of an orbital hemangioma could lead to severe complications. Superficially located orbital hemangiomas are easily diagnosed clinically; however, hemangiomas that involve multiple compartments of the orbit or those that are located in the deeper portions of the orbit without a skin or subcutaneous component can be difficult to differentiate from other lesions such as rhabdomyosarcoma, neuroblastoma, and venous lymphatic malformation. Thus, diagnostic studies need to be used, and the best of these is magnetic resonance imaging. High-resolution thin-section T2-weighted (T2W) MR images with fat suppression and T1-weighted (T1W) MR images with gadolinium enhancement provide excellent depictions of the morphology and internal architecture of the lesion and its relationship to the adjacent structures (Figs. 1–5). On T1W imaging, a hemangioma is similar to or slightly higher in intensity compared with muscles. Signal voids caused by vessels can be seen within and on the periphery of the lesion. The internal lobular character of the hemangioma is well demonstrated on T2W MR images with fat suppression, which has increased intensity, with septae and vessels having lower intensity. After an intravenous injection of gadolinium contrast material, there is marked contrast enhancement. On CT scanning, a hemangioma appears as a homogeneous contrast-

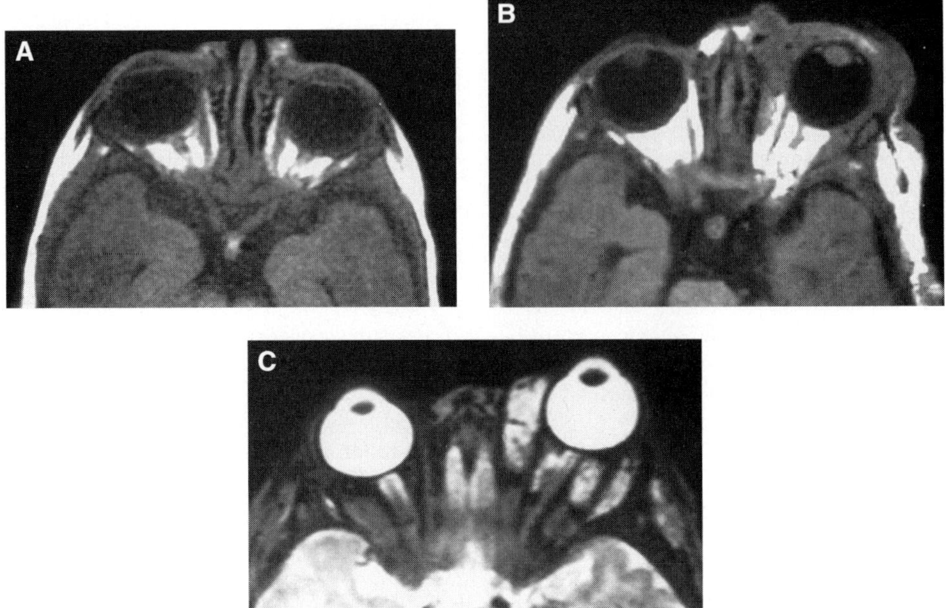


Fig. 1. Hemangioma showing prominent growth in an interval of 4 months. (*A*) Axial T1W MR image shows barely perceptible fullness with one slightly prominent flow void in the left medial canthal region. The 11-day-old patient was referred because of an erythematous macule noted on physical examination. (*B*) At 4 months of age, the patient presented with a large multilobulated mass noted on both sides of the left globe, extending into the extraconal spaces. More prominent signal voids are noted in the medial aspect of the mass. (*C*) Axial fast spin-echo T2W MR image with fat saturation shows the hemangioma in both the extraconic and intraconic spaces of the left orbit. Note the characteristically increased intensity and multilobulated pattern of the tumor.

enhancing mass that often has a lobulated, irregular margin; however, the internal structure of the lesion is not well demonstrated (Figs. 4D, 4E, 5A, and 5C). On CT scans, a hemangioma can appear similar to rhabdomyosarcoma (Fig. 5). Some rhabdomyosarcoma masses may be so vascularized that on MR imaging they are shown to contain prominent signal voids and thus mimic the hemangioma (Fig. 6). Often, differential diagnosis is not a problem because infants have a much higher incidence of hemangioma than of rhabdomyosarcoma, and the mean age of onset for rhabdomyosarcoma is 6 years.

On ultrasonography, hemangiomas have a characteristic pattern, but their extent and delineation are shown much better with MR imaging. However, after the diagnosis has been made, ultrasonography can be used in a follow-up of lesions to monitor changes such as growth or involution. The variation in internal reflectivity seen on the B-scan corresponds to the variation in the internal structure of the tumor. Involution-related changes in the hemangioma can also be well demonstrated with MR imaging (Fig. 4).

Just as with any enlarging orbital tumor in the very young patient, large hemangiomas can markedly expand the orbital cavity (Figs. 1B, 1C, 4, and 5B). Smaller lesions can produce focal scalloping of the adjacent bone. These changes can be well appreciated on both CT and MR imaging.

When the lesion is large and is in its proliferative phase, the enlargement of arteries such as the ophthalmic artery and branches of the external carotid artery can be well demonstrated on MR angiography. However, in the rare circumstance in which an intravascular therapy is being considered with sclerosing agents, conventional arteriography needs to be performed to obtain a detailed anatomy of the vasculature.

Although hemangiomas involute spontaneously, if they are located in the lids or orbit, they often require some form of therapy. If the tumor obstructs the visual axis or produces rapid proptosis with stretching of the optic nerve and causes exposure of the cornea, some form of therapy needs to be instituted promptly. A wide spectrum of therapies can be used, including amblyopic therapy, surgery, radiotherapy, systemic corticosteroids, intralesional corticosteroids, interferon injections [34], and laser therapy [28]. Corticosteroids can be injected into the lesion or used

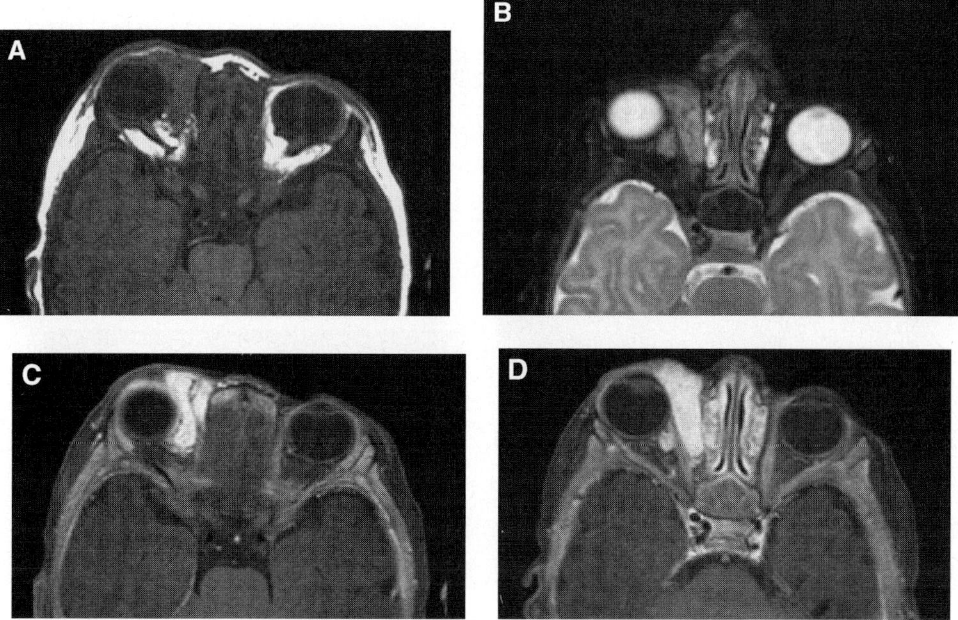

Fig. 2. Hemangioma in the medial aspect of the right orbit. (*A*) Axial T1W MR image shows peripherally lobulated and irregular mass in the medial aspect of the right orbit, displacing the right globe laterally. Small signal voids are present within the mass. (*B*) T2W fat-saturated MR image shows a slightly heterogeneous, moderately increased intensity in the hemangioma. A lobule of the tumor extending intraconally behind the globe is well demonstrated. (*C*) Contrast-enhanced fat-saturated T1W MR image shows marked enhancement of the mass. Several linear flow voids are noted within the mass. (*D*) T1W contrast-enhanced fat-saturated MR image obtained at a slightly lower plane than in (*C*) demonstrates well the extent of the mass and its affects on the medial rectus muscle and the globe.

systemically. Intralesional injections of corticosteroids have proved effective in preventing amblyopia, have resulted in the reversal of astigmatism, and have been found to be a safe procedure without complications [35–37]. However, the long-term follow-up of patients treated with corticosteroids may require management of refractive amblyopia with glasses and patching [37]. If there is danger of the development of amblyopia, then the normal eye is patched intermittently, and optical correction is prescribed. Stra-

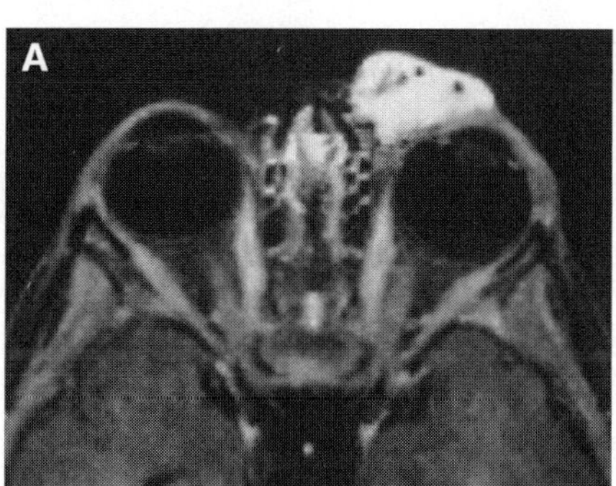

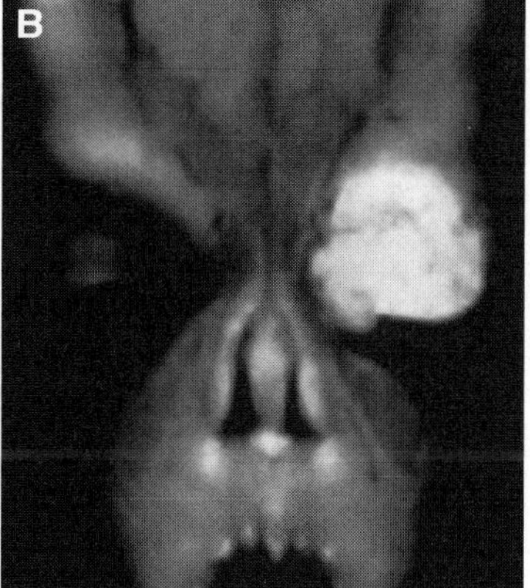

Fig. 3. Hemangioma in a 16-month-old male patient. (*A*) Axial contrast-enhanced fat-saturated T1W MR image shows a multilobulated contrast-enhancing mass with signal voids anterior to the medial aspect of the left globe. (*B*) Coronal contrast-enhanced fat-saturated T1W MR image shows the large mass obstructing the visual axis.

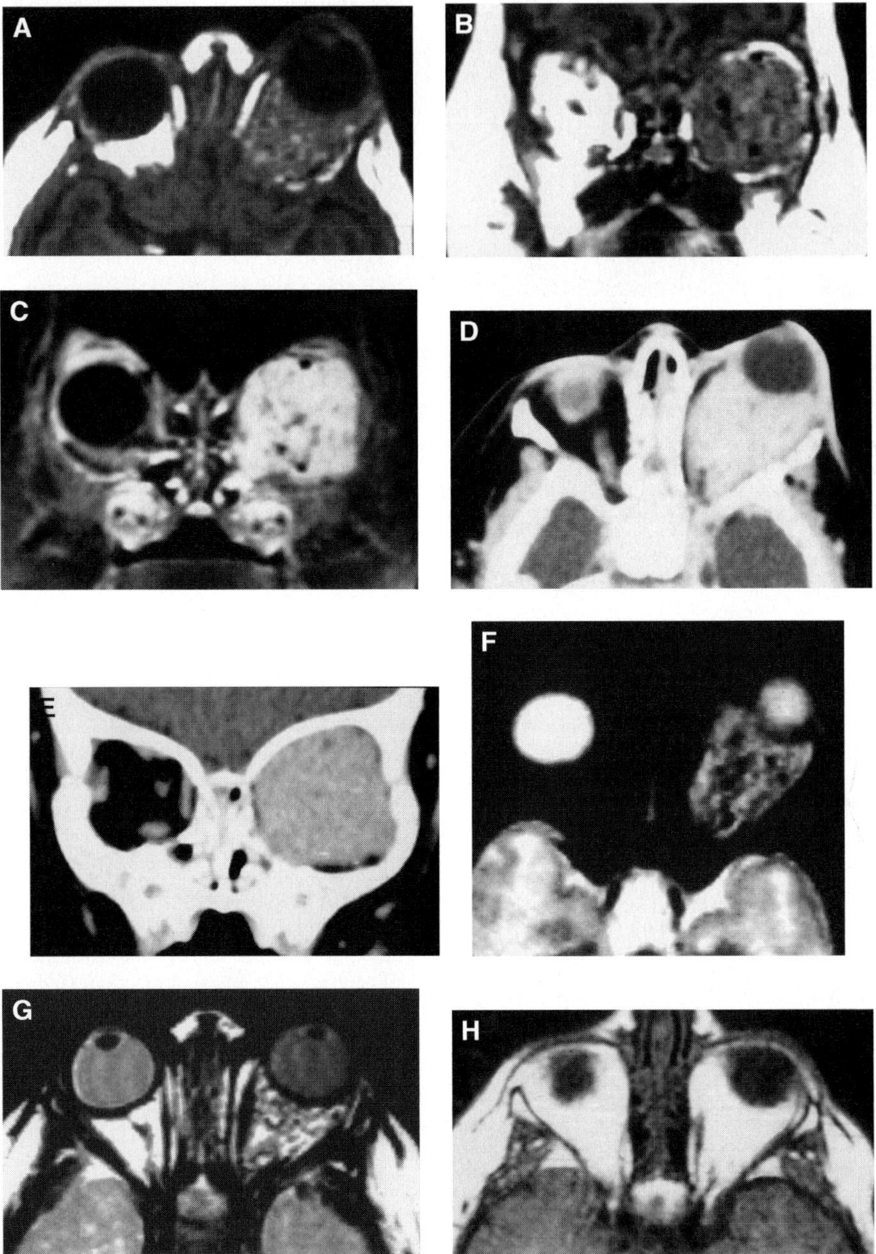


Fig. 4. Large retroconal hemangioma producing marked proptosis in a 2-month-old patient. (*A*) An axial T1W MR image shows a large retroglobar heterogeneous mass consisting of lobules and signal voids. (*B*) A coronal T1W MR image shows the mass with prominent signal voids expanding the left orbit. (*C*) A coronal contrast-enhanced T1W MR image with fat saturation shows prominent enhancement of the mass. Obtained at 4 months of age, axial (*D*) and coronal (*E*) contrast-enhanced CT images show an interval increase in the size of the mass. The mass shows prominent homogeneous enhancement. The bony orbit is markedly expanded. (*F*) A T2W MR image obtained at 4 months of age shows the large mass with prominent signal voids. (*G*) A follow-up T2W MR image with no fat saturation obtained at 10 months of age shows a significant decrease in the size of the mass and in the signal voids. There is fat interspersed between the tumor lobules. (*H*) A follow-up axial T1W MR image obtained at 28 months of age reveals complete involution of the left orbital mass. (*I*) A coronal T1W MR image obtained at 28 months of age no longer shows a mass, but asymmetric orbital contour with enlargement of the left orbit is noted.

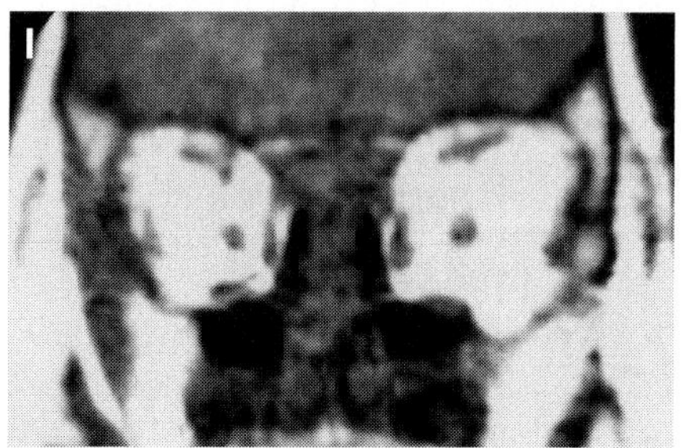

Fig. 4 (*continued*).

bismus that develops may resolve in parallel with tumor involution, but in some cases, muscle surgery may be necessary eventually. In all of the situations, whether before or during therapy, MR imaging is particularly invaluable because it can show the tumor involving and enlarging the eyelid and obstructing vision, displacing or distorting the globe or the extraocular muscles, and the affect of the tumor on the optic nerve (Figs. 1–5). By demonstrating all these changes, MR imaging can be used to plan patient management and to evaluate the effectiveness of therapy. In addition to the complications related to the mass effect of the hemangioma, there can be dermatologic complications if the lesion is superficial or has a superficial component.

## Venous lymphatic malformations

Of all of the vascular lesions of the orbit, the most controversy surrounds the origin and nature of the lesions that contain both lymphatic and venous components. Traditionally, these lesions have been referred to as lymphangiomas. First, the term *lymphangioma* does not reflect the histologic spectrum of the lesions, which may include, in addition to lymphatic channels, blood vessels with venous characteristics, smooth muscle fibers, lymphocytic tissue, and blood or blood products [8,23,24,38–42].

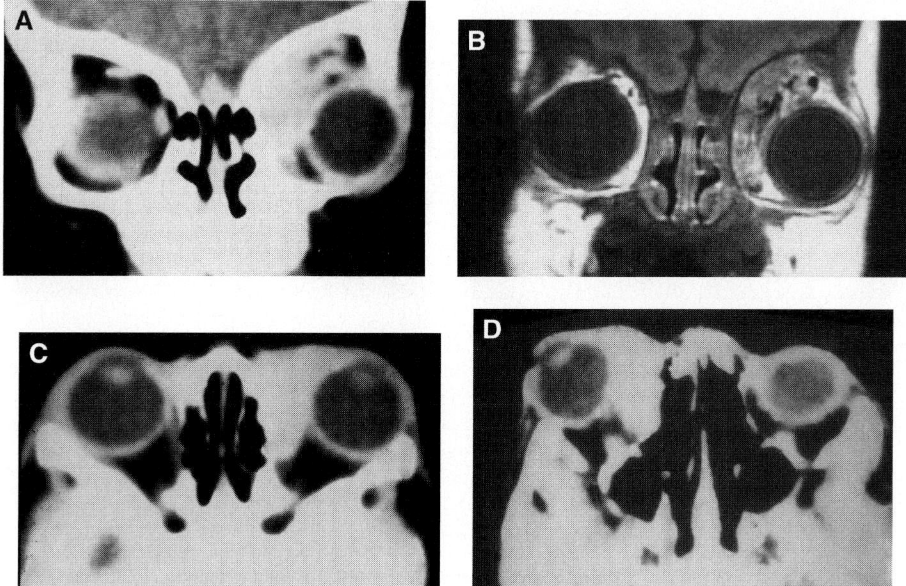

Fig. 5. Hemangioma and rhabdomyosarcoma may appear similar on CT scans. (*A*) Coronal contrast-enhanced CT scan shows an enhancing mass displacing the left globe. (*B*) Coronal T1W MR image performed on the same patient (*A*) reveals a characteristic pattern of a hemangioma. There are multiple lobulations and signal voids, and the left orbit is enlarged. (*C*) Axial contrast-enhanced CT scan obtained from the same patient (*A*, *B*) reveals a homogeneously enhancing mass in the medial aspect of the left orbit that displaces the globe. (*D*) Axial contrast-enhanced CT scan showing a rhabdomyosarcoma in the medial aspect of the right orbit, which appears similar to the image of hemangioma shown in (*C*). There is homogeneous enhancement of the rhabdomyosarcoma.

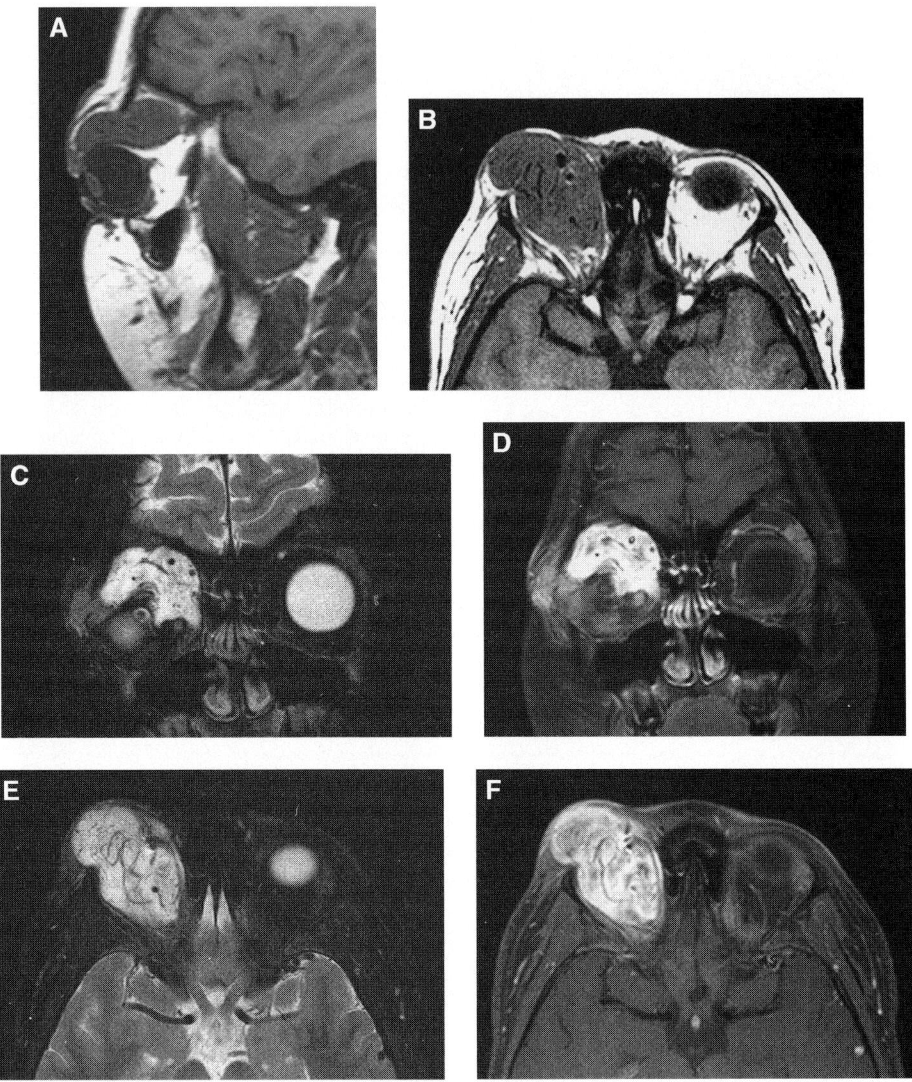


Fig. 6. Vascular embryonal cell rhabdomyosarcoma in a 12-year-old child that mimics a hemangioma. (*A*) Sagittal T1W MR image shows a bilobed mass with prominent signal voids within it, in the superior portion of the orbit. (*B*) Axial T1W MR image shows the large mass with prominent signal voids within it. (*C*) Coronal T2W MR image shows a peripherally lobulated mass with prominent signal voids. The mass is primarily extraconal but extends intraconally. (*D*) Coronal T1W fat-saturated contrast-enhanced MR image again demonstrates the lobulated margin and the vascularity and prominent enhancement of the rhabdomyosarcoma. (*E*) Axial T2W MR image again demonstrates a highly vascular mass with increased signal intensity. The mass lacks internal lobulations seen typically in a hemangioma. (*F*) There is prominent enhancement of the tumor shown on a postconstrast axial T1W fat-saturated MR image.

Second, because the term lymphangioma has the suffix *-oma* there is an incorrect connotation that the lesion is a neoplasm with proliferating cells. Some investigators classify lymphangiomas in the same group as other vascular neoplasms and not with vascular malformations [26]. Mulliken and Glowacki [19] and Mulliken [21] believe that a term with the suffix oma should be reserved for lesions that truly have replicating cells such as hemangiomas (hemangiomas but not cavernous hemangiomas, which are actually malformations) [42]. Therefore, the term "venous lymphatic malformation" has been suggested to replace the term *lymphangioma* because it is more reflective of the nature of the lesion. This term has been accepted by some, but many practitioners continue to use the traditional term *lymphangioma*. Still others consider lymphangiomas as orbital venous anomalies [24,43]. These investigators argue that there are no lymphatics in the deeper portions of the orbit to give rise to such lesions and that they have in their examinations of orbital lesions detected lymphatic channels and lymphatic malformations only in the superficial orbital tissues. They state that, in their experience, they have found lymphangiomas to have frequent connections to the orbital venous system, and they have phleboliths, both of which are characteristics that support a venous origin [24]. Thus, these investigators consider the lymphangiomas and orbital varices to represent a spectrum of the same orbital vascular lesion, the orbital venous anomaly. This grouping of the solely venous lesions with lesions that contain both lymphatic and venous components is not accepted by other investigators who consider the orbital varices to be distinct from the venous lymphatic malformations. Those investigators who disagree characterize these lesions hemodynamically, on the basis of clinical or investigative evidence of communication to the systemic venous system or lack of it, the characteristic of hemodynamic isolation [23,42].

Venous lymphatic malformations of the orbit are congenital vascular malformations that arise from the venous anlage [42]. It is believed that this anlage is pluripotential and can develop into venous and lymphatic structures. Rootman et al [23] classified these lesions on the basis of the location as superficial, deep, or combined. Venous lymphatic malformations are considered to be vascular hamartomas showing a spectrum of characteristics on clinical, radiologic, hemodynamic, and histologic evaluation that indicate both their lymphatic and venous nature. Rootman et al [23] consider these lesions distinct from varices. Although venous lymphatic malformations arise from a venous anlage, they demonstrate both lymphatic and venous differentiation and thus differ from varices. Also, their hemodynamic characteristics are different from those of varices; however, this is disputed by Wright et al [24].

Venous lymphatic malformations are unencapsulated multicompartmental lesions that tend to insinuate themselves between normal orbital structures, often having both intraconal and extraconal components. Therefore, they are difficult or impossible to resect completely. On histopathologic evaluation, the venous lymphatic malformations lack a capsule and consist of a network of endothelial-lined irregularly branching, delicate channels filled with pale-staining fluid. Between these channels there are septae and lymphocytic aggregates.

Most patients who have orbital venous lymphatic malformations present with proptosis, but many of these patients have had some evidence of an orbital lesion such as eyelid fullness from birth. The venous lymphatic malformations of the orbit generally present early in life, during infancy or childhood. In the series by Wright et al [24], 43% of patients were less than 6 years of age, and 60% were less than 16 years of age. The behavior of the venous lymphatic malformations varies, and this is reflected in their presentation. Some of these lesions may remain clinically silent for a long period of time and may only enlarge slowly, producing progressive proptosis, or globe displacement. These slowly developing lesions may be seen on imaging and at surgery to mimic clinically a low-flow malformation (cavernous hemangioma) [44]. Most of the venous lymphatic malformations present abruptly, caused by hemorrhage. They are also reported to enlarge when the lymphoid tissue within them increases in response to an upper respiratory infection. When there is a massive hemorrhage, there may be restriction of eye movement and a loss of vision. The larger and more deeply located the venous lymphatic orbital malformation is, the more significant and common will be the visual loss [42]. Similar to the findings of Wright et al [24], Katz et al [42] found that the more superficially located the venous lymphatic malformation is, the larger the lymphatic component is.

Management of the venous lymphatic lesions depends on the symptoms and signs that they produce, which, in turn, are related to the size, location, and morphology of the lesions and how rapidly change has occurred. Conservative management is recommended and is effective in many situations [45]; however, surgery is indicated when there is marked compression or stretching of the optic nerve, anisometropy in case of strabismus, or significant cosmetic deformity. Recently, a technique has been proposed for the sclerotherapy of orbital venous lymphatic malformations in which both navigational assistance for precise needle placement and intralesional contrast medium injection to assess venous drainage are used [46].

Magnetic resonance imaging is considered the imaging procedure of choice for evaluating venous lymphatic malformations because it is most accurate in delineating and demonstrating the various components of these malformations (Figs. 7–9). T1- and T2W MR images, inversion recovery pulse sequences, and the use of gadolinium-based contrast

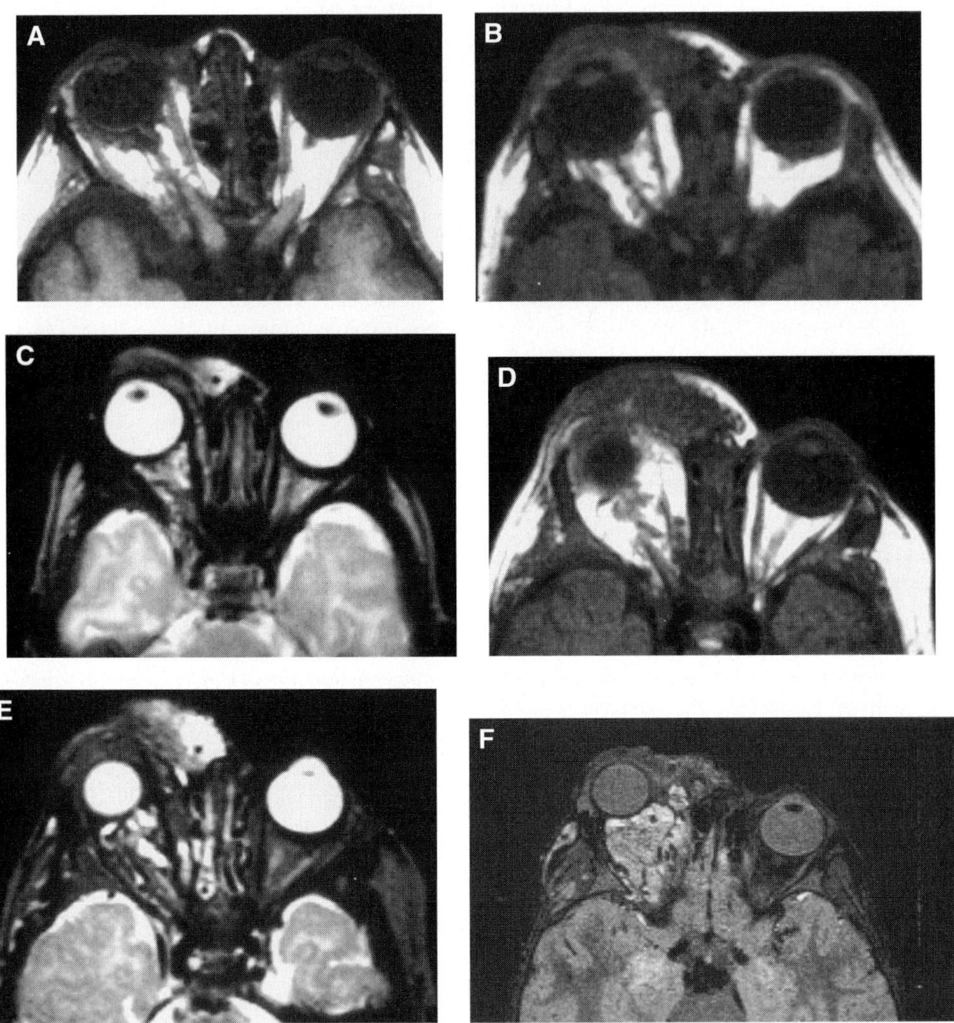


Fig. 7. Venous lymphatic malformation of the orbit was monitored with MR imaging since the patient's birth. The patient also has two additional venous lymphatic malformations. (*A*) Axial T1W MR image performed shortly after the patient's birth shows fullness in the medial canthal region of the right orbit and serpigenous structures in the retroglobar region. (*B*) Axial T1W MR image obtained from the patient at 2 months of age reveals thickening of the tissue anterior to the right globe and some irregularity in the tissue planes in the retroglobar region. (*C*) T2W MR image obtained at the same time as (*B*) reveals both the superficial and the deeper components of the malformation, including the extent of invasion through the superior orbital fissure into the right cavernous sinus. (*D*) Obtained 9 months later, a T1W MR image shows that the venous lymphatic malformation has increased in size. This image was obtained when the patient had an upper respiratory infection. (*E*) Axial T2W MR image performed at the same time as the image shown in (*D*) shows a better view of both the superficial and deep components of the lesion. (*F*, *G*) Axial proton density images performed when the patient was 6 years of age and presented again with proptosis. There is a large heterogeneous mass both in the retroglobar region and in the medial superficial portion of the orbit, with both intraconic and extraconic components. The right optic nerve sheath complex is stretched. (*H*) Coronal T2W MR image performed slightly posterior to the globe shows again the extensive mass in the retroglobar region and a lymphatic malformation in the right temporalis region and in the inferior right cheek.

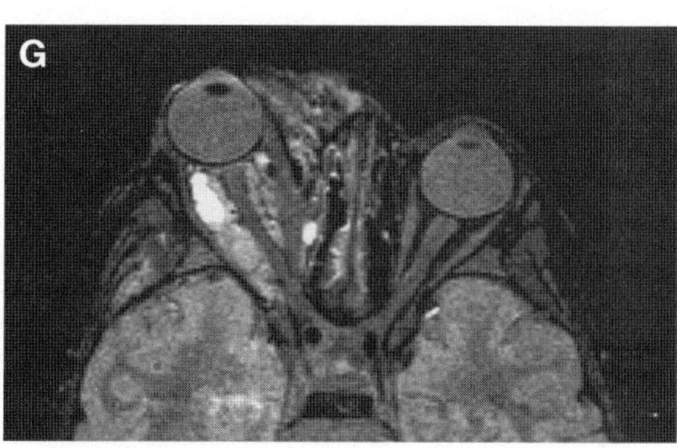

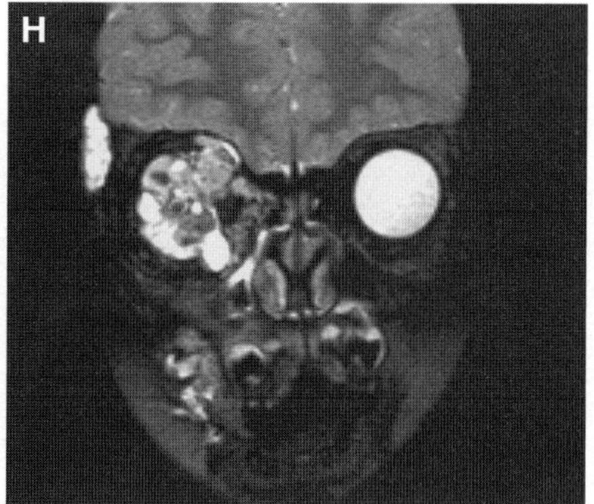

Fig. 7 (*continued*).

medium are all helpful in localizing and characterizing the lesions. The intensity of the lesion depends on the type of fluid within the cystic components of the lesion, whether the lesion is nonhemorrhagic or hemorrhagic, and on the age of the hemorrhage. T1W MR images without fat saturation will demonstrate components containing lymphatic or proteinaceous fluid, whereas those containing blood or blood products are best shown on fat-saturated T1W MR images (Fig. 9). On T2W MR images, fat saturation improves the visibility of channels and cysts that contain nonhemorrhagic fluid (Figs. 7C, 7E, 7H, 8B, and 9E); however, structures containing intracellular methemoglobin may show a hypointensity similar to that of saturated fat. The use of contrast material with fat saturation may help in identifying and locating venous components and in indicating where the solid vascular tissue is located. In many instances, the use of contrast material provides no additional information about the lesion [47], although a nonenhancing lesion confirms the lymphangetic component of the lesion [48]. CT imaging can be useful in identifying the lesion, but it does not provide good soft tissue discrimination and, therefore, is not as accurate as MR imaging in delineating the lesion. Also, CT imaging is a less desirable technique because it involves radiation; however, CT scans are fast and may be easier to use when the orbit is imaged during the Valsalva maneuver, in search of a distensible component, or in the evaluation of a patient who has a vascular lesion such as a varix (Fig. 10). Positioning the patient for a coronal CT scan can increase the patient's venous pressure enough to distend the varix and make it evident on

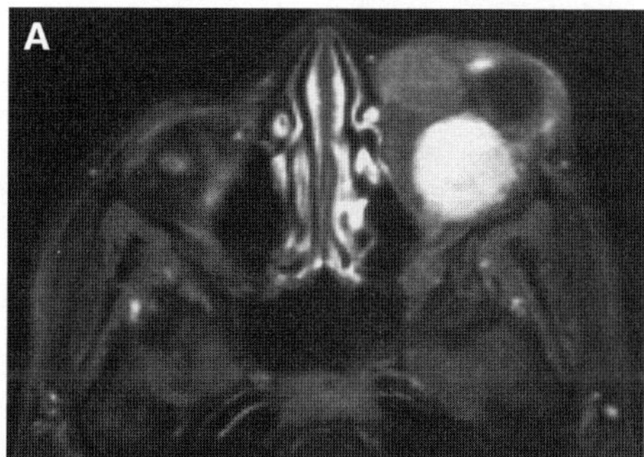

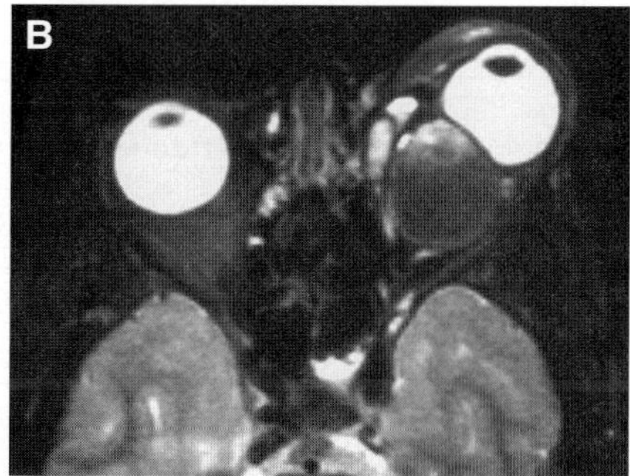

Fig. 8. Large venous lymphatic malformation that presented with marked left proptosis. (*A*) Axial T1W fat-saturated MR image reveals a multicystic mass having cysts of various intensities that displaces the left globe anterolaterally. (*B*) Axial T2W MR image shows that the large retroglobar cystic component has decreased in intensity, consistent with intracellular methemoglobin, producing deformity of the left optic globe. Medially located in the orbit are smaller cystic components with fluid-fluid levels.

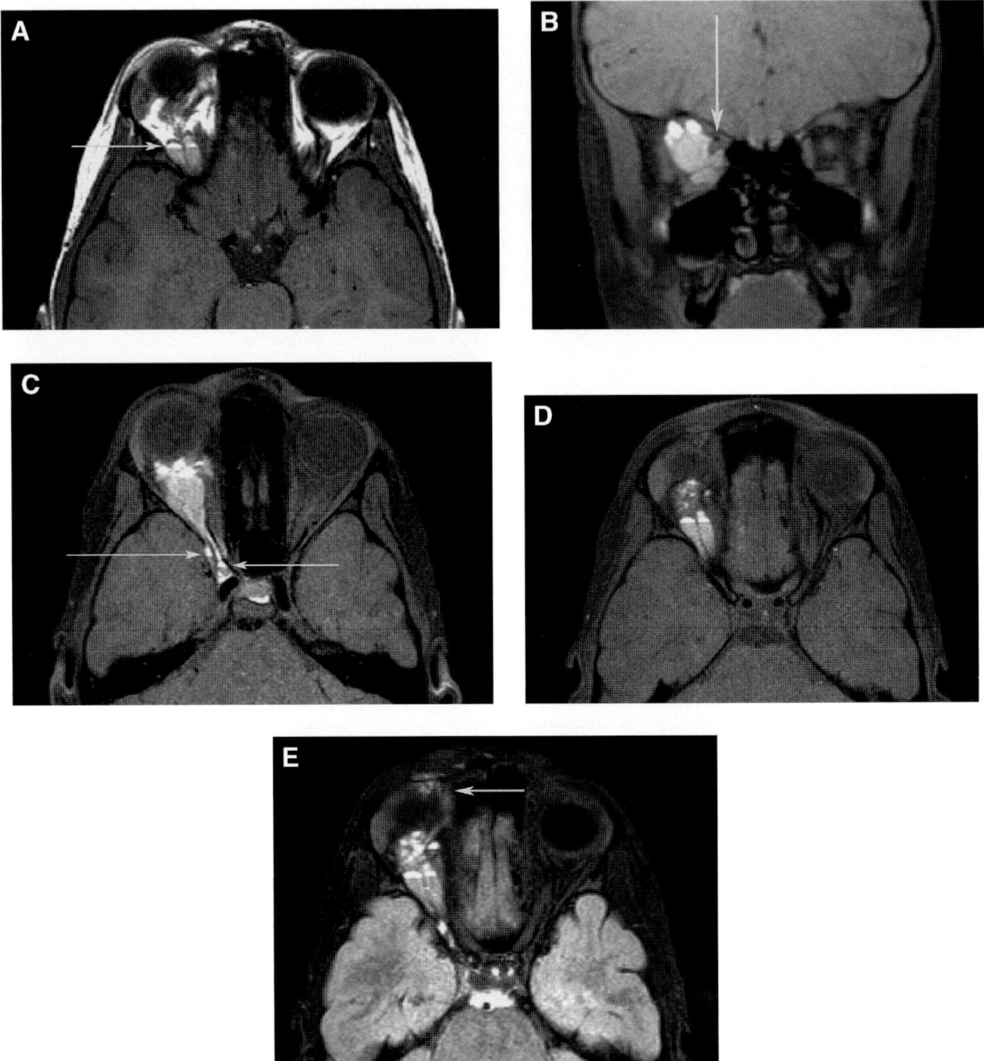


Fig. 9. Venous lymphatic malformation presenting with proptosis. CT and MR performed at an outside institution was misinterpreted as an infiltrative neoplasm. (*A*) Axial nonenhanced T1W MR image reveals proptosis on the right, irregularity of retroglobar tissues, and two small fluid-fluid levels (*arrow*) within elongated cystic structures that are slightly increased in intensity. (*B*) Coronal nonenhanced fat-saturated T1W MR image reveals a multicompartmented cystic lesion in the right orbit. The optic nerve (*arrow*) is displaced superomedially. The fluid within the cystic components of the lesion is of increased intensity, consistent with blood or blood products. (*C*) Axial nonenhanced fat-saturated T1W MR image shows the lesion to be of increased intensity. The posterior extent of the lesion through the superior orbital fissure is demonstrated. Two small fluid-fluid levels (*arrows*) are identified within the intracranial portion of the venous lymphatic malformation. (*D*) Axial nonenhanced fat-saturated T1W MR image obtained through the upper portion of the orbit reveals two elongated cystic structures with fluid-fluid levels. Additionally, more anteriorly there is a heterogeneous component of the venous lymphatic malformation. Note that the lesion was not shown as well on a non–fat-saturated T1W MR image (*A*). (*E*) An inversion recovery fat-saturated MR image demonstrates the multicystic nature of the retroglobar mass and its intracranial extent. It also shows slightly irregular channels of the malformation in the anteromedial portion of the right orbit (*arrow*). Note the multiple fluid-fluid levels in the retroglobar cysts.

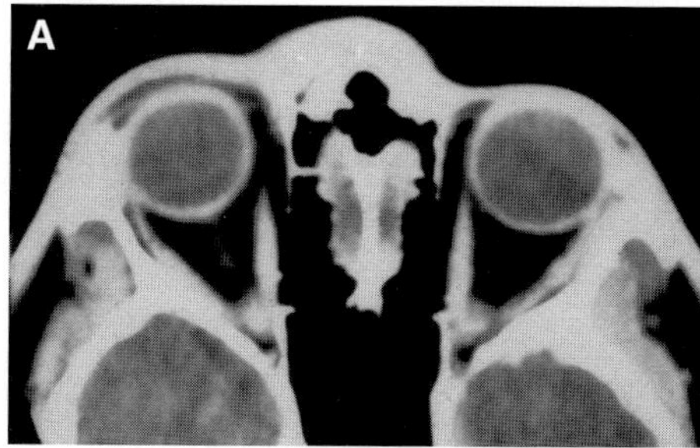


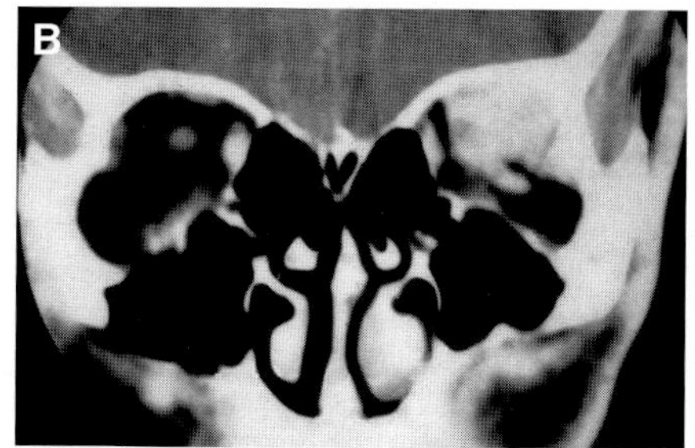


Fig. 10. A left orbital varix that caused marked proptosis whenever the patient's head was in a dependent position. (*A*) Axial CT scan reveals slight anopthalmos on the left. (*B*) With the patient positioned for coronal imaging, the left superolateral extraconic varix becomes evident.

images (Fig. 10). True orbital varices are not common in the pediatric age group.

The information that MR imaging provides about the venous lymphatic malformations is invaluable for surgical planning. Also, in cases of extensive orbital venous lymphatic malformations, the brain can be evaluated better for noncontiguous intracranial vascular anomalies. Recent reports [42] have described associated brain vascular anomalies when there is an orbital venous lymphatic malformation.

## References


[1] Mafee MM, Putterman A, Valvassori G, et al. Orbital space-occupying lesions: role of computed tomography and magnetic resonance imaging. An analysis of 145 cases. Radiol Clin North Am 1987;25:529–59.

[2] Armington WG, Bilaniuk LT. The radiologic evaluation of the orbit: conal and intraconal lesions. Semin Ultrasound CT MR 1988;9:455–73.

[3] Bilaniuk LT, Zimmerman RA, Newton RH. Magnetic resonance imaging: orbital pathology. In: Newton TH, Bilaniuk LT, editors. Radiology of the eye and orbit. New York: Raven Press; 1990. p. 5.1–5.84.

[4] Bilaniuk LT. Imaging of the pediatric orbit. In: Katowitz JA, editor. Pediatric oculoplastic surgery. New York: Springer-Verlag; 2002. p. 365–406.

[5] Bilaniuk LT. Orbital vascular lesions. Role of imaging. Radiol Clin North Am 1999;37:169–83.

[6] Bond JB, Haik BG, Taveras JL, et al. Magnetic resonance imaging of orbital lymphangioma with and without gadolinium contrast enhancement. Ophthalmology 1992;99:1318–24.

[7] Kazim M, Kennerdell JS, Rothfus W, et al. Orbital lymphangioma: correlation of magnetic resonance images and intraoperative findings. Ophthalmology 1992;99:1588–94.

[8] Rootman J. Vascular malformations of the orbit: hemodynamic concepts. Orbit 2003;22:103–20.

[9] Gallione CJ, Pasyk KA, Boon LM, et al. A gene for familial venous malformations maps to chromosome 9p in a second large kindred. J Med Genet 1995;32:197–9.

[10] Vikkula M, Boon LM, Mulliken JB. Molecular genetics of vascular malformations. Matrix Biol 2001;20:327–35.

[11] Razon MJ, Kraling BM, Mulliken JB, et al. The increased apoptosis coincides with onset of involution in infantile hemangioma. Microcirculation 1998;5:189–95.

[12] Boye E, Yu Y, Paranya G, et al. Clonality and altered behavior of endothelial cells from hemangiomas. J Clin Invest 2001;107:745–52.

[13] Iliff WJ, Green WR. Orbital tumors in children. In: Jakobiec FA, editor. Ocular and adnexal tumors. Birmingham (AL): Aesculapius Publishing Company; 1978. p. 669–84.

[14] Crawford JS. Diseases of the orbit. In: Crawford JS, Morin JD, editors. The eye in childhood. New York: Grune & Straton; 1983. p. 361–94.

[15] Shields JA, Bakewell B, Augsburger JJ, et al. Space occupying orbital masses in children: a review of 250 consecutive biopsies. Ophthalmology 1986;93:379–84.

[16] Rootman J. Frequency and differential diagnosis of orbital disease. In: Diseases of the orbit. Philadelphia: J.B. Lippincott Co; 1988. p. 119–39.

[17] Kodst SR, Shetlar DJ, Campbell RJ, et al. A review of 340 orbital tumors in children during a 60-year period. Am J Ophthalmol 1994;117:177–82.

[18] Kazim M, Fries PD, Katowitz JA. Classification and evaluation of orbital disorders in children. In: Katowitz JA, editor. Pediatric oculoplastic surgery. New York: Springer-Verlag; 2002. p. 359–64.

[19] Mulliken JB, Glowacki J. Hemangiomas and vascular malformations in infants and children: a classification based on endothelial characteristics. Plast Reconstr Surg 1982;69:412–20.

[20] Finn MC, Glowacki J, Mulliken JB. Congenital vascular lesions: clinical application of a new classification. J Pediatr Surg 1983;18:894–900.

[21] Mullike JB. Diagnosis and natural history of hemangiomas. In: Mullike JB, Young AE, editors. Vascular

birthmarks: hemangiomas and malformations. Philadelphia: WB Saunders; 1988. p. 24–62.

[22] Young AE. Pathogenesis of vascular malformations. In: Mulliken JB, Young AE, editors. Vascular birthmarks: hemangiomas and malformations. Philadelphia: WB Saunders; 1988. p. 107–13.

[23] Rootman J, Hay E, Graeb D, et al. Orbital-adnexal lymphangiomas: a spectrum of hemodynamically vascular hamartomas. Ophthalmology 1986;93:1558–70.

[24] Wright JE, Sullivan TJ, Garner A, et al. Orbital venous anomalies. Ophthalmology 1997;104:905–13.

[25] Harris GJ. Orbital vascular malformations: a consensus statement on terminology and its clinical implications. Orbital Society. Am J Ophthalmol 1999; 127:453–5.

[26] Gunalp I, Gunduz K. Vascular tumors of the orbit. Documenta Ophthalmologica 1995;89:337–45.

[27] Haik BG, Jacobiec FA, Ellsworth RM, et al. Capillary hemangioma of the lids and orbit: an analysis of the clinical features and therapeutic results in 101 cases. Ophthalmology 1979;86:760–89.

[28] Haik BG, Karcioglu ZA, Gordon RA, et al. Capillary hemangioma (infantile periocular hemangioma). Surv Ophthalmol 1994;38:399–426.

[29] Boon LM, Enjolras O, Mulliken B. Congenital hemangioma: evidence of accelerated involution. J Pediatr 1996;128:329–35.

[30] Glowacki J, Mulliken JB. Mast cells in hemangioma and vascular malformations. Pediatrics 1982;70:48–51.

[31] Robb RM. Refractive errors associated with hemangiomas of the eyelids and orbit in infancy. Am J Ophthalmol 1977;83:52–8.

[32] Stigmar G, Crawford JS, Ward CM, et al. Ophthalmic sequelae of infantile hemangiomas of the eyelids and orbit. Am J Ophthalmol 1978;85:806–13.

[33] White WL, Mumma JV, Tomasovic JJ. Congenital oculomotor nerve palsy, cerebellar hypoplasia and facial capillary hemangioma. Am J Ophthalmol 1992; 113:497–500.

[34] Ezekowitz RAB, Mulliken JB, Folkman J. Interferon alpha-2a therapy for life-threatening hemangiomas of infancy. N Engl J Med 1992;326:1456–63.

[35] Kushner BJ. Intralesional corticosteroid injection for infantile adnexal hemangioma. Am J Ophthalmol 1982;93:496–506.

[36] Willshaw HE, Deady JP. Vascular hamartomas in childhood. J Pediatr Surg 1987;22:281–3.

[37] O'Keefe M, Lanigan B, Byrne SA. Capillary hemangioma of eyelids and orbit: a clinical review of the safety and efficacy of intralesional steroids. Acta Ophthalmol Scand 2003;81:294–8.

[38] Jones IS. Lymphangiomas of the ocular adnexa: an analysis of sixty-two cases. Am J Ophthalmol 1961; 51:481–509.

[39] Iliff WJ, Green WR. Orbital lymphangiomas. Ophthalmology 1979;86:914–29.

[40] Graeb DA, Rootman J, Robertson WD, et al. Orbital lymphangiomas: clinical, radiologic, and pathologic characteristics. Radiology 1990;175:417–21.

[41] Harris GJ, Sakol PJ, Bonavolonta G, et al. An analysis of thirty cases of orbital lymphangioma: pathophysiologic considerations and management recommendations. Ophthalmology 1990;97:1583–92.

[42] Katz SE, Rootman J, Vangveeravong S, et al. Combined venous lymphatic malformations of the orbit (so-called lymphangiomas): association with noncontiguous intracranial vascular anomalies. Ophthalmology 1998;105:176–84.

[43] Lloyd GAS, Wright JE, Morgan G. Venous malformations in the orbit. Br J Ophthalmol 1971;55:505–16.

[44] Selva D, Fraco DS, Bonavoconta G, et al. Orbital venous-lymphatic malformations (lymphangiomas) mimicking cavernous hemangiomas. Am J Ophthalmol 2001;131:364–70.

[45] Wilson ME, Parker PL, Chavis RM. Conservative management of childhood orbital lymphangioma. Ophthalmology 1989;96:484–9.

[46] Ermann U, Westendorff C, Troitzsch D, et al. Navigation-assisted sclerotherapy of orbital venolymphatic malformation: a new guidance technique for percutaneous treatment of low-flow vascular malformations. AJNR Am J Neuroradiol 2004;25: 1792–5.

[47] Bond JB, Haik BG, Taveras JL, et al. Magnetic resonance imaging of orbital lymphangioma with and without gadolinium contrast enhancement. Opthalmology 1992;99:1318–24.

[48] Mafee MF. Orbit. In: Mafee MF, Valvassori GE, Becker M, editors. Imaging of the head and neck. Stuttgart: Thieme; 2004. p. 196–294.

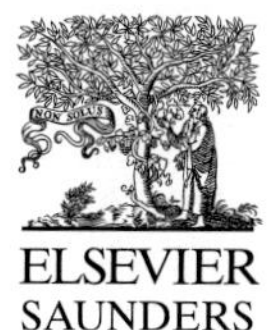
ELSEVIER
SAUNDERS

Neuroimag Clin N Am 15 (2005) 121 – 136

NEUROIMAGING
CLINICS OF
NORTH AMERICA

# Orbital Rhabdomyosarcoma and Simulating Lesions

Mark F. Conneely, MD*, Mahmood F. Mafee, MD

*Department of Radiology, University of Illinois at Chicago Medical Center, MC 931, 1740 West Taylor Street, Chicago, IL 60612, USA*

Rhabdomyosarcoma is the most common mesenchymal tumor of childhood. Common primary sites include the head and neck (45%); trunk (40%); and extremities (15%) [1]. Orbital rhabdomyosarcoma accounts for 25% to 35% of head and neck rhabdomyosarcomas. Parameningeal sites, such as the nasopharynx, paranasal sinuses, and middle ear, account for 50%, and the rest occur in other locations, such as the scalp, face, buccal mucosa, oropharynx, larynx, and elsewhere in the neck [2].

Rhabdomyosarcoma occurs most commonly in patients between the ages of 2 and 5, [3,4]; however, cases have been reported in all age groups, from birth [5] to adulthood. The age distribution is bimodal, reflecting the age prevalence of the different subtypes. The embryonal subtype (Fig. 1) presents in childhood, whereas the pleomorphic type occurs in adults [6]. Other subtypes include the alveolar subtype, which occurs in older children and young adults, and is associated with a poor prognosis [7]. The botryoid variant of the embryonal subtype has been associated with specific findings on imaging, as is discussed later.

* Corresponding author.
*E-mail address:* mconne3@uic.edu (M.F. Conneely).

## Orbital rhabdomyosarcoma

This discussion is meant to focus on primary orbital rhabdomyosarcoma (Fig. 2) and its simulating lesions. It is, however, probably relevant briefly to address the other forms of rhabdomyosarcoma that can occur in and around the orbit. Primary ocular rhabdomyosarcoma is a rare tumor that can arise from the conjunctiva, iris, or ciliary body. Rhabdomyosarcoma arising in the eyelid has also been reported [8], although it has been suggested that some of the reported cases may actually represent subcutaneous extension of primary orbital rhabdomyosarcoma [2]. Secondary orbital rhabdomyosarcoma (Figs. 3 and 4) is a term that applies when there is direct extension to the orbits from the adjacent paranasal sinuses, pterygopalatine fossa, infratemporal fossa, or nasopharynx. Finally, rhabdomyosarcoma can metastasize to the orbits from primary tumors in the head and neck, trunk, and extremities. Although metastatic rhabdomyosarcoma to the orbits carries an extremely poor prognosis, patients can nevertheless benefit from prompt diagnosis and palliative radiotherapy [3].

Primary orbital rhabdomyosarcoma (see Fig. 2) usually occurs in young children, with a mean age of 8 years. Patients can present, however, at any age. In a recent study reviewing 1264 consecutive patients with orbital tumors and simulating lesions, the 35 biopsy-proved cases of rhabdomyosarcoma ranged from 0 to 68 years of age [9]. The prevalence is slightly higher in males, with a male to female ratio of 5:3. Embryonal rhabdomyosarcoma is the most

1052-5149/05/$ – see front matter 
doi:10.1016/j.nic.2005.02.006

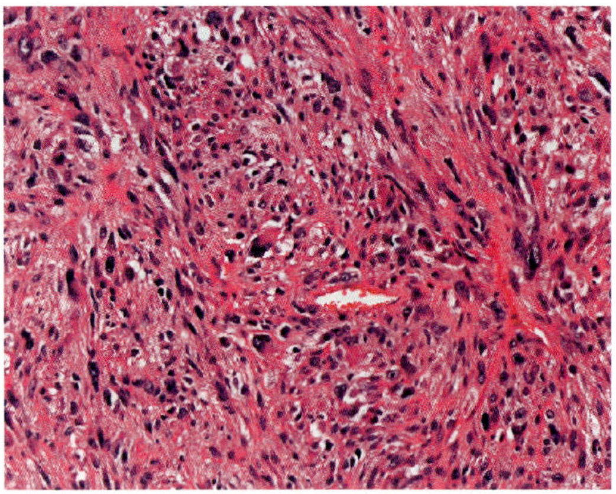

Fig. 1. Rhabdomyosarcoma: embryonal pattern. Note the fascicles of pleomorphic, spindle-shaped cells with hyperchromatic nuclei. Also of note are the eosinophilic myoblasts (hematoxylin–eosin, original magnification ×20).

common histologic subtype occurring in the orbit. It originates not from preformed striated extraocular muscles, but instead from rests of primitive undifferentiated mesenchymal cells. Primary orbital rhabdomyosarcoma can arise from any location within the orbit: extraconal (37%); intraconal (17%); or both (47%). There is a predilection for the upper inner quadrant, which is involved in 67% of cases [10].

The advent of cross-sectional imaging, improved access to medical care, and advances in chemotherapy and radiotherapy has improved the average survival of patients with rhabdomyosarcoma from 30% in the early 1970s [11] to greater than 90% in recent years. The appropriate diagnosis and treatment of orbital rhabdomyosarcoma requires close cooperation and communication between a numbers of specialists: the radiologist, the ophthalmologist, and the medical and radiation oncologists.

Clinically, patients present with rapidly developing unilateral proptosis (80%–100%); globe displacement (80%); ptosis (30%–50%) (often the first sign in a superior orbital tumor); conjunctival and eyelid swelling (60%); palpable mass (25%); and pain (10%) [12,13]. Proptosis develops most rapidly in infants. In older children and adults, it tends to have a slower course [2].

On imaging, the tumors typically have moderately well-defined to ill-defined margins and an irregular shape, with mild to moderate contrast enhancement. They exhibit soft tissue attenuation values on CT. Calcification is infrequent but can occur [10]. On MR imaging, the tumors are generally isointense to muscle on T1- and hyperintense to muscle on T2-weighted images. Adjacent bone destruction is common, occurring in up to 40% of cases. The globe is often displaced and distorted by the tumor but rarely is invaded [10]. Invasion of paranasal sinuses and intracranial extension can also occur [2,7]. Because of the absence of lymphatics about the orbit, regional lymph nodes do not become involved until advanced local tumor spread has occurred.

CT and MR imaging can be complimentary in evaluation and staging of orbital rhabdomyosarcoma. MR imaging, with its superior soft tissue contrast, multiplanar capability, and lack of ionizing radiation, is well suited for tumor staging. The authors' imaging recommendations for patients' orbital rhabdomyosarcoma have been previously published [14]. Conversely, CT offers superior resolution and better demonstrates the extent of bone involvement. In infants and young children, dynamic postcontrast CT may obviate the need for biopsy by confirming the diagnosis of capillary hemangioma, as is discussed later.

Rarely, orbital rhabdomyosarcoma can present a confusing picture on imaging. It has been reported to simulate subperiosteal abscess, with peripheral enhancement and concomitant sinus disease [15]. It can appear as multiple grouped ring-enhancing lesions resembling bunches of grapes, a finding that has been associated with the botryoid variant of the embryonic histologic subtype, and has been deemed the "botryoid sign" [16]. Rhabdomyosarcoma can be masked by orbital trauma, resulting in delay of diagnosis and appropriate management [17].

When orbital rhabdomyosarcoma is suspected on the basis of imaging, tissue sampling is necessary to confirm the diagnosis. Open biopsy is preferred for most lesions, to ensure an adequate sample. Deeply seated tumors that are technically difficult to reach surgically may be approached and aspirated under CT guidance with minimal risk and morbidity [14]. Biopsy may be excisional or incisional, depending on the extent of the tumor and its proximity to vital orbital structures. Postsurgical management consists of radiation and chemotherapy.

Cross-sectional imaging plays an important role in staging and monitoring of patients following surgery. In addition to detecting residual tumor following excision, serial MR imaging examinations are useful to evaluate for recurrent disease in the months and years following excision. Serial examinations are necessary because it is often difficult to distinguish between enlarging recurrent tumor and scarring and fibrosis in the surgical bed. CT is useful in docu-

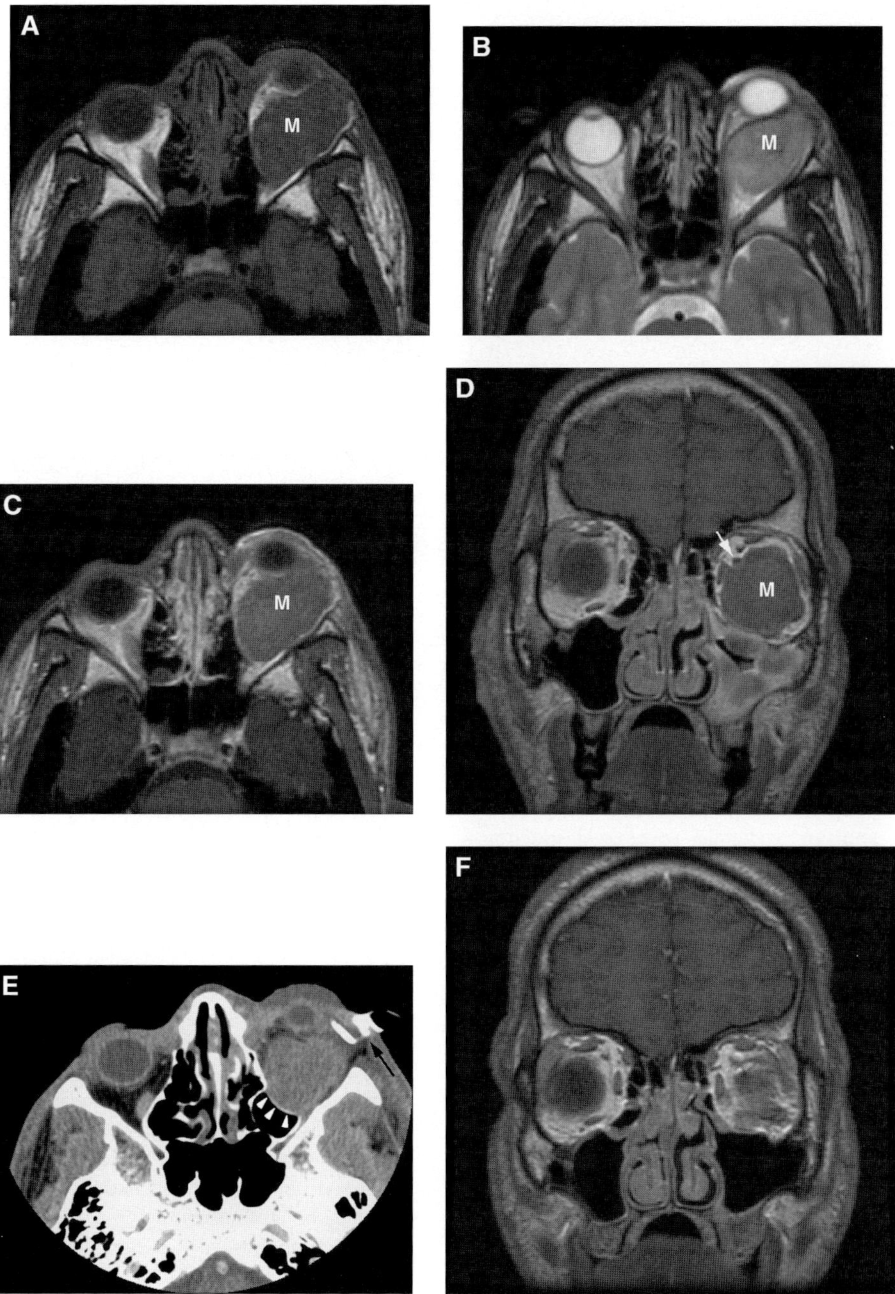


Fig. 2. Primary orbital rhabdomyosarcoma in an 18-year-old man. (*A*) T1-weighted image (500/14, repetition time/echo time [TR/TE]) shows an intraconal mass (M) isointense to muscle. (*B*) Axial T2-weighted image (4000/88, TR/TE). The mass (M) has heterogeneously hyperintense internal signal. Axial (*C*) and coronal (*D*) T1 following gadolinium infusion show heterogeneous enhancement. The optic nerve (*arrow* in *D*) is displaced superiorly and medially. (*E*) Axial CT section through the orbit reveals soft tissue attenuation mass (M) with associated bony remodeling of the inferior orbital wall (*arrowheads*). A surgical drain, form recent incisional biopsy, is in place (*arrow*). (*F*) Coronal T1 postinfusion section from follow-up MR image 2 months later, after incisional biopsy and radiation therapy. Unfortunately, this patient's tumor had recurred when he was imaged 1 year later.

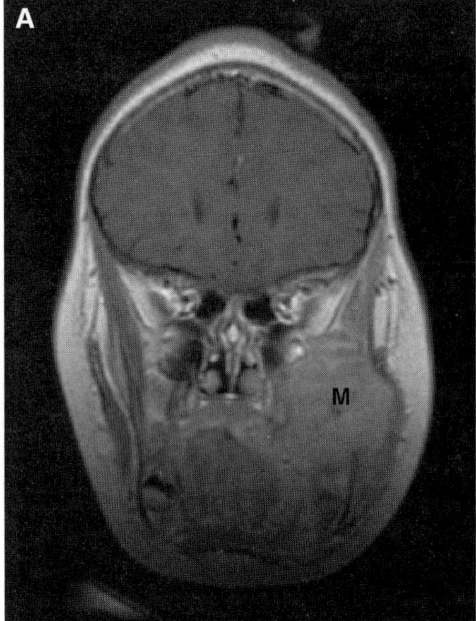


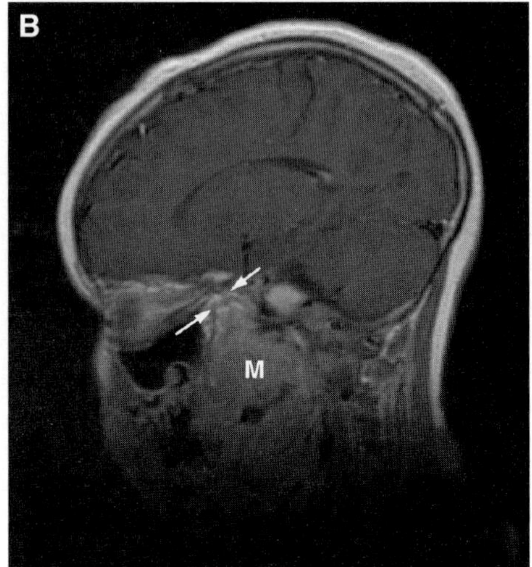


Fig. 3. Rhabdomyosarcoma arising in the infratemporal fossa in a 5-year-old girl. (*A*) Coronal T1-weighted image performed following infusion reveals a multilobulated heterogeneously enhancing mass (M) arising in the left infratemporal fossa. (*B*) Postcontrast sagittal T1-weighted image, revealing extension of the mass superiorly into the inferior orbital fissure (*arrows*).

menting healing or worsening of bony destruction, which can also help to establish the effectiveness of therapy [14].

The most widely accepted staging system for rhabdomyosarcoma was first set forth by the Intergroup Rhabdomyosarcoma Study (IRSG) in 1972 [18]. It applies to rhabdomyosarcoma arising from any location throughout the body, and was intended to create a uniform standard by which the effectiveness of different treatment regimens could be measured. Since then, a number of studies have been published using the IRSG standards, including several focusing on orbital rhabdomyosarcoma [2,19,20].

The IRSG divides patients into four major groups. Group I includes patients who had localized disease that was completely resected, without microscopic or gross evidence of residual or recurrent tumor. Group II consists of patients with microscopic disease remaining after biopsy, without residual tumor visualized during surgery or on imaging. Group III includes those patients whose tumors could not be completely resected during biopsy, or in whom residual tumor was demonstrated on imaging following biopsy. Group IV is reserved for patients in whom distant metastases were present at the onset. More detailed information regarding the IRSG guidelines is provided in Box 1.

## Simulating lesions

### *Subperiosteal hematoma*

Rhabdomyosarcoma can be masked in the setting of acute trauma [16]. This is particularly true on CT, where the tumors may be mistaken for subperiosteal hemorrhage and underlying bone destruction may be attributed to trauma. The same is true in reverse: subperiosteal hematomas can be associated with rapid-onset proptosis and can be mistaken for tumors on CT, leading to unnecessary biopsy. Clinical information, such as a history of trauma, coagulopathy, or anticoagulation, can be crucial to making the correct diagnosis on CT. In the weeks and months following the initial injury, subperiosteal hematomas can be associated with erosive changes and periosteal reaction, and can easily be mistaken for an aggressive process, especially in the absence of a good clinical history [21]. On MR imaging, subperiosteal he-

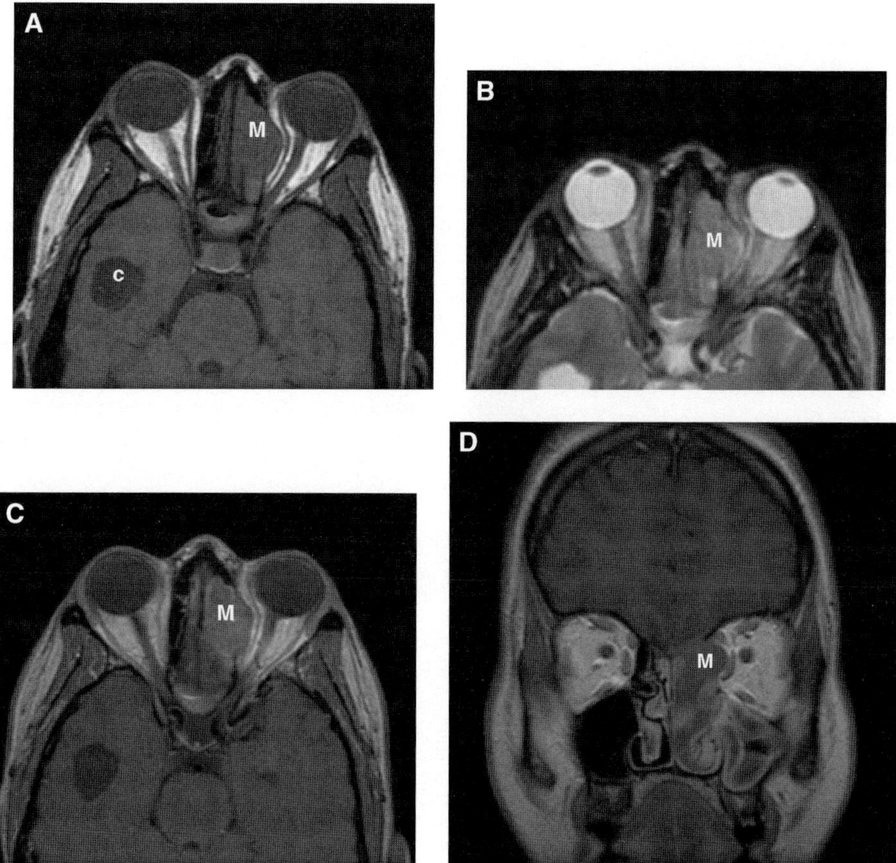


Fig. 4. A 31-year-old woman with rhabdomyosarcoma arising from the left ethmoid sinuses, with secondary involvement of the left orbit. (*A*) Axial T1-weighted image (600/17, TR/TE) shows a mass (M) in the left ethmoid complex with extension into the medial left orbit. The mass is hyperintense on T2-weighted images (3700/96, TR/TE). A cerebrospinal fluid–containing cystic structure (c) in the right temporal lobe, an unrelated finding, remained stable on serial examinations. (*B*) Axial T1-weighted fat-saturated (400/15, TR/TE) image (*C*) and coronal T1-weighted (400/16, TR/TE) image (*D*) following contrast infusion show heterogeneous enhancement.

matomas are usually easily recognized by the presence of T1 hyperintense methemoglobin and T1 and T2 hypointense hemosiderin (Fig. 5). MR imaging is indicated in equivocal cases, before biopsy.

### *Orbital cellulitis and abscess*

Orbital cellulitis most commonly occurs as a result of local spread from frontal or ethmoid sinusitis. Clinical findings include the rapid onset of proptosis, fever, and leukocytosis. Subperiosteal abscess of the orbital bone, most often involving the medial wall, is a common associated finding. Although orbital cellulitis is typically associated with inflammation of the orbital fatty reticulum and sinusitis, occasionally a discrete abscess occurs in the absence of sinusitis or systemic toxicity, simulating rhabdomyosarcoma on nonenhanced CT and MR imaging [22]. Although orbital cellulitis is far more common than rhabdomyosarcoma, this tumor-like presentation is relatively rare; in a recent series of 1264 orbital tumors and simulating lesions, tumor-like infectious processes only accounted for 1% of lesions [9].

Conversely, orbital rhabdomyosarcoma has been reported to simulate subperiosteal abscess on im-

**Box 1. Intergroup Rhabdomyosarcoma Study classification system**

**Group I:** Completely localized disease, implying both gross impression resection and microscopic confirmation of complete resection and absence of regional lymph node involvement
**Group Ia:** Confined to muscle or organ of origin
**Group Ib:** Contiguous involvement outside the muscle or organ of origin
**Group II:** Contiguous involvement ouside the mucle or organ of origin
**Group IIa:** Grossly resected localized tumor with microscopic residual disease and no evidence of gross residual tumor or regional lymph node involvement
**Group IIb:** Completely resected regional disease with no microscopic residual tumor
**Group IIc:** Grossly resected regional disease with microscopic residual tumor
**Group III:** Incomplete resection with biopsy proven or gross residual disease
**Group IV:** Distant metastatic disease present at onset

*Data from* Refs. [18,23–25].

aging, presenting as a ring-enhancing lesion in a patient with acute sinusitis. Because of the overlap in imaging characteristics, it is occasionally necessary to obtain a biopsy in patients with orbital cellulitis [14].

### *Vasculogenic tumors*

The two most common vasculogenic tumors of the orbit that present in childhood are capillary hemangiomas and vascular malformations. Vascular malformations can be venular; venous (previously known as *cavernous hemangiomas*); or venolymphatic (previously termed *lymphangiomas* or *lymphangiohemangiomas*). The rationale behind this change in terminology is intended to reflect the distinction between capillary hemangiomas, in which there is abnormal proliferation of endothelial cells, and vascular malformations, which enlarge only because of dilatation of existing vascular structures. The most common vasculogenic tumors to simulate orbital rhabdomyosarcoma are capillary hemangiomas and venolymphatic malformations.

Capillary hemangioma (Fig. 6) is a hamartomatous proliferation of vascular endothelial cells that usually presents in infancy, whereas rhabdomyosarcoma more typically presents in early childhood. The natural history of capillary hemangiomas occurs in two phases: a proliferative phase, which typically lasts from 8 to 18 months of age, and an involutional phase, in which there is regression of the hemangioma. Most capillary hemangiomas begin to involute by 2 to 3 years of age, and by age 7 completely resolve [26,27]. Because most tumors involute spontaneously, only complications justify active treatment. Treatment consists of steroid injection or surgical excision [28,29].

On imaging, capillary hemangiomas present as multilobulated, intensely enhancing masses that can involve any portion of the orbit, and may involve multiple contiguous areas. The most common sites involved are the superonasal extraconal orbit, eyelid, and superonasal periorbita [30]. Contrast enhancement is intense and homogenous. Rapid wash-in of contrast on dynamic CT can be useful in differentiating capillary hemangiomas from other tumors (see Fig. 6) [14,31]. On MR imaging, capillary hemangiomas are slightly hyperintense to muscle on T1-weighted and heterogeneously hyperintense on T2-weighted images, frequently with internal flow voids [30]. As on CT, there is diffuse, intense enhancement on postinfusion images. Enhancement is diffusely homogenous during the proliferative phase, but during involution may become heterogeneous [30].

Venolymphatic malformations (Fig. 7), also known as lymphangiomas, orbital lymphatic-venous malformations, and lymphangiohemangiomas are benign hamartomatous tumors that arise from vascular mesenchymal anlage. Unlike capillary hemangiomas, the endothelial cells divide at a normal rate, and tumor growth occurs only as a result of dilatation of pre-existing vascular channels. The terms *cystic hygroma* and *lymphangioma simplex* are still widely used to describe tumors that consist exclusively of lymphangitic tissue.

On imaging, venolymphatic malformations present as multilobulated, poorly circumscribed masses, often with internal fluid-fluid levels from hemorrhage into the cystic components. Variable signal on T1-weighted images is caused by internal blood and

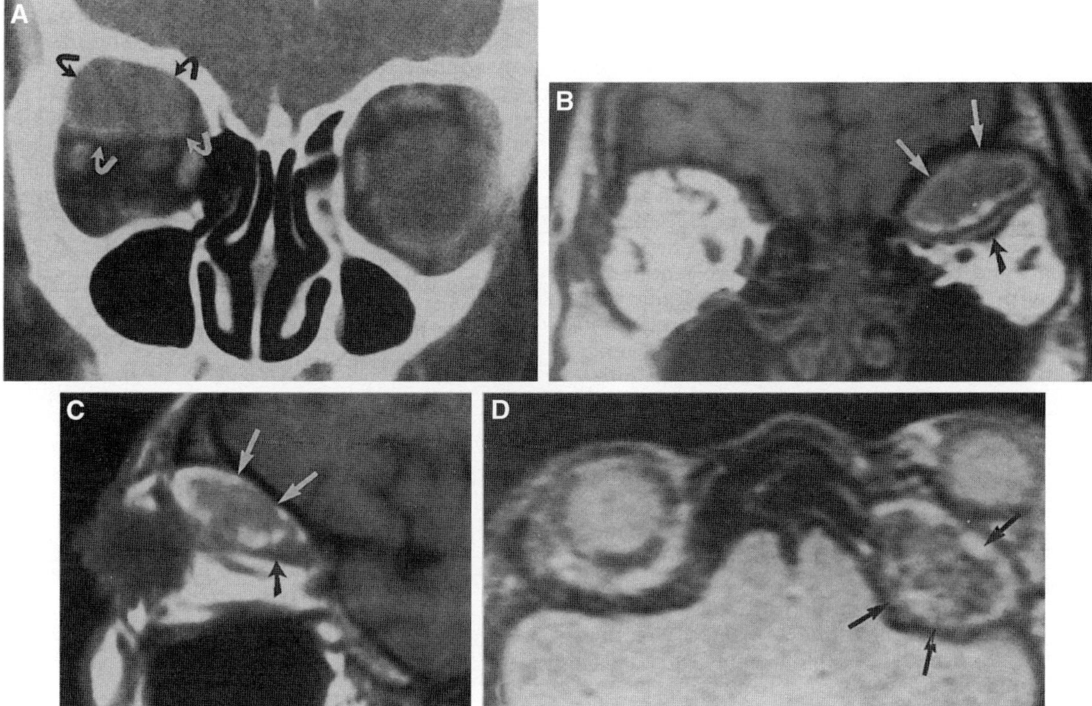


Fig. 5. Acute subperiosteal hematoma. (*A*) Coronal CT scan through the orbit showing a hyperdense acute subperiosteal hematoma (*arrows*) extending along the roof of the orbit and displacing the orbital contents inferiorly. (*B*) Coronal T1-weighted (500/20, TR/TE) MR image in another patient showing the intermediate signal intensity of an acute subperiosteal hematoma (*white arrows*). Note the displaced periosteum (*black arrow*). (*C*) Sagittal T1-weighted (600/20, TR/TE) MR image of the same patient in *B* showing the acute subperiosteal orbital hematoma (*white arrows*). Note the displaced periosteum (*black arrow*). (*D*) Axial T2-weighted (200/80, TR/TE) MR image of same patient in *B* through the orbit. Note the low signal intensity of the acute hematoma in T2-weighted image. (*From* Dobben GD, Philip B, Mafee MF, et al. Orbital subperiosteal hematoma, cholesterol granuloma, and infection. Radiol Clin North Am 1998;36:1188.)

blood product of different ages. High signal on T2-weighted images reflects a high fluid content. Unlike capillary hemangiomas, no flow voids are present on T2-weighted images. On postcontrast images, there is variable enhancement. The cystic lymphatic components typically have peripheral rim enhancement, whereas the venous components demonstrate heterogenous internal enhancement [32].

### *Inflammatory pseudotumor*

Inflammatory pseudotumor (Fig. 8) is an idiopathic inflammatory phenomenon that accounts for 8% of biopsied orbital lesions [9]. Although orbital inflammatory pseudotumor more typically occurs in middle-aged patients, it can occur in patients of any age and is part of the differential for primary orbital rhabdomyosarcoma [33]. The clinical course is characterized by acute onset of exopthalmos and pain, which can be severe.

On imaging, pseudotumor typically presents as a moderately enhancing mass, often with adjacent inflammation of the orbital fat and extraocular muscles. Uveal and scleral thickening is seen in 33%, and is considered a specific sign for inflammatory pseudotumor [34]. Bone destruction and intracranial extension are rare but have been reported [34,35].

On MR imaging, inflammatory pseudotumors are typically (but not always) hypointense on T2-weighted images compared with other tumors, including rhabdomyosarcoma. Like rhabdomyosarcoma, they are isointense to muscle on T1-weighted images and exhibit variable contrast enhancement [33].

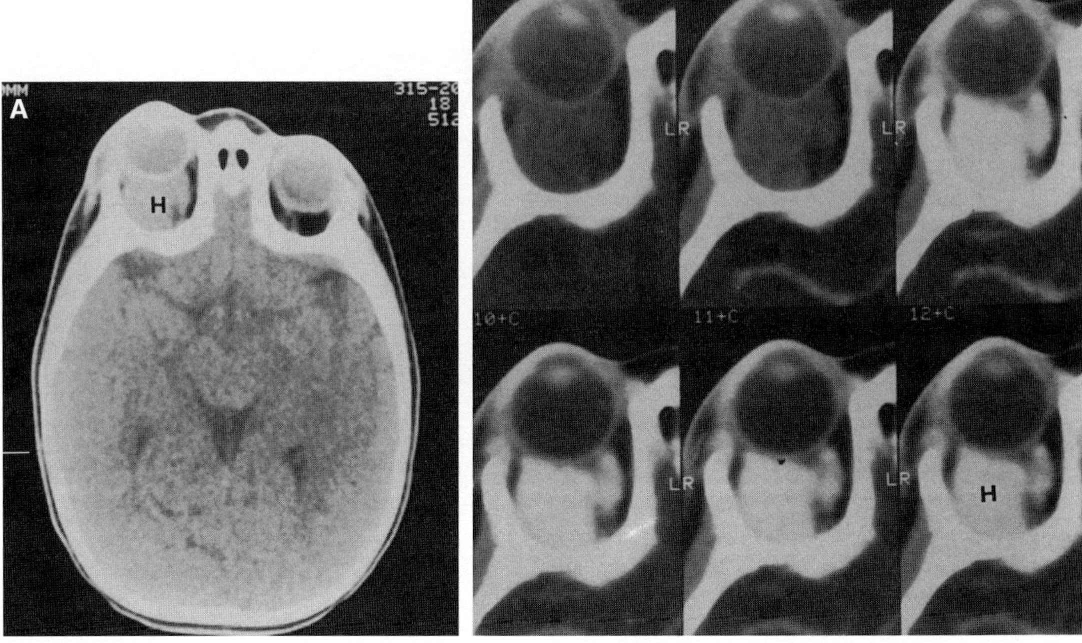


Fig. 6. Capillary hemangioma. (*A*) Enhanced CT scan showing a large retrobulbar mass compatible with a capillary hemangioma (H). (*B*) Dynamic CT scanning reveals rapid wash-in of contrast in hemangioma (H). (*From* Mafee MF, Pai E, Philip B. Rhabdomyosarcoma of the orbit. Radiol Clin North Am 1998;36:1224.)

*Dermoid cyst*

Dermoid cysts are the most common orbital masses in childhood. They are developmental in origin, resulting from abnormal sequestration or implantation of surface ectoderm along embryonic lines of closure that form the eyes, ears, and face [36]. These tumors are lined with squamous epithelium and skin appendages (hair follicles, sweat glands, sebaceous glands). It is the presence of skin appendages that differentiate dermoids from epidermoid cysts, which are lined only with squamous epithelial cells. Orbital dermoids typically arise in the vicinity of sutures, especially the zygomaticofrontal and frontoethmoidal sutures [37]. Dermoids become symptomatic by one of two mechanisms: they can enlarge until they begin to exert compressive forces on adjacent nerves and vascular structures, or they can spontaneously rupture, spilling their contents and inciting an intense inflammatory response.

On imaging, dermoids often exhibit a characteristic appearance, with internal fat density on CT, high signal on T1-weighted and T2-weighted MR images, and a well-defined, thin wall. Calcification and fluid levels are occasionally seen. Bone involvement occurs in 85% [37].

Occasionally, dermoid cysts do not contain fat. These lesions often cannot be differentiated from epidermoid cysts on imaging. Less commonly, they can present with multicompartmental or heterogeneous attenuation and signal or with a thickened, irregular wall (Fig. 9).

Dermoid cysts can usually be distinguished from orbital rhabdomyosarcoma and other tumors because of internal fat attenuation on CT and bright signal on T1-weighted MR images [38]. Rarely, in atypical cases, biopsy may be required to confirm the diagnosis.

*Langerhans' cell histiocytosis*

Histiocytic lesions account for just over 1% of biopsied orbital tumors [9]. The most important histiocytic tumor that can simulate orbital rhabdomyosarcoma is Langerhans' cell histiocytosis (Fig. 10).

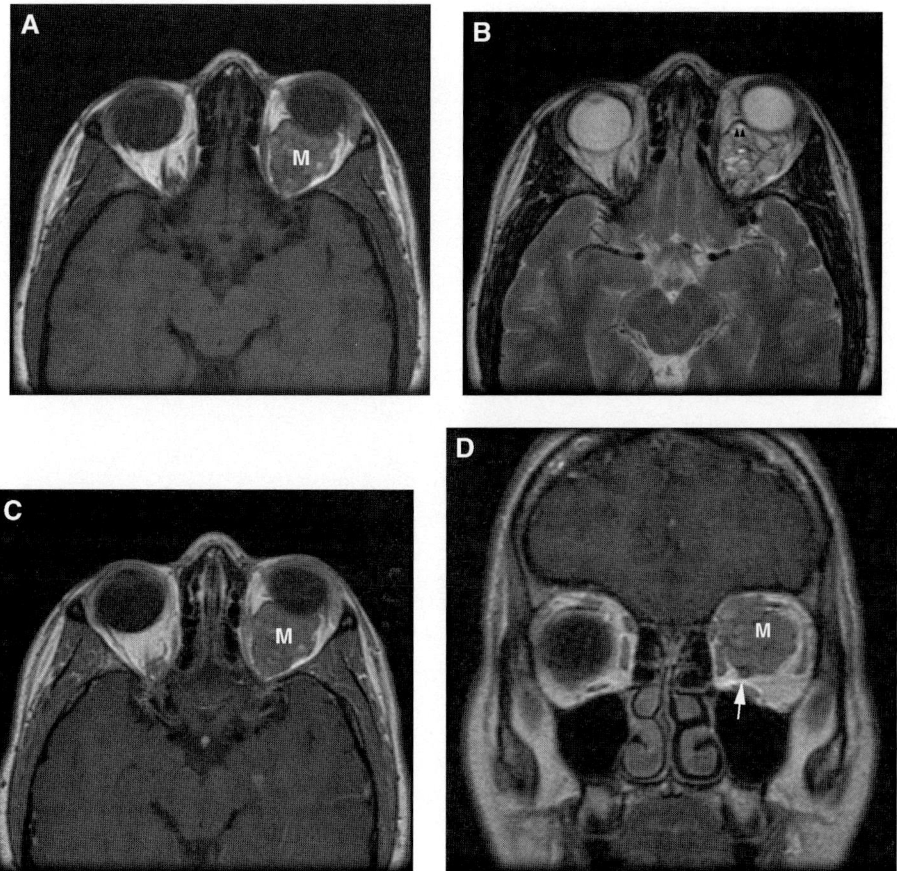


Fig. 7. Presumed venolymphatic malformation (lymphangioma) in a 25-year-old woman. Axial T1-weighted (466/13, TR/TE) (*A*), T2-weighted (4000/99, TR/TE) (*B*), and postinfusion axial and coronal T1- weighted images (*C,D*) reveal a multiseptated, primarily intraconal mass (M) with an internal fluid-fluid level (*arrowheads*) and minimal enhancement following gadolinium infusion. The optic nerve (*arrow*) is displaced inferomedially by the mass.

Orbital involvement occurs in approximately 23% of patients with Langerhans' cell histiocytosis [39]. As in orbital rhabdomyosarcoma, most patients are children. The lesions typically arise in bone or bone marrow, and spread to the orbits by direct extension. This appearance can simulate a primary orbital rhabdomyosarcoma with bone involvement. The superior and superotemporal orbital region is most commonly involved. Extension into the epidural space and temporal fossa commonly occurs, and additional lesions may be detected in the facial bones and base of the skull. Infrequently, the lesion may be entirely extraosseous.

Management of Langerhans' cell histiocytosis of the orbit depends on the presence or absence of symptoms. Because many lesions spontaneously involute, smaller lesions may be observed following biopsy, or managed with partial curettage or intralesional steroid injection [39]. Extensive lesions with optic nerve involvement, proptosis, and bone destruction are managed with radiation therapy. Acute vision loss caused by optic nerve involvement warrants emergent radiation therapy; vision may be spared if patients are treated within 24 to 48 hours following the onset of visual symptoms.

### *Leukemia and lymphoma*

Lymphoid and leukemic lesions of the orbits together account for approximately 10% of orbital tumors. The two most important lesions in this category that can simulate orbital rhabdomyosarcoma are orbital granulocytic sarcoma and non-Hodgkin's lymphoma.

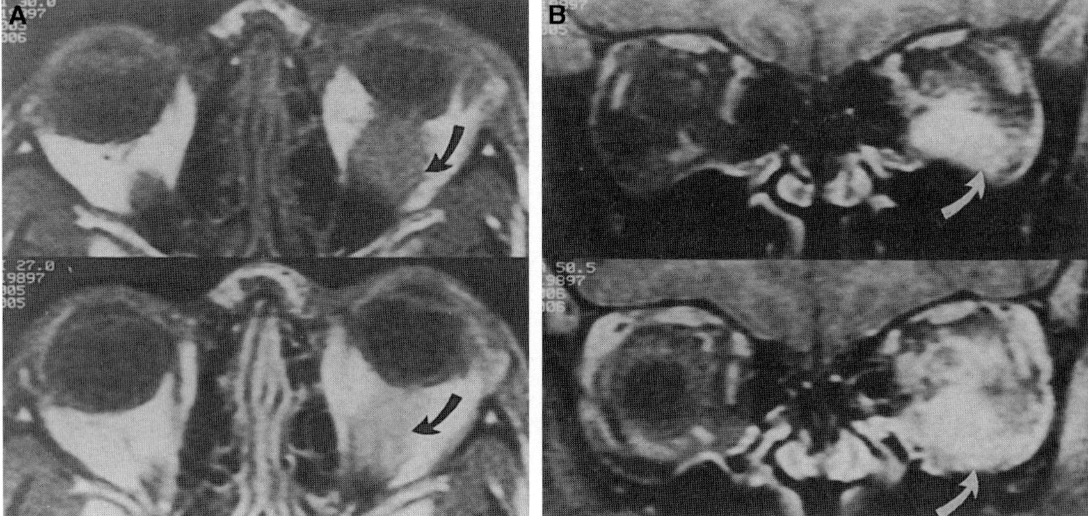

Fig. 8. Pseudotumor. (*A*) Nonenhanced (*top*) and enhanced (*bottom*) T1-weighted MR images show thickening and enhancement of the left inferior rectus. (*B*) Enhanced fat-suppressed T1-weighted image shows marked enhancement within the lesion (*arrows*). (*From* Mafee MF, Pai E, Philip B. Rhabdomyosarcoma of the orbit. Radiol Clin North Am 1998;36:1222.)

Orbital granulocytic sarcomas (Fig. 11), also known as chloromas, occur in the setting of myelogenous leukemia and other myeloproliferative disorders. These rare tumors consist of granulocytic cell precursors, such as myeloblasts, promyelocytes, and myelocytes. Occasionally, they can be the first manifestation of acute myelogenous leukemia. The masses typically demonstrate similar attenuation to muscle on CT, and enhance on postinfusion images. They are slightly hypointense to muscle on T2-weighted images, a characteristic that can be useful in distinguishing them from rhabdomyosarcoma [40]. Biopsy is necessary to confirm the diagnosis in most cases.

Lymphoma of the orbit (Fig. 12) may occur as a primary tumor or may be secondary to systemic lymphoma. Non-Hodgkin's lymphoma is by far the most common lymphomatous neoplasm to affect the orbit, and low-grade mucosa-associated lymphoid tissue lymphoma is the most common subtype [41]. Although it is typically a disease of older adults with an average age of presentation of 50 to 70 years, it can occur in young adults and children. Although any portion of the orbit can be involved, there is a predilection for the lacrimal gland, which is often enlarged [40].

On imaging, lymphoma is highly variable in appearance, ranging from a diffuse infiltrative process in high-grade lesions to a solid tumor with discrete lobulated margins in less aggressive tumors. Orbital lymphoma can closely simulate orbital rhabdomyosarcoma. Like rhabdomyosarcoma, the tumors are similar in intensity to muscle on T1-weighted images and have variable (moderate to marked) contrast enhancement. One distinguishing feature is the relatively hypointense signal on T2-weighted images, which is related to the hypercellular nature of these tumors. Another is the tendency of lymphomas to mold themselves around structures they come into contact with, such as the globe and the orbital wall. Lymphomas cause less extensive bony destruction than rhabdomyosarcomas, and almost never result in indentation of the globe, regardless of size [40].

### *Metastatic neuroblastoma*

Neuroblastoma metastasizes to the orbits from primary tumors arising in the adrenal medulla (35%); extra-adrenal retroperitoneum (30%–35%); posterior mediastinum (20%); neck (1%–5%); and pelvis (2%–3%) [42,43]. The typical presentation is a rapidly progressive orbital mass, with frequent involvement of the skull base [30]. The presence of multiple lesions or a pre-existing diagnosis of neu-

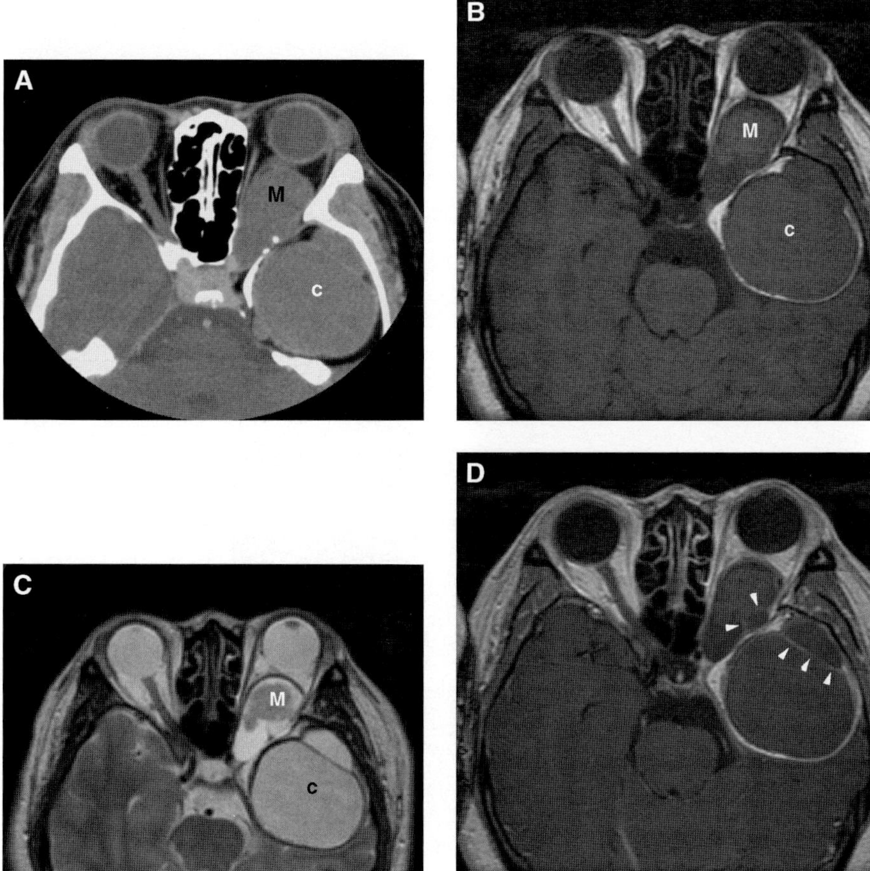


Fig. 9. Dermoid cysts in a 38-year-old woman. (*A*) Axial CT section reveals an intraconal cystic mass (M) and an intracranial cyst (C). Both are compatible with dermoid cysts. Axial T1-weighted (*B*) and T2-weighted (*C*) images better establish the cystic nature of the masses, with heterogeneous signal on T1-weighted images and hyperintense signal on T2-weighted images. (*D*) Postinfusion T1-weighted image shows peripheral enhancement of the cysts. Enhancing septa (*arrowheads*) are present in both dermoids.

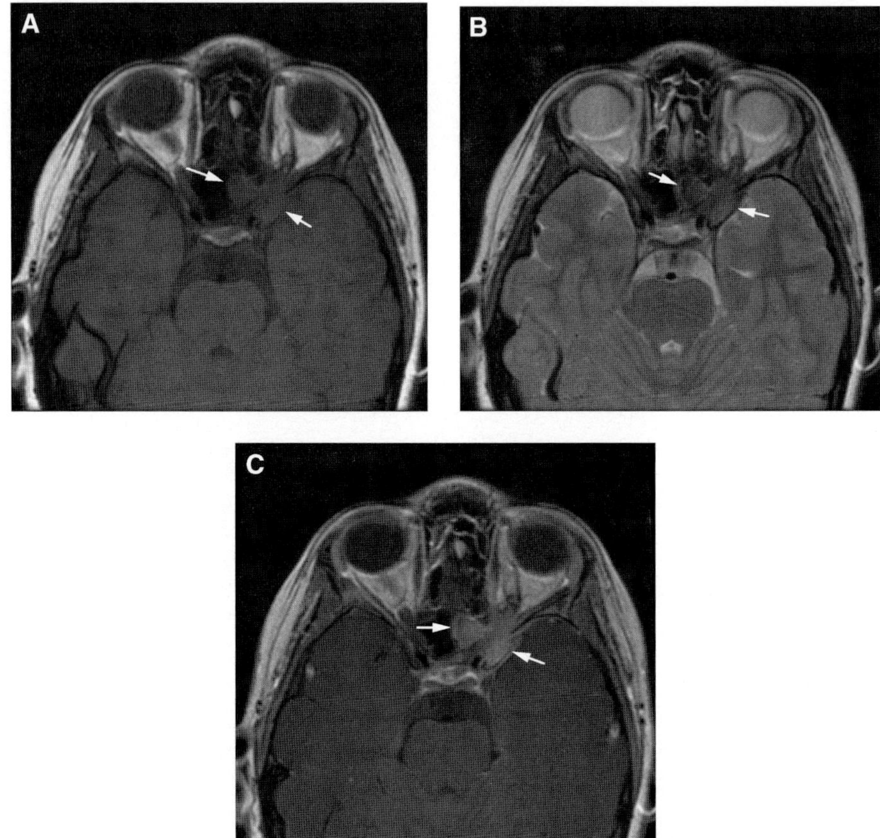


Fig. 10. Langerhans' cell histiocytosis in a 10-year-old boy who presented with acute onset of impaired vision in the left eye. Axial T1-weighted (466/13, TR/TE) (*A*) and T2-weighted (4000/99, TR/TE) (*B*) images reveal a mass (*arrows*) arising from the lesser wing of the sphenoid with extension into the orbital apex. There is relatively low internal signal on the T2-weighted image, an important factor differentiating this lesion from rhabdomyosarcoma. (*C*) On the postinfusion axial T1-weighted image (500/13, TR/TE) there is avid enhancement of the mass.

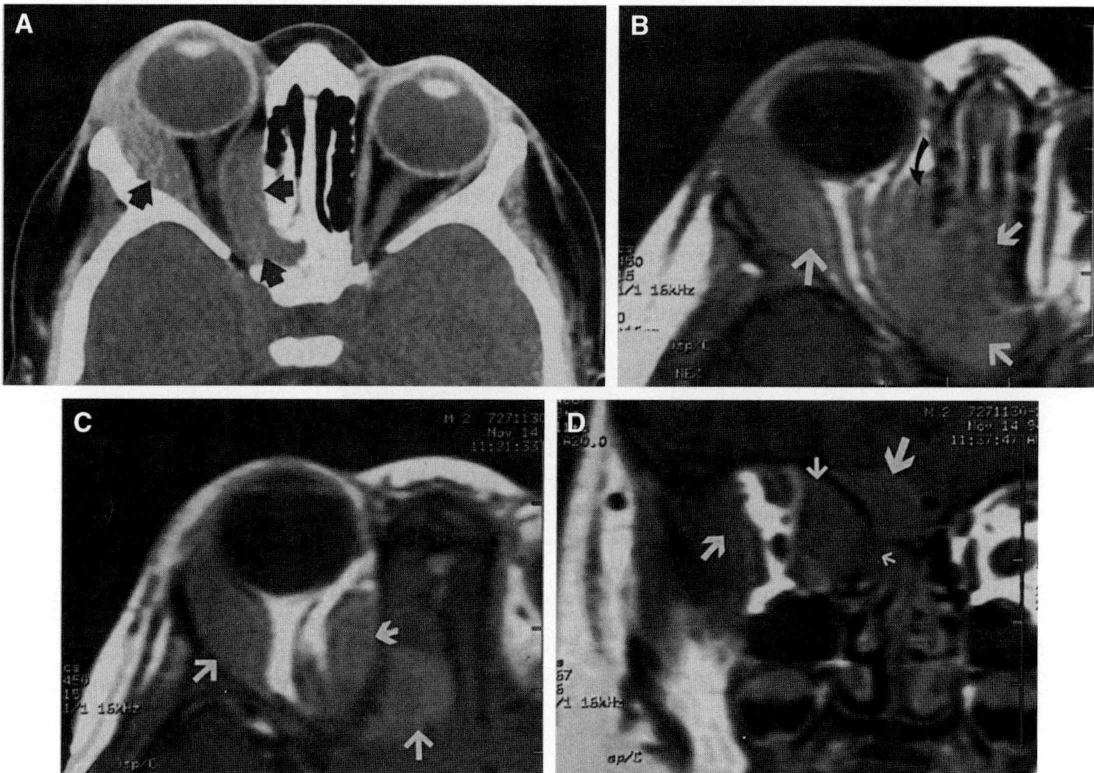


Fig. 11. Granulocytic sarcoma (leukemia). Axial CT (*A*), postcontrast axial T1-weighted (*B, C*), and postcontrast coronal T1-weighted (*D*) MR images demonstrate an extraconal infiltration involving both the medial and lateral aspect of the orbit (*arrows*). The lesion erodes into the ethmoid air cells and erodes the cribriform plate, with extension into the anterior cranial fossa. (*From* Valvassori GE, Sabnis SS, Mafee RF, et al. Imaging of orbital lymphoproliferative disorders. Radiol Clin North Am 1999;37:138.)

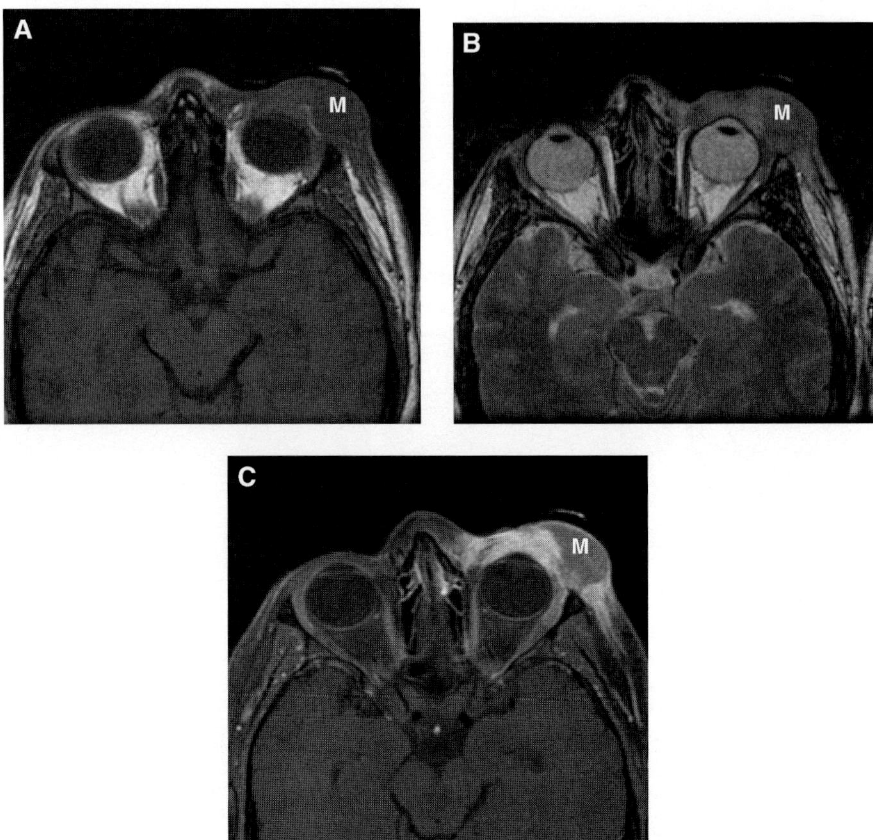


Fig. 12. A 16-year-old boy with high-grade B-cell lymphoma. Axial T1-weighted (400/14, TR/TE) (*A*) and T2-weighted (3000/101, TR/TE) (*B*) images reveal a preseptal superotemporal mass (M) with low internal T2 signal. (*C*) Axial T1-weighted image following gadolinium infusion shows homogeneous enhancement in the mass and enhancement of the adjacent soft tissues (400/14, TR/TE).

roblastoma can help establish this diagnosis, which otherwise must be made by tissue sampling.

## Summary

Rhabdomyosarcoma is the most common primary orbital malignancy in children. It is rare in neonates and in the adult population, but can occur at any age. It arises from rests of primitive embryonic tissue that can occur at any location within the orbit, not from preformed striated muscle tissue. CT and MR imaging are the most important modalities for diagnosis, tumor staging, and surgical planning. An awareness of imaging characteristics of rhabdomyosarcoma and of the common simulating lesions is essential in forming a sensible differential diagnosis, and in recommending appropriate additional imaging or tissue sampling.

## Acknowledgments

The authors would like to thank Reema Lamba and Dr. Deepak Edward for their help in procuring pathology slides. We also thank Yassir Aich for his assistance in preparing images for this article.

## References

[1] Weiss SW, Goldblum JR. Rhabdomyosarcoma. In: Weiss SW, Goldblum JR, editors. Enzinger and Weiss's soft tissue tumors. 4th edition. St. Louis: CV Mosby; 2001. p. 785–835.

[2] Shields JA, Shields CL. Rhabdomyosarcoma. Review for the ophthalmologist. Ophthalmology 2003;48: 39–57.

[3] Walton RC, Ellis GS, Haik BG. Rhabdomyosarcoma presumed metastatic to the orbit. Ophthalmology 1996; 103:1512–6.

[4] MacArthur CJ, McGill TJ, Healy GB. Pediatric head and neck rhabdomyosarcoma. Clin Pediatr 1992;31: 66–70.

[5] Sheilds JA, Shields CL. Rhabdomyosarcoma of the orbit. Int Ophthalmol Clin 1993;33:203–10.

[6] Volpe NJ, Jakobiec FA. Pediatric orbital tumors. Int Ophthalmol Clin 1992;32:201–21.

[7] Folpe AL, McKenney JK, Bridge JA, et al. Sclerosing rhabdomyosarcoma in adults: report of four cases of hyalinizing, matrix-rich variant of rhabdomyosarcoma that may be confused with osteosarcoma, chondrosarcoma, or angiosarcoma. Am J Surg Pathol 2002;26: 1175–83.

[8] Kwan B. Rhabdomyosarcoma of the eyelid with enophthalmos. Ann Ophthalmol 1980;12:540–3.

[9] Shields JA, Shields CL, Scartozzi R. Survey of 1264 patients with orbital tumors and simulating lesions. Ophthalmology 2004;111:997–1008.

[10] Sohaib SA, Moseley I, Wright JE. Orbital rhabdomyosarcoma: the radiological characteristics. Clin Radiol 1998;53:357–62.

[11] Knowles DM, Jakobiec FA, Potter GD, et al. Ophthalmic striated muscle neoplasms. Surv Ophthalmol 1976;21:219–61.

[12] Jones IS, Reese AB, Kraut J. Orbital rhabdomyosarcoma. Am J Ophthalmol 1966;61:721–36.

[13] Jones IS, Reese AB, Kraut J. Orbital rhabdomyosarcoma: an analysis of sixty-two cases. Trans Am Ophthalmol Soc 1965;63:223–55.

[14] Mafee MF, Pai E, Philip B. Rhabdomyosarcoma of the orbit: evaluation with MR imaging and CT. Radiol Clin North Am 1998;36:1215–27.

[15] Seedat RY, Hamilton PD, de Jager LP, et al. Orbital rhabdomyosarcoma presenting as an apparent orbital subperiosteal abscess. Int J Pediatr Otorhinolaryngol 2000;52:177–81.

[16] Hagiwara A, Inoue Y, Nakaymara T, et al. The botryoid sign: a characteristic feature of rhabdomyosarcomas in the head and neck. Neuroradiology 2001;43: 331–5.

[17] Backhouse OC, Cove P, Bowen DI. Rhabdomyosarcoma masked by orbital trauma. Int J Oral Maxillofac Surg 1997;26:374–5.

[18] Mauerer HM, Beltangady M, Gehan EA, et al. The Intergroup Rhabdomyosarcoma study—I. A final report. Cancer 1988;61:209–20.

[19] Shields CL, Shields JA, Honavar SG, et al. Clinical spectrum of primary orbital rhabdomyosarcoma. Ophthalmology 2001;108(12):2284–92.

[20] Wharam M, Beltangady M, Hays D, et al. Localized orbital rhabdomyosarcoma: an interim report of the Intergroup Rhabdomyosarcoma Study Committee. Ophthalmology 1987;94:251–4.

[21] Morón FE, Morriss MC, Jones JJ, et al. Lumps and bumps on the head in children: use of CT and MR imaging in solving the clinical diagnostic dilemma. Radiographics 2004;24:1655–74.

[22] Cota N, Chandna A, Abernathy LJ. Orbital abscess masquerading as a rhabdomyosarcoma. J AAPOS 2000; 4:318–20.

[23] Maurer HM, Gehan EA, Beltangady M, et al. The Intergroup Rhabdomyosarcoma Study—II. Cancer 1993;71:1904–22.

[24] Crist W, Gehan EA, Ragab AH, et al. The Third Intergroup Rhabdomyosarcoma Study. J Clinical Oncol 1995;13:610–30.

[25] Crist WM, Anderson JR, Meza JL, et al. Intergroup Rhabdomyosarcoma study—IV: results for patients with nonmetastatic disease. J Clin Oncol 2001;19: 3091–102.

[26] Castillo Jr BV, Kaufman L. Pediatric tumors of the eye and orbit. Pediatr Clin North Am 2003;50:149–72.

[27] Haik BG, Karcioglu ZA, Gordon RA, et al. Capillary hemangioma (infantile periocular hemangioma). Surv Ophthalmol 1994;38:399–426.

[28] Weiss AH. Adrenal suppression after corticosteroid injection of periocular hemangiomas. Am J Ophthalmol 1989;107:518–22.

[29] O'Keefe M, Lanigan B, Byrne SA. Capillary haemangioma of the eyelids and orbit: a clinical review of the safety and efficacy of intralesional steroid. Acta Ophthalmol Scand 2003;81:294–8.

[30] Harnsberger HR, Wiggins RH, Hudgins PA, et al. Head and neck. 1st edition. Salt Lake City (UT): Amirsys; 2004.

[31] Mafee MF, Miller MT, Tan W, et al. Dynamic computed tomography and its application to ophthalmology. Radiol Clin North Am 1987;25:715–31.

[32] Bilaniuk LT. Orbital vascular lesions: role of imaging. Radiol Clin North Am 1999;37:169–86.

[33] Narla LD, Newman B, Spottswood SS, et al. Inflammatory pseudotumor. Radiographics 2003;23: 719–29.

[34] Frohman LP, Kupersmith ML, Lang J, et al. Intracranial extension and bone destruction in orbital pseudotumor. Arch Ophthalmol 1986;104:380–4.

[35] Harr DL, Qenier RM, Abrams GW. Computed tomography and ultrasound in the evaluation of orbital infection and pseudotumors. Radiology 1982;142: 395–401.

[36] Hicks J, Flaitz C. Rhabdomyosarcoma of the head and neck in children. Oral Oncol 2002;38:450–9.

[37] Chawda SJ, Moseley IF. Computed tomography of orbital dermoids: a 20 year review. Clin Radiol 1999; 54:821–5.

[38] Grossman RI, Yousem DM. Neuroradiology: the requisites. 2nd edition. Philadelphia: Mosby; 2003.

[39] Hidayat AA, Mafee MF, Laver NV, et al. Langerhans' cell histiocytosis and juvenile xanthgranuloma of the orbit: clinicopathologic, CT, and MR imaging features. Radiol Clin North Am 1998;36:1229–40.

[40] Valvassori GE, Sabnis SS, Mafee RF, et al. Imaging

of orbital lymphoproliferative disorders. Radiol Clin North Am 1999;37:135–50.
[41] Galieni P, Polito E, et al. Localized orbital lymphoma. Haematologica 1997;82:436.
[42] Morris JA, Shcochat SJ, Smith EI, et al. Biological variables in thoracic neuroblastoma: a Pediatric Oncology Group study. J Pediatr Surg 1995;30:296–302 [discussion: 302–3].
[43] Lonergan GL, Schwab CM, Suarez ES, et al. From the archives of the AFIP: neuroblastoma, ganglioneuroblastoma, and ganglioneuroma: radiologic-pathologic correlation. Radiographics 2002;22:911–34.

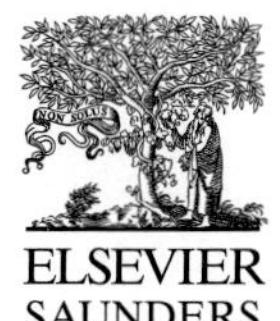
ELSEVIER
SAUNDERS

Neuroimag Clin N Am 15 (2005) 137 – 158

NEUROIMAGING
CLINICS OF
NORTH AMERICA

# Orbital Cavernous Hemangioma: Role of Imaging

Sameer A. Ansari, MD, PhD[a], Mahmood F. Mafee, MD[b,*]

[a]*Department of Radiology, University of Illinois Hospital at Chicago, University of Illinois College of Medicine, 1801 West Taylor Street, MC 711, Chicago, IL 60612, USA*
[b]*Department of Radiology, University of Illinois at Chicago Medical Center, 1740 West Taylor Street, MC 931, Chicago, IL 60612, USA*

Vascular disorders of the orbit encompass vascular malformations and vascular tumors. According to recent literature, orbital vascular malformations include type 1 venous-lymphatic malformations (lymphangiomas), type 2 venous malformations (varices), type 3 arterial-venous malformations, carotid-cavernous fistulas, and aneurysms, whereas orbital vascular tumors are limited to capillary hemangiomas, hemangiopericytomas, hemangioendotheliomas, and angiofibromas (Box 1) [1,2]. Interestingly, orbital cavernous hemangiomas have eluded definitive classification because of overlapping clinical, histologic, and radiologic features [2–4]. In this article, we provide an extensive review of orbital cavernous hemangioma and the role of diagnostic imaging. We aim to elucidate its differentiating features with respect to CT, MR imaging, ultrasonography, nuclear scintigraphy, and conventional digital subtraction angiography (DSA). In addition, it is our hope to provide some insight into the vascular nature of this lesion and its classification as a type 3 low-flow arterial-venous malformation (AVM) [2].

Cavernous hemangioma has often been cited as the most common primary orbital tumor in adults [5–7], and specifically in the histopathologically proven series by Shields et al [8], as the most common orbital vascular lesion. However, the incidence is infrequent, with only 0.6 to 2.0 cases identified per year at major referral institutions [9], and many asymptomatic hemangiomas are not characterized histologically because they are exempt from biopsy or surgical excision. Therefore, the incidence statistics of orbital vascular lesions are prone to sample error and selection bias but may differ depending on geographic location, because capillary hemangiomas were noted to be respectively more common in the separate clinical-pathologic series by Kennedy [10] and in a recent study from Turkey [11].

## Clinical presentation

Orbital cavernous hemangiomas demonstrate a predilection to affect middle-aged women (60%–70%), with a mean age of 43 to 48 years and range of 18 to 72 years based on several large series. Because they exhibit slow progressive enlargement, the most common presenting sign and symptom is painless proptosis (mean: 5–6 mm; range: 0–15 mm). Hence, the average duration of symptoms before presentation may last for several years (mean: 4 years; range: weeks to decades). Less common symptoms include pain, lid swelling, diplopia, lump, and recurrent obscured vision [3,12–14].

Objectively, a significant number of patients with progressive exophthalmos also present with impaired vision and a field cut corresponding to the size and location of the lesion, presumably secondary to optic nerve compression. Most orbital cavernous hemangiomas are identified in the retrobulbar muscle cone, predominantly in the lateral aspect of the intraconal space. On physical examination, enlarging intraconal lesions may cause optic disc papilledema with desaturation to red color and Marcus-Gunn pupils; indent the posterior pole of the globe, producing choroidal folds or anisometric hyperopia; or affect

* Corresponding author.
*E-mail address:* mmafee@uic.edu (M.F. Mafee).

1052-5149/05/$ – see front matter 
doi:10.1016/j.nic.2005.02.009

**Box 1. Orbital vascular lesions**

*Vascular malformations*

Type 1: no flow
  Venous-lymphatic malformation (lymphangioma)
Type 2: venous flow
  Venous malformation (varix)
    Distensible
    Nondistensible
Combined types 1 and 2:
  Distensible venous-lymphatic malformation
Type 3: arterial flow
  AVM
    High flow
    Low flow (cavernous hemangioma)
Carotid-cavernous fistula
Aneurysm

*Vascular tumors*

Capillary hemangioma
Hemangioperictyoma
Hemangioendothelioma
Angiofibroma

extraocular muscle function, resulting in diplopia [12–15]. Smaller lesions within the orbital apex and, rarely, in the optic canal [13,15,16] can compress the optic nerve at an earlier stage with minimal proptosis, resulting in monocular vision loss or transient gaze-evoked amaurosis fugax by compromising the optic nerve's blood supply [17–19]. Moreover, dilated episcleral vessels and optic disc atrophy, thought to be related to prolonged (years) or severe (>8 mm) proptosis, may be observed [11,13]. An associated bruit or pulsation has been noted in the literature, but this finding is unlikely in most cases because of the low-flow arterial hemodynamics and thick outer capsule of orbital cavernous hemangiomas [2,12,13].

In contrast to the frequent hemorrhage of intracranial cavernous hemangiomas [20,21], orbital cavernous hemangiomas present less commonly with spontaneous intraorbital hemorrhage from an occult site [22]. The respective absence of hemorrhage in orbital lesions may be a result of the interposition of rich fibrous tissue, which bestows a firm tumor texture unlike that of the friable intracranial lesions [23]. Other unusual presentations include several reports of intraosseous cavernous hemangiomas of the orbital rim [13,24,25] and a single case of lacrimal gland involvement [26]. Although orbital cavernous hemangiomas are predominantly unifocal and unilateral, multifocal unilateral [12,14,27] and bilateral [28–31] lesions have been described. Interestingly, two of the six reported cases of bilateral orbital cavernous hemangiomas occurred in syndromes predisposed to hemangiomas: Maffucci's syndrome [32], a nonhereditary disease characterized by cutaneous hemangiomas and enchondromas, and the blue rubber bleb nevus syndrome [33,34], a vascular disorder characterized by multiple cutaneous and gastrointestinal hemangiomas.

In the past, orbital cavernous hemangiomas were invariably resected, because differentiation from potentially malignant hemangiopericytoma could not be conclusively discerned clinically or radiologically [14]. Current imaging modalities have evolved to deliver high sensitivity and specificity in diagnosing these vascular lesions, however. Recent literature supports observation as an alternative to surgical excision for asymptomatic orbital cavernous hemangiomas, even in cases presenting solely with exophthalmos [35,36]. Asymptomatic orbital cavernous hemangiomas usually demonstrate absent or slow growth and are only incidentally discovered on CT or MR imaging for unrelated indications. The role of diagnostic imaging is then crucial for an accurate diagnosis and correct treatment planning. We begin to examine the histopathologic findings and classification of orbital cavernous hemangiomas so as to understand their differentiating features on multiple diagnostic imaging modalities.

## Histopathology and classification

On gross examination, orbital cavernous hemangiomas are benign noninfiltrative masses that appear as dark "plum" or purplish-colored ovoid lesions within a well-defined fibrous pseudocapsule consisting of trabeculations and septae. The surface of the mass is spongy or rubbery and may demonstrate purplish lobulations between the pale white fibrous septae (Fig. 1A) [7,12,13].

Histologically, they are classically defined as large dilated vascular channels, containing blood and occasional thrombus and lined by flattened or attenuated endothelial cells. Immediately outside these vascular channels and endothelial cells, the fibrous interstitium varies from being devoid of trabeculae to containing a collagenous matrix that may include myxomatous connective tissue or short strands or bundles of smooth muscle cells indicative of myofibroblasts

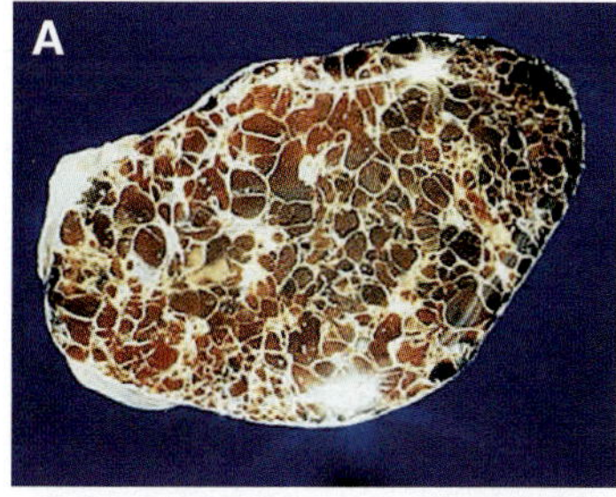


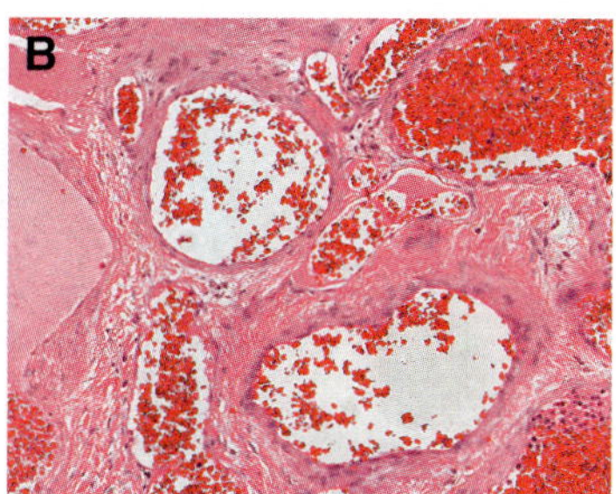


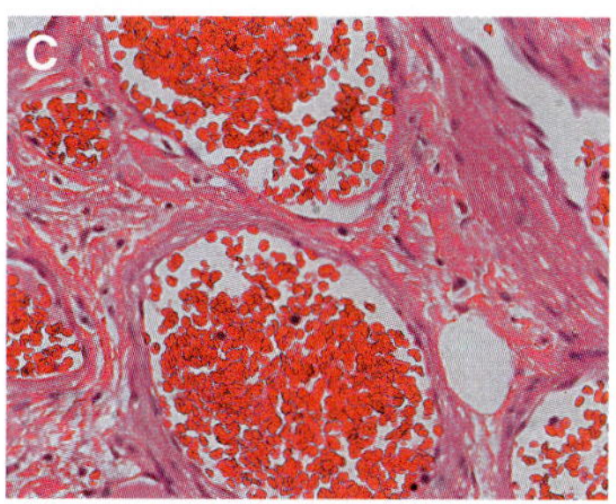


Fig. 1. Orbital cavernous hemangioma. (*A*) Gross pathologic specimen of an orbital cavernous hemangioma demonstrates a purple lobulated mass composed of dilated vascular spaces and intervening fibrous septae within a pseudocapsule. (*B*, *C*) Histologic photomicrographs show blood-filled dilated vascular spaces lined by flattened endothelial cells and surrounded by collagenous trabeculae and smooth muscle cells (*B*, hematoxylin–eosin, ×20 original magnification; *C*, hematoxylin–eosin, original magnification ×40). (Courtesy of D. Edwards, MD, Chicago, IL.)

(Fig. 1B and C). Moreover, small capillaries may be seen extending from the main cavernous spaces into the interstitium [7,12,37]. These "capillary proliferations" may initiate the slow enlargement of cavernous hemangiomas, with progressive ectasia and peripheral smooth muscle differentiation beyond the capsule, as predecessors of the dilated vascular channels and interstitium [12,13]. Others have postulated that a preexisting vascular hamartoma or malformation is induced, perhaps by hemodynamic demand, toward dilatation of the vascular channels. Subsequent expansion may occur through incorporation of these preexisting and dilated vascular spaces by the outermost portion of the capsule [38].

The neoplastic potential of cavernous hemangiomas is minimal, and, to our knowledge, there is no evidence of malignant transformation in the literature. Orbital cavernous hemangiomas do not demonstrate the rapid endothelial proliferation seen in capillary hemangiomas, arguing against classification as a vascular tumor [3,12,39]. The infrequency of cavernous hemangiomas found in children or adolescents also counters against induced endothelial proliferation within a congenital vascular hamartoma [13]. Orbital cavernous hemangiomas have been thought to arise from a venous origin and classified as encapsulated venous malformations [3,12,40]. Nevertheless, an arterial origin is suggested anatomically and physiologically because vascular malformations preferentially occur in arterial-rich environments within the lateral half of the orbit along the posterior ciliary arteries, entering the globe in the region of the macula [41]. Interestingly, solitary choroidal hemangiomas also demonstrate a preference lateral to the optic nerve head and adjacent to the dense entry zone of the posterior ciliary arteries [42]. These arterial regions may be more conducive to allow capillary proliferation and ectasia, expanding the dilated vascular channels seen histologically. The occasional findings of small feeding arteries and delayed contrast pooling using prolonged conventional DSA techniques are described in detail elsewhere in this article and support a low-flow arterial-venous origin. Therefore, these lesions may be better classified as AVMs (arterial low-flow type) rather than as true neoplasms or proliferating hamartomas. Local hemodynamic disturbances and hypoxia from low blood flow or ischemia have been implicated in the etiology or angiogenesis of orbital cavernous hemangiomas through intrapapillary endothelial hyperplasia and capillary formation [13,43]. In addition, hormonal or cytokine-mediated angiogenic factors may complement their growth, because there is a higher incidence in women, reports of rapid proptosis during puberty and pregnancy [13,44], and progesterone receptor expression in endothelial and smooth muscle cells derived from orbital cavernous hemangiomas [45].

Orbital cavernous hemangiomas have recently been classified as type 3 low-flow AVMs with a direct arterial in-flow and venous out-flow mechanism [2]. This low-flow mechanism is probably affected by the small caliber of feeding arteries, dilated vascular channels within the lesion, or slow circulation secondary to thrombosis [20]. However, some investigators still contend that vascular lesions expanding by any type of cellular proliferation, including capillary and cavernous hemangiomas, are exempt from this classification of vascular malformations [4].

## Diagnostic imaging

### *CT*

CT and MR imaging are the primary diagnostic imaging methods used to evaluate orbital tumors and vascular lesions. The superior cross-sectional, multiplanar, and contrast enhancement properties of CT and MR imaging have resulted in higher diagnostic sensitivity for most orbital lesions, surpassing ultrasound in spatial resolution and contrast. In fact, MR imaging often supersedes CT because of its inherent high-contrast resolution and improved spatial resolution, providing more specific tissue characterization [46]. The specificity of these imaging modalities to differentiate orbital cavernous hemangiomas from other vascular malformations, vascular tumors, and simulating orbital tumors remained in question until the introduction of multiphase dynamic contrast CT [3,47–50] and MR [23,51,52] scanning techniques, however.

Axial and coronal thin-section (1–3 mm) scanning and multiplanar reformatted imaging are standard CT protocols to study the orbit [48]. Through faster acquisition times, helical multidetector CT has dramatically improved multiphase dynamic contrast scanning by better delineating the arterial and venous phases, increasing resolution with thinner sections, decreasing volume averaging and motion artifacts, and reducing radiation exposure. Despite no recent standardized protocols to evaluate orbital cavernous hemangiomas using multiphase dynamic contrast CT,

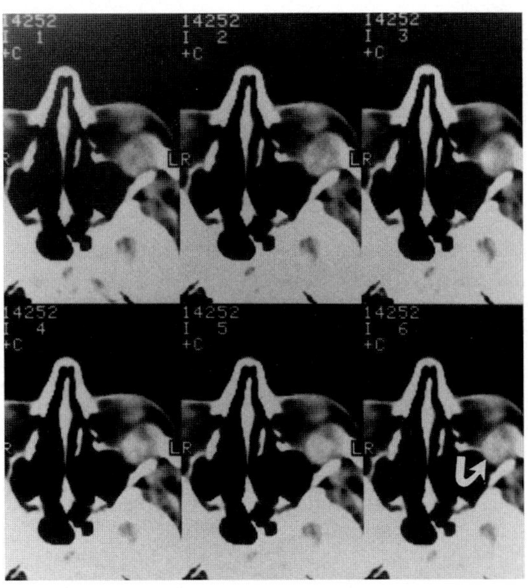


Fig. 3. Orbital cavernous hemangioma. Using dynamic contrast CT, serial axial postcontrast CT scans demonstrate an intraconal mass with heterogeneous and increasing enhancement through the early/late venous phase consistent with the delayed enhancement characteristics of a pathologically proven orbital cavernous hemangioma. (*From* Mafee MF, Valvassori GE, Becker M. Imaging of the head and neck. Stuttgart (Germany): Thieme; 2004. p. 254; with permission.)

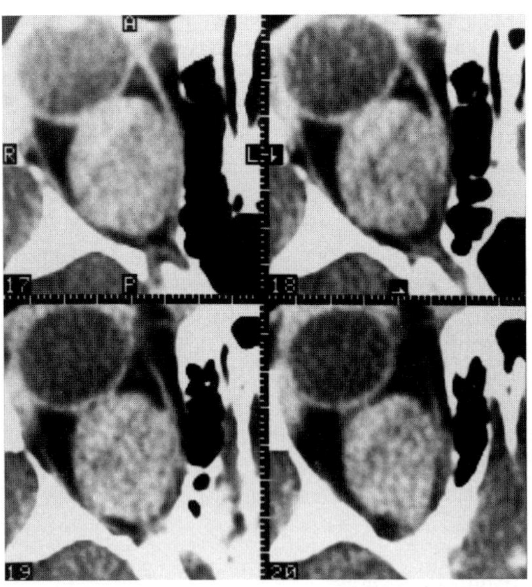


Fig. 2. Orbital cavernous hemangioma. Using single-phase contrast CT, contiguous axial postcontrast CT scans show a retrobulbar, intraconal, well-defined, and enhancing mass consistent with a pathologically proven orbital cavernous hemangioma.

four-phase dynamic techniques have been well documented for studying hepatic cavernous hemangiomas [53,54] and may be paralleled with consideration of blood transit time through the orbit. After a baseline noncontrast CT scan, a dynamic intravenous 100-mL (4–5 mL/s) bolus of iodinated contrast is administered and multiple serial postcontrast CT scans are acquired in the early arterial or angiographic phase (20–30-second delay), early venous phase (50–70-second delay), late venous phase (2–10-minute delay), and delayed equilibrium phases (10–60-minute delay).

Earlier studies have extensively characterized the CT appearance of orbital cavernous hemangiomas [15,55–59]. Predominantly located in the retrobulbar intraconal space, they are described as ovoid or round, lobulated when enlarged, well-circumscribed, and smoothly marginated lesions with homogeneous soft tissue density (Fig. 2). Microcalcifications (or phleboliths) and orbital bone expansion may be present. These findings are unusual, but best visualized by noncontrast CT using bone window algorithms [15,48]. Variable degrees of contrast enhancement are observed using single-phase contrast CT, probably related to variable scan times after contrast infusion. On multiphase dynamic contrast CT, orbital cavernous hemangiomas enhance poorly and heterogeneously in the early arterial and early venous phases because of their low-flow arterial supply (Fig. 3), analogous to the peripheral globular enhancement seen in hepatic cavernous hemangiomas. However, slow progressive accumulation of contrast continues within the dilated vascular spaces filling in centrally during the late venous phase. Subsequently, homogeneous contrast enhancement occurs and persists in the delayed equilibrium phases [2,3,47–49], correlating with late blood pool uptake in nuclear scintigraphy and delayed contrast pooling in angiography as described elsewhere in this article.

### MR imaging

Multiplanar spin echo T1-weighted imaging and fast spin echo T2-weighted imaging with the use of paramagnetic (gadolinium–diethylenetriamine penta-acetic acid [DTPA]) contrast enhancement and fat suppression MR pulse sequences are standard MR imaging protocols to study the orbit. Advances in MR imaging technology with higher field strengths (1.5–3.0 T) and an increased signal-to-noise ratio

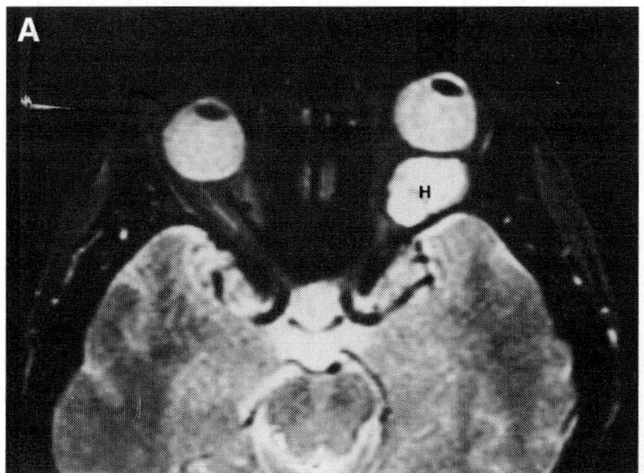


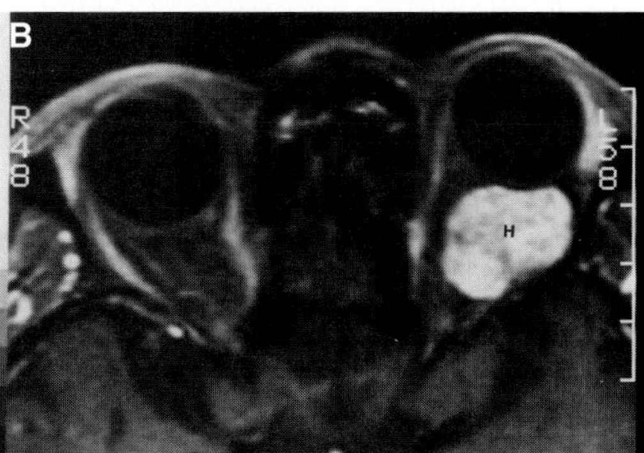


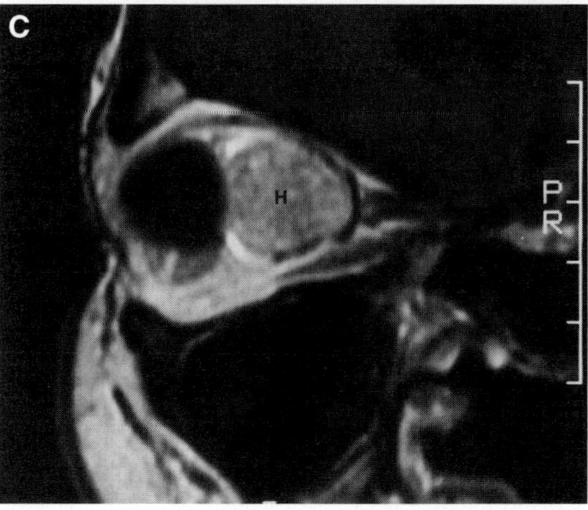


Fig. 4. Orbital cavernous hemangioma. Using single-phase contrast MR imaging, axial T2-weighted (*A*), axial T1-weighted (repetition time [TR]/echo time [TE]: 550/20 ms) post–gadolinium (Gd)-diethylenetriamine penta-acetic acid (DTPA) contrast fat-suppressed (*B*), and sagittal T1-weighted (TR/TE: 600/30 ms) post–Gd-DTPA contrast (*C*) MR imaging scans show an intraconal, lobulated, and well-defined mass exhibiting T2 hyperintensity and near-homogeneous contrast enhancement on T1-weighted imaging consistent with a pathologically proven left orbital cavernous hemangioma in a 51-year-old patient. (B *and* C *from* Mafee MF, Valvassori GE, Becker M. Imaging of the head and neck. Stuttgart (Germany): Thieme; 2004. p. 255; with permission.)

have allowed a decrease in slice thickness (3 mm), volume averaging artifact, and scan times, improving spatial and temporal resolution. In the past, the use of a surface coil was advocated for evaluating orbital lesions [60], but with higher field strengths, the head coil is now preferred to adequately cover the orbital apex using a 16- to 20-cm field of view, 256 × 256 matrix (512 × 512 matrix or 512 × 382 matrix at 3 T), and multiple excitations [48]. Combining these improvements in MR imaging with multiphase dynamic contrast MR scanning, orbital cavernous hemangiomas may be differentiated with virtually pathognomonic imaging features. Several multiphase dynamic contrast MR imaging protocols have been reported for studying hepatic [61–63] and orbital [23,51,52] cavernous hemangiomas. After all non-contrast MR scanning, an intravenous bolus of gadolinium-DTPA contrast (0.1 mmol/kg) is administered and multiple serial axial T1-weighted images are obtained throughout the arterial-venous delayed phases as described for multiphase dynamic contrast CT.

On MR imaging, orbital cavernous hemangiomas exhibit a morphology identical to that seen on CT as homogeneous and well-defined intraconal lesions (Figs. 4–6) but can also involve the orbital apex (Fig. 7) or extraconal space (Figs. 8 and 9). They appear hypointense to fat and isointense to muscle on T1-weighted imaging and hyperintense to muscle and fat on T2-weighted imaging (Figs. 5A and B, 6A and B, and 9A–C) [3,46,64,65]. Although noncontrast CT and MR imaging findings are nonspecific, noncontrast MR imaging may offer some advantage in the differentiation of orbital cavernous hemangiomas by demonstrating internal septations on T2-weighted imaging, a hypointense circumferential rim corresponding to the fibrous pseudocapsule, and chemical shift artifact in the frequency-encoded direction secondary to high water content within the lesion surrounded by orbital fat [3,23,46,65]. The multi-

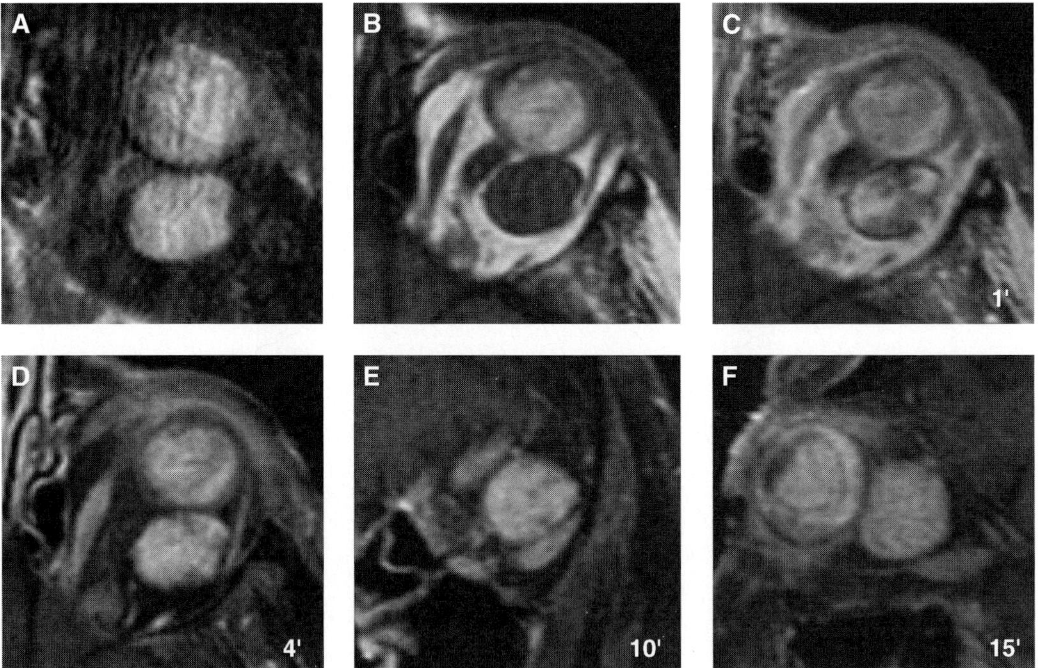


Fig. 5. Orbital cavernous hemangioma. Using multiphase dynamic contrast 1.5-T MR imaging, axial T2-weighted (TR/TE: 3500/82 ms) (*A*), axial T1-weighted (TR/TE: 450/14 ms) (*B*), axial T1-weighted (TR/TE: 450/14 ms) post–Gd-DTPA contrast (*C*), axial T1-weighted (TR/TE: 400/14 ms) post–Gd-DTPA contrast fat-suppressed (*D*), coronal T1-weighted (TR/TE: 450/20 ms) post–Gd-DTPA contrast fat-suppressed (*E*), and sagittal T1-weighted (TR/TE: 400/14 ms) post–Gd-DTPA contrast fat-suppressed (*F*) MR images demonstrate a pathologically proven intraconal orbital cavernous hemangioma. Heterogeneous contrast enhancement is observed in the early/late venous phase (1–4 min in *C* and *D*) with subsequent contrast filling and homogeneous enhancement by the late venous/delayed equilibrium phases (10 min in *E*, 15 min in *F*).

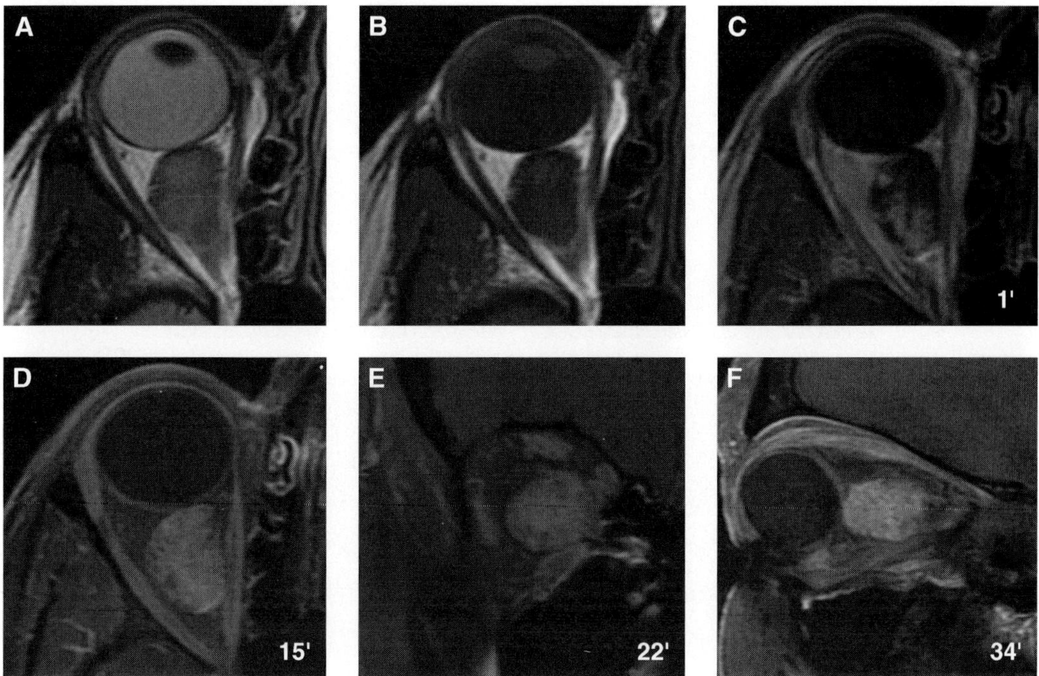


Fig. 6. Orbital cavernous hemangioma. Using multiphase dynamic contrast 3-T MR imaging, axial T2-weighted (TR/TE: 2566/88 ms) (*A*), axial T1-weighted (TR/TE: 400/12 ms) (*B*), axial T1-weighted (TR/TE: 400/12 ms) post–Gd-DTPA contrast (*C*), axial T1-weighted (TR/TE: 516/12 ms) post–Gd-DTPA contrast fat-suppressed (*D*), coronal T1-weighted (TR/TE: 600/12 ms) post–Gd-DTPA contrast fat-suppressed (*E*), and sagittal T1-weighted (TR/TE: 450/12 ms) post–Gd-DTPA contrast fat-suppressed (*F*) MR imaging scans demonstrate a presumed intraconal orbital cavernous hemangioma followed for several years in a 57-year-old patient. Heterogeneous contrast enhancement is observed in the early arterial/early venous phase (1 min in *C*) with accumulation of contrast and homogeneous enhancement by the late venous/delayed equilibrium phases (15 min in *D*). Homogeneous enhancement persists throughout the delayed equilibrium phases (22 min in *E*, 34 min in *F*).

phase dynamic contrast MR imaging findings parallel the multiphase dynamic contrast CT findings and confirm the diagnosis of orbital cavernous hemangiomas with patchy heterogeneous enhancement in the early arterial and early venous phases, contrast filling in centrally during the late venous phase, and persisting homogeneous enhancement in the delayed equilibrium phases (Figs. 5C–F, 6C–F, and Fig. 10) [23,51,52].

### *CT angiography and MR angiography and/or venography*

Dynamic CT angiography (CTA) and time-of-flight MR angiography (MRA) and/or MR venography (MRV) with maximum intensity projections are promising imaging modalities with the potential to replace conventional DSA in the evaluation of high-flow vascular lesions. In fact, at some institutions, improved CTA imaging with multidetector helical CT technology and three-dimensional arterial reconstruction has replaced conventional DSA in the primary screening of high-flow AVMs, carotid-cavernous fistulas, and aneurysms. Nevertheless, conventional DSA remains the "gold standard" and offers an expanding base of therapeutic options in the field of interventional neuroradiology. Delayed scanning may be performed with dynamic CTA to emulate multiphase dynamic contrast CT techniques for the evaluation of low-flow AVMs (cavernous hemangiomas), venous malformations, and vascular tumors. In contrast, orbital cavernous hemangiomas demonstrate no observable MRA or MRV flow enhancement, because the sensitivity is insufficient to detect low-velocity and delayed vascular flow through the lesion's small feeding arteries and dilated draining veins (Fig. 9D–F). Surprisingly, MRA flow enhance-

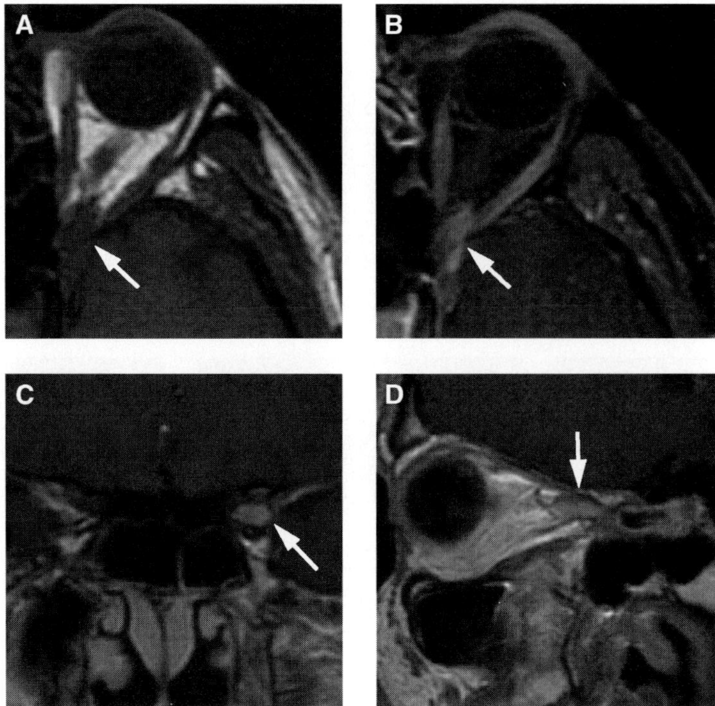


Fig. 7. Orbital apex cavernous hemangioma. Axial T1-weighted (TR/TE: 400/8 ms) (*A*), axial T1-weighted (TR/TE: 416/8 ms) post–Gd-DTPA contrast fat-suppressed (*B*), coronal T1-weighted (TR/TE: 500/20 ms) post–Gd-DTPA contrast (*C*), and sagittal T1-weighted (TR/TE: 400/14 ms) post–Gd-DTPA contrast (*D*) MR images demonstrate a small pathologically proven cavernous hemangioma within the left orbital apex (*arrows*). The lesion shows contrast enhancement and extends into the optic canal inferior to the optic nerve (*C*, *D*).

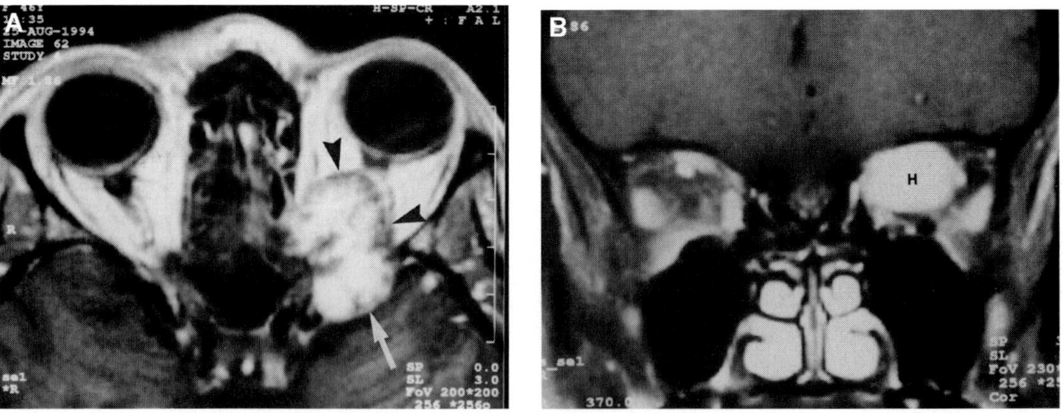


Fig. 8. Orbital cavernous hemangioma with extraconal extension. Axial T1-weighted post–Gd-DTPA contrast (*A*) and coronal T1-weighted post–Gd-DTPA contrast (*B*) MR images demonstrate a large contrast-enhancing intraconal mass (*black arrowheads*, H) in the left orbit with atypical extension into the posterior extraconal space (*white arrow*) consistent with a pathologically proven cavernous hemangioma in a 46-year-old patient. (*A* courtesy of R. Hewlett, MD, Cape Town, South Africa.)

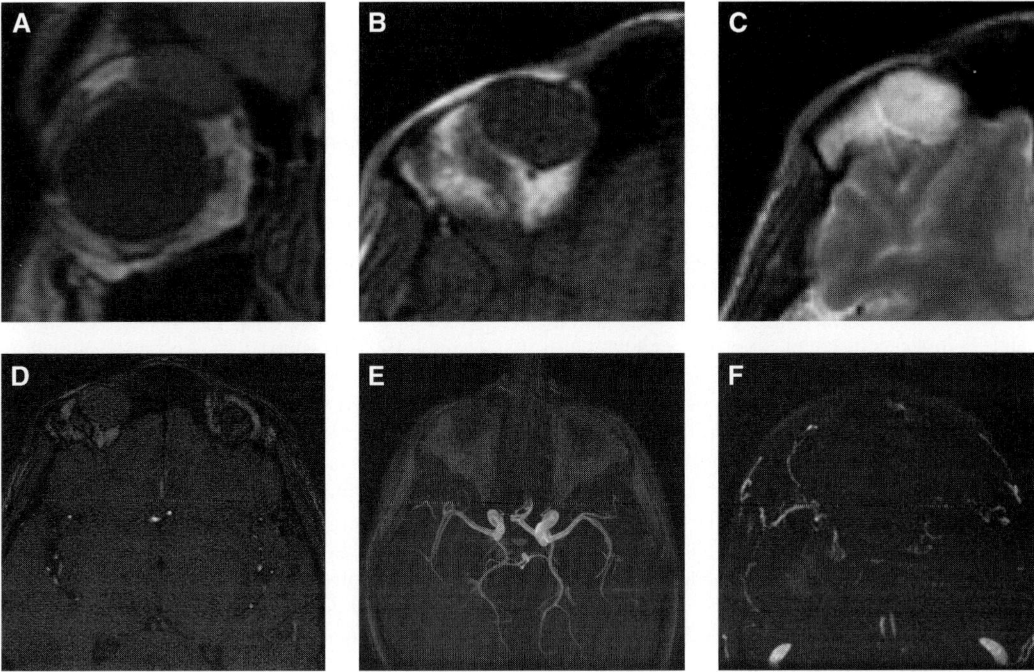

Fig. 9. Extraconal orbital cavernous hemangioma. Coronal T1-weighted (TR/TE: 666/20 ms) (*A*), axial T1-weighted (TR/TE: 316/8 ms) (*B*), and axial T2-weighted (TR/TE: 4000/88 ms) (*C*) MR imaging scans demonstrate a pathologically proven extraconal cavernous hemangioma in the right orbit. Axial three-dimensional (3D) time-of-flight (TOF) MR angiography source image (*D*), axial 3D TOF collapsed MR angiography image (*E*), and axial two-dimensional TOF flight collapsed MR venography image (*F*) show no detectable arterial or venous flow enhancement. The MR venography was obtained with the patient in the prone position to evaluate the possibility of a distensible orbital varix.

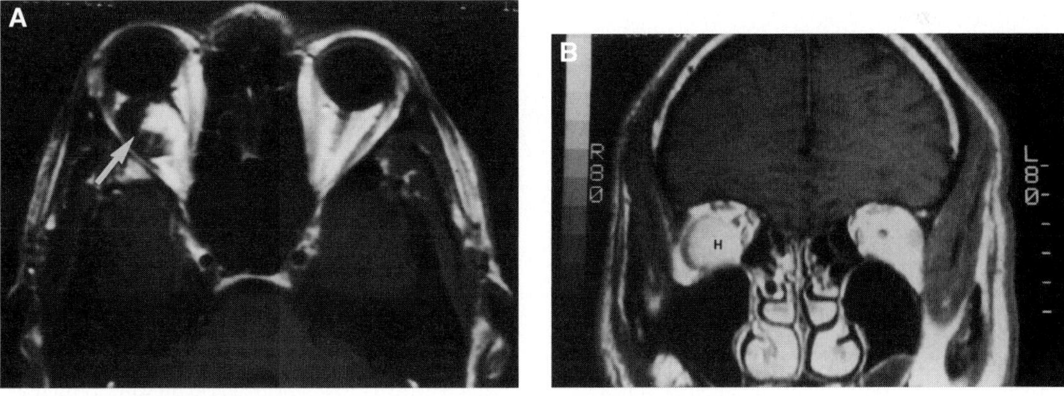

Fig. 10. Orbital cavernous hemangioma. Using multiphase dynamic contrast MR imaging, axial T1-weighted post–Gd-DTPA) contrast (*A*) and coronal T1-weighted post–Gd-DTPA contrast (*B*) MR imaging scans demonstrate a right intraconal mass (*arrow*, H) with partial and heterogeneous contrast enhancement in the early arterial/early venous phase (1 min in *A*). Subsequent contrast filling and homogeneous enhancement in the late venous/delayed equilibrium phases (10 min in *B*), compatible with a presumed orbital cavernous hemangioma. (A *from* Mafee MF, Valvassori GE, Becker M. Imaging of the head and neck. Stuttgart (Germany): Thieme; 2004. p. 255; with permission.)

ment is even absent in some high-flow vascular tumors (capillary hemangiomas and hemangiopericytomas). A prominent ectopic draining vein may be identified using MR venography and suggests the presence of a venous malformation.

*Ultrasonography*

Before the advent of CT and MR imaging, orbital cavernous hemangiomas were detected, localized, and diagnosed with a high degree of accuracy using A- and B-mode ultrasound. A-mode echographic patterns are specific and reveal well-defined borders related to the fibrous pseudocapsule (distinct surface spikes), moderate to high internal reflectivity from the surfaces of large vascular spaces (80%–90% spike height), moderate acoustic attenuation from intravascular blood (decreasing spikes posteriorly), and a honeycomb-like structure (alternating long and short spikes) [66]. In fact, A-mode echographic patterns have been reported to be nearly pathognomonic for orbital cavernous hemangiomas and venous-lymphatic malformations (lymphangiomas), with diagnostic hypoechoic regions corresponding to the vascular or wider lymphatic channels, respectively [55,56,67].

B-mode ultrasound supplements A-mode echography by offering a visual image with moderate spatial resolution, characterizing the size and location of the lesion, and differentiating encapsulated masses from infiltrative lesions. The B-mode imaging findings of orbital cavernous hemangiomas include a round well-defined outline, sharp anterior acoustic border, and low to moderate acoustic absorption (moderate to high sound transmission) [56,68].

Color Doppler ultrasound is a valuable adjunct to B-mode ultrasound in the evaluation and differentiation of orbital vascular lesions by detecting and quantifying blood flow. Low velocity or absent flow is consistent with more benign lesions, such as orbital cavernous hemangiomas and venous-lymphatic malformations (lymphangiomas) [69–73]. In contrast, orbital vascular tumors (capillary hemangiomas and hemangiopericytomas) and other less benign or malignant orbital tumors (schwannomas, meningiomas, fibrosarcomas, choroidal melanomas, and metastases) demonstrate moderate to marked vascularity with high-velocity flow on color Doppler imaging, but variable nonspecific reflective patterns on conventional ultrasound [69,72–74]. Reversal of high-velocity Doppler flow in the superior ophthalmic vein suggests the presence of a carotid-cavernous fistula, whereas postural or Valsalva-induced flow reversal is more compatible with distensible venous malformations (varices) [72,75,76]. In addition, color Doppler ultrasound may localize vasculature for surgical planning, guide endovascular or percutaneous embolization, and evaluate radiation treatment efficacy in high-flow malignant lesions [73].

*Nuclear scintigraphy*

Technetium-99m–labeled red blood cell scintigraphy is an established diagnostic method for hepatic cavernous hemangiomas, approaching 94% sensitivity and 100% specificity [77]. Recent studies have corroborated these findings with respect to orbital cavernous hemangiomas using three-phase radionuclide scintigraphy [56,77–81]. No abnormal radiotracer uptake is seen in the dynamic angiographic phase (< 1 minute), and variable mild radiotracer uptake may be observed during the early blood pool phase (1–5 minutes). After a delay (20 minutes–2 hours), prominent focal uptake is identified during the late blood pool phase after intravenous infusion. This perfusion–late blood pool mismatch is a characteristic finding of cavernous hemangiomas because of their low-flow arterial supply [80]. In addition, because the resolution of planar imaging presents challenges in diagnosing orbital cavernous hemangiomas attributable to their small size and high background of intravascular activity, some have advocated single photon emission computed tomography (SPECT) imaging for enhanced sensitivity [78].

Technetium-99m–labeled red blood cell scintigraphy can assist in differentiating between relatively avascular lesions (venous-lymphatic malformations or lymphangiomas, rhabdomyosarcomas, lymphomas, and pseudotumors) and early-uptake/moderate-flow lesions (meningiomas, schwannomas, neurofibromas, malignant fibrous histiocytomas, and metastatic melanomas) that may simulate the late-uptake/low-flow orbital cavernous hemangiomas on CT or MR imaging, especially when multiphase dynamic contrast scanning is not available. Even more dramatic than early-uptake/moderate-flow lesions, high-flow vascular tumors (capillary hemangiomas and hemangiopericytomas) and high-flow AVMs are expected to demonstrate intense radiotracer uptake in both perfusion phases (angiographic and early blood pool phases) with no evidence of a perfusion–late blood pool mismatch. However, in diagnosing orbital cavernous hemangiomas using nuclear scintigraphy, the specificity may be decreased in comparison to that of hepatic cavernous hemangiomas, because a subset of low-flow orbital vascular tumors, venous malformations, and AVMs may present as false-positive findings, notably if angiographic uptake is absent, with

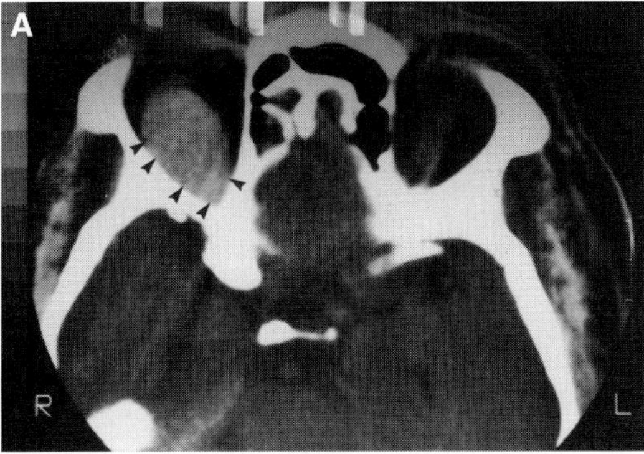


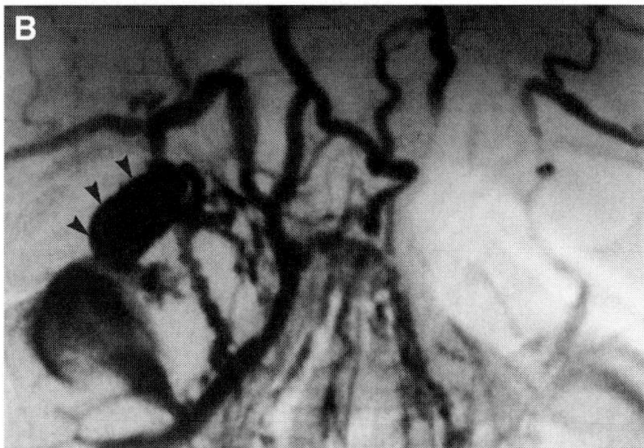


Fig. 11. Venous malformation (orbital varix). (*A*) Axial postcontrast CT scan shows a well-defined and homogeneously enhancing mass (*arrowheads*) in the superior intraconal space simulating an orbital cavernous hemangioma but consistent with a pathologically proven orbital varix. (*B*) Venography in another patient confirms the massive dilatation of orbital veins consistent with an orbital varix (*arrowheads*). (*A* courtesy of J.D. Bullock, MD, Dayton, OH.)

early blood pool uptake as the only discriminating factor.

*Digital subtraction angiography*

Because orbital cavernous hemangiomas may escape angiographic detection entirely, conventional DSA is rarely required for preoperative evaluation or embolization. Usually, incidental findings on carotid angiography, displacement of the ophthalmic artery, small feeding arteries, a modest to faint tumor blush, and dilated draining veins may usually be identified [1,56,82,83]. Despite reports of being angiographically occult with limited opacification or blush [12,13], prolonged injection angiography has been

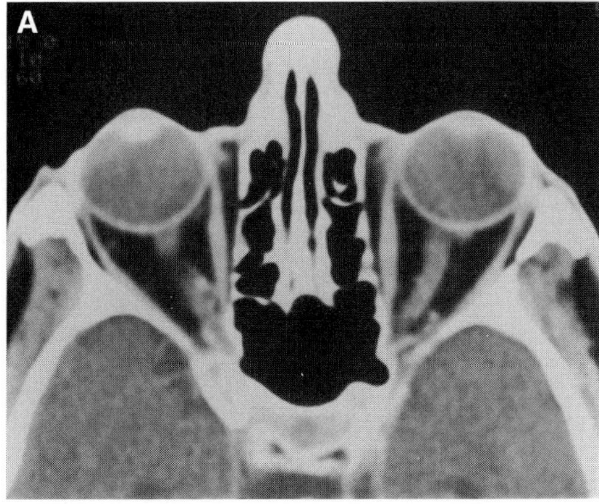


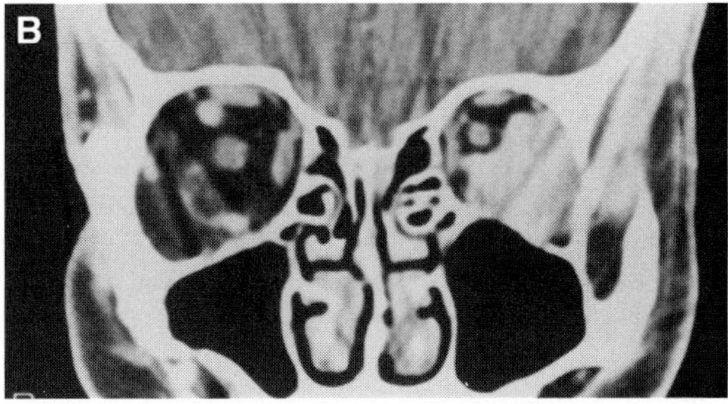


Fig. 12. Distensible venous malformation. (*A*) Axial postcontrast CT scan shows normal orbital anatomy with no evidence of an orbital lesion during imaging with the patient in the supine position. (*B*) Coronal postcontrast CT scan demonstrates a large well-defined mass with interval contrast filling and expansion as a result of imaging with the patient in the prone position, compatible with a distensible venous malformation. (*From* Mafee MF, Valvassori GE, Becker M. Imaging of the head and neck. Stuttgart (Germany): Thieme; 2004. p. 259; with permission.)

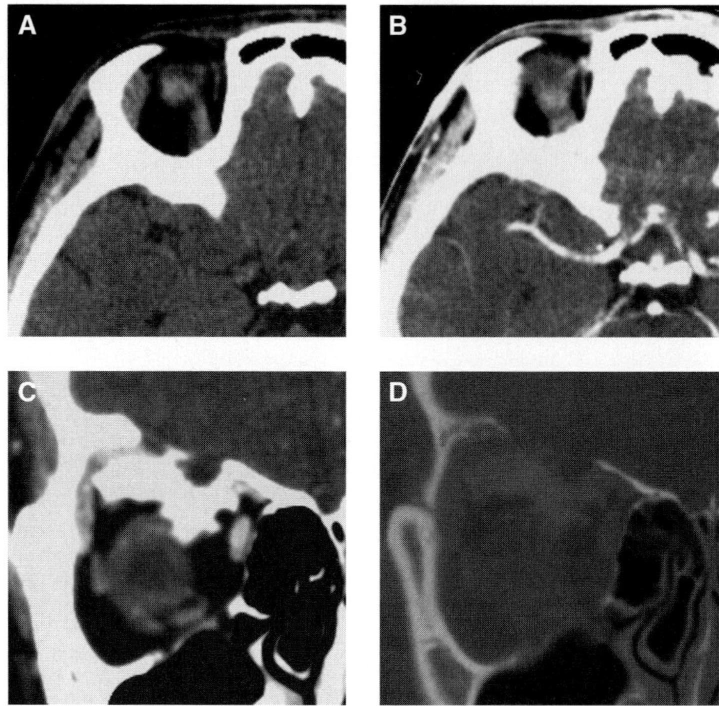


Fig. 13. Distensible venous malformation. Axial precontrast (*A*) and axial postcontrast (*B*) CT scans show no evidence of a contrast-enhancing lesion during imaging with the patient in the supine position. *C, D*, Coronal postcontrast CT scans demonstrate an enhancing orbital lesion, induced with prone positioning, along with bone erosion of the adjacent superior orbital rim (*D*).

shown to increase detection sensitivity of intracranial and orbital cavernous hemangiomas [20,84], with small areas of contrast pooling or "puddles" accumulating in the delayed arterial phase [2,3,57,83]. This finding allows differentiation from the early arterial enhancing vascular tumors (capillary hemangiomas and hemangiopericytomas), high-flow AVMs, aneurysms, and carotid-cavernous fistulas with prominent feeding arteries, early draining veins, and a marked tumor blush. Other simulating orbital tumors (meningiomas, schwannomas, neurofibromas, malignant fibrous histiocytomas, fibrosarcomas, and metastases) also demonstrate increased arterial vascularity relative to orbital cavernous hemangiomas, although with a more extended or delayed tumor blush [1,15]. Interestingly, intraosseous cavernous hemangiomas involving the bony orbit demonstrate greater vascularity than intraconal lesions through supply from the branches of the external carotid artery, explaining the role of endovascular embolization in this subset before surgical resection [57,85].

Venography has also been used with mixed results, because low blood flow through the lesion facilitates retrograde opacification of dilated draining veins and the cavernous hemangioma itself. Nevertheless, mass effect and displacement of the superior ophthalmic vein may be the only finding [82,83,86]. Although venography can aid in differentiating orbital cavernous hemangiomas from distensible venous malformations (varices) (Fig. 11), this is rather easily done using postural or Valsalva-induced clinical and cross-sectional imaging findings (Figs. 12 and 13) [57].

## Discussion

### *Diagnostic imaging*

The differentiation of orbital cavernous hemangiomas from related vascular malformations and vascular tumors can be diagnostically challenging based on imaging criteria alone. High-flow vascular malformations (AVMs, carotid-cavernous fistulas, and aneurysms) are distinctly recognized by their serpiginous vasculature or nidus with early enhancing feeding arteries and draining veins on CT angiography, MR angiography, and conventional DSA (Fig. 14). Similar findings are appreciated on noncontrast MR imaging because of characteristic flow voids. Using multiphase dynamic contrast CT and/or MR imaging, these lesions demonstrate early arterial phase enhancement and early venous washout [1]. Although high-flow vascular malformations are

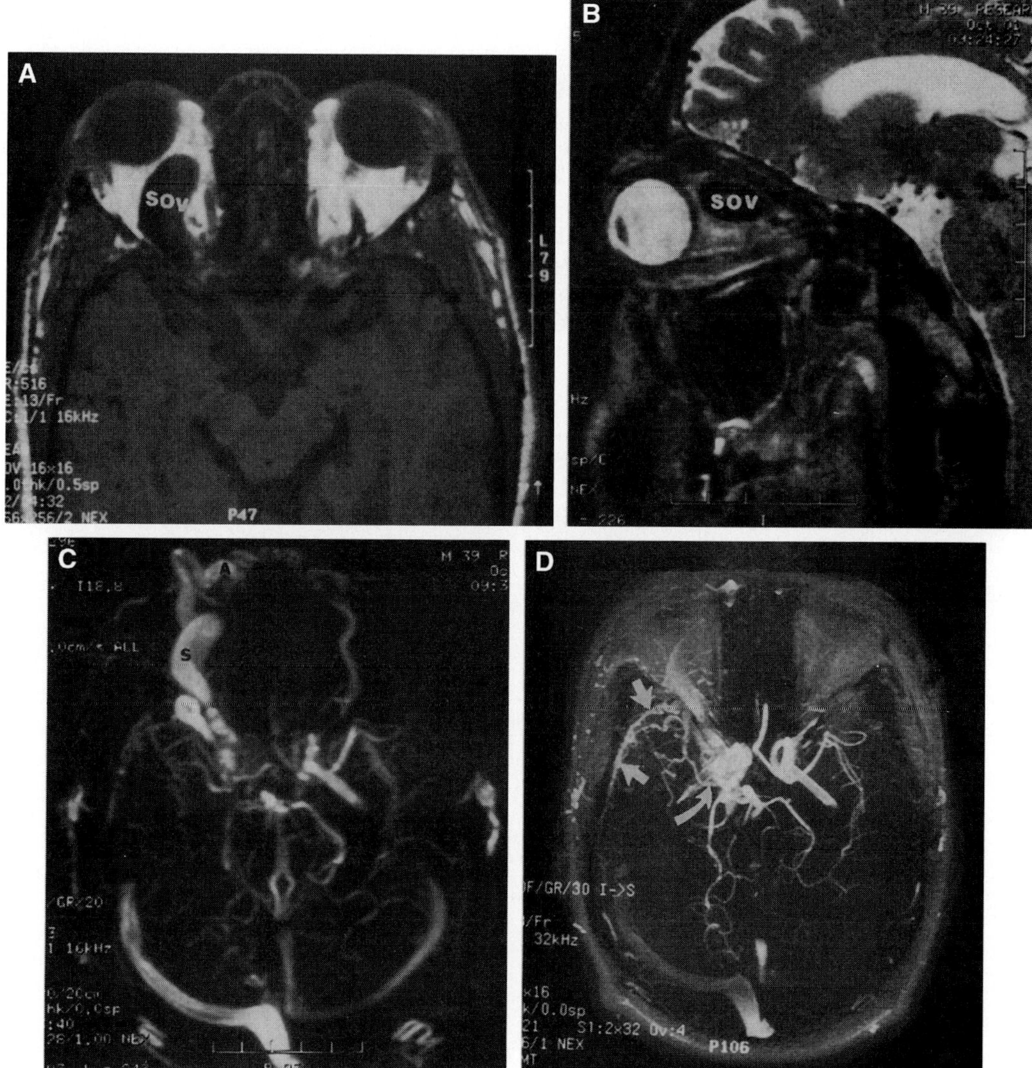


Fig. 14. Dural cavernous sinus vascular malformation. T1-weighted (TR/TE: 516/13 ms) (*A*) and T2-weighted (TR/TE: 3000/15 ms) (*B*) MR images show a large superior ophthalmic vein (SOV). (*C*) Three-dimensional (3D) phase contrast collapsed MRA image shows a large superior ophthalmic vein (S) and large angular vein (A). (*D*) Axial 3D time-of-flight collapsed MRA image shows abnormal dural vessels (*straight arrows*) and increased vascularity adjacent to the right cavernous sinus along with a large feeding vessel (*curved arrow*). (*From* Mafee MF, Inoue Y, Mafee RF. Ocular and orbital imaging. Neuroimaging Clin North Am 1996;6(2):291–318.)

easily distinguished by morphology and imaging features, an ophthalmic artery aneurysm can mimic an intraconal cavernous hemangioma in the absence of multiphase dynamic contrast scanning (Fig. 15).

Orbital vascular tumors (capillary hemangiomas, hemangiopericytomas, hemangioendotheliomas, and orbital extension of angiofibromas) appear morphologically irregular, less defined, and more commonly extraconal in comparison to orbital cavernous hemangiomas, but these criteria are not absolute, and noncontrast or single-phase contrast CT findings are nonspecific. In fact, orbital cavernous hemangiomas may also occur or extend into the extraconal space (see Figs. 8 and 9). Despite the sensitivity of MR imaging to detect the internal architecture of capillary hemangiomas and the infiltration of adjacent tissues, MR angiography has proved to be nonspecific in depicting the vascular nature of these lesions. Multiphase dynamic contrast CT and/or MR imaging may prove to be more useful in differentiating capillary hemangiomas from simulating lesions by demonstrating their intense vascularity and rapid contrast enhancement in the early arterial phase and/or early venous phase (Fig. 16). Aggressive vascular tumors, such as hemangiopericytomas are notorious for resembling orbital cavernous hemangiomas as homogeneous masses with or without associated bone erosion (Fig. 17A and B). Similar to capillary hemangiomas, hemangiopericytomas are described as having a prominent arterial supply and an intense tumor blush on conventional DSA (Fig. 17C), which translates into rapid contrast enhancement in the early arterial/early venous phase using multiphase dynamic contrast CT and/or MR imaging [3,15]. Capillary hemangiomas and hemangiopericytomas exhibit marked early arterial phase/early venous phase enhancement followed by rapid washout by the delayed equilibrium phases, as opposed to the findings for orbital cavernous hemangiomas [15,47]. Color Doppler ultrasound and conventional DSA have also been used to differentiate these lesions based on vascularity as described [1,69].

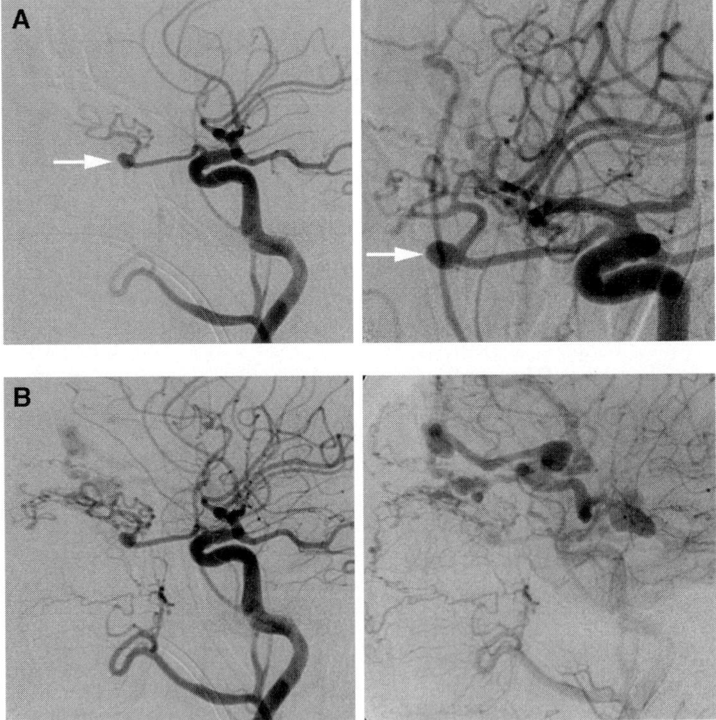


Fig. 15. Ophthalmic artery aneurysm and high-flow AVM. (*A*) Lateral and oblique DSA images from a right common carotid artery injection demonstrate an aneurysm (*arrows*) arising from the ophthalmic artery. (*B*) Two serial DSA images show early contrast opacification of several feeding arteries and draining veins just distal to the aneurysm consistent with a high-flow AVM.

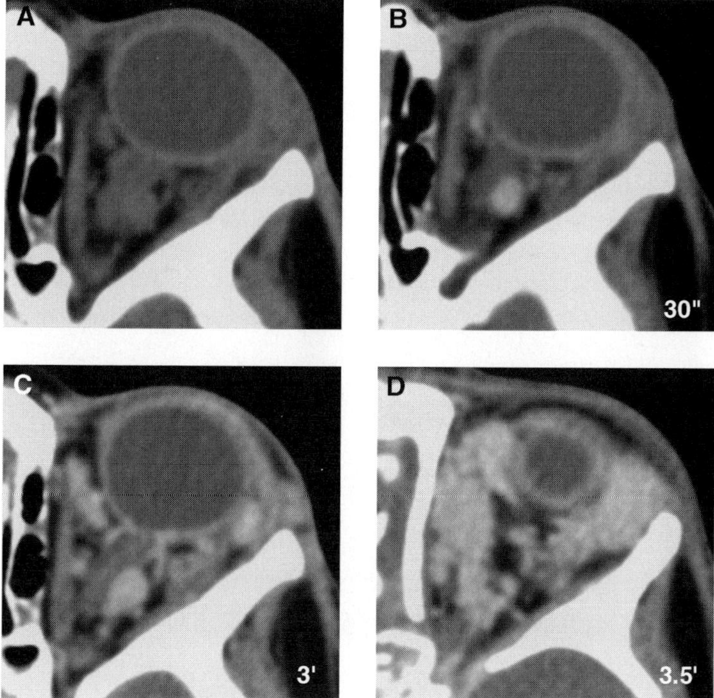


Fig. 16. Capillary hemangioma. Using multiphase dynamic contrast CT, axial precontrast (*A*) and serial axial postcontrast (*B–D*) CT scans demonstrate an irregular and infiltrative mass exhibiting rapid contrast enhancement in the early arterial/early venous phase (30 seconds in *B*) compatible with a presumed capillary hemangioma in a 9-month-old boy. Complete homogeneous enhancement is seen by the start of the late venous phase (3–3.5 min in *C* and *D*).

Some benign and malignant orbital tumors (meningiomas, schwannomas, neurofibromas, malignant fibrous histiocytomas, fibrosarcomas, and metastases) may appear morphologically identical to orbital cavernous hemangiomas on noncontrast or single-phase contrast CT and/or MR imaging. Using conventional DSA or multiphase dynamic contrast imaging, these moderately vascular simulating lesions are also excluded by their homogeneous enhancement patterns in the early arterial phase and/or early venous phase, extended angiographic tumor blush (probably correlating with late venous phase enhancement), and eventual washout by the delayed equilibrium phases.

A subset of type 1 (no flow) venous-lymphatic and type 2 (venous flow) venous malformations can present some difficulty in differentiating type 3 (arterial low flow) AVMs or cavernous hemangiomas. Typical venous-lymphatic malformations (lymphangiomas) are extraconal, heterogeneously infiltrating, and multiloculated hemorrhagic lesions that are easily distinguishable based on T1 and T2 hyperintense MR imaging findings [3,15]. Despite classification as no-flow vascular malformations, venous-lymphatic malformations (lymphangiomas) are embryologically derived from a venous origin, explaining the occasional delayed contrast enhancement pattern seen more consistently in pure venous malformations (varices) and orbital cavernous hemangiomas during the early venous phase and/or late venous phase, although orbital cavernous hemangiomas may be separated by their initial patchy heterogeneous enhancement [2,3,47,48]. A few venous-lymphatic malformations (Fig. 18) and most venous malformations (Fig. 19A–C) also mimic orbital cavernous hemangiomas with respect to morphology on noncontrast or single-phase contrast CT and/or MR imaging [37], requiring multiphase dynamic contrast imaging for accurate diagnosis. The multiphase dynamic contrast CT and/or MR imaging technique may require some cautious modification to demonstrate complete washout from these venous-lymphatic and venous malformations (Fig. 19D–F) during the

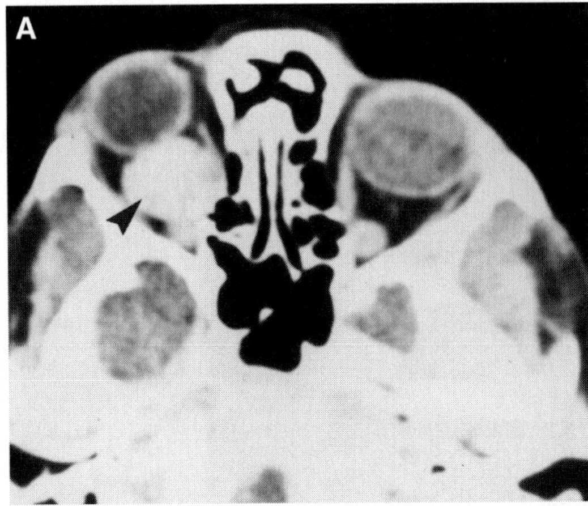


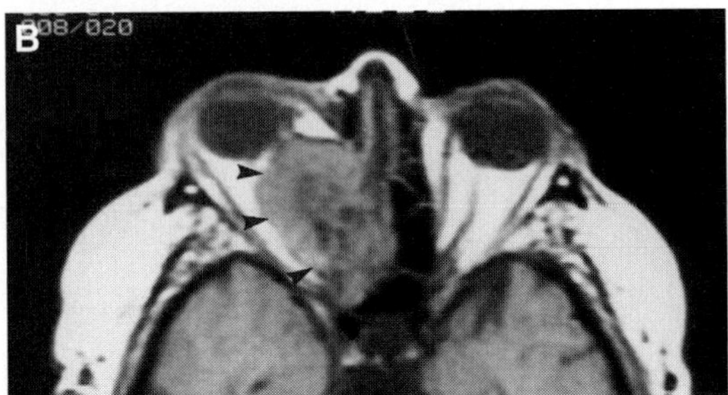


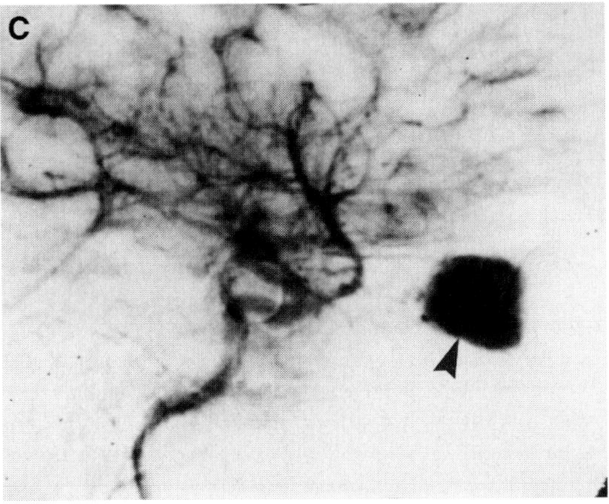


Fig. 17. Hemangiopericytoma. (*A*) Axial postcontrast CT scan shows a well-defined homogeneously enhancing mass (*arrowhead*) simulating an orbital cavernous hemangioma but pathologically proven to be a hemangiopericytoma. (*B*) Axial T1-weighted post–Gd-DTPA contrast MR image demonstrates a more aggressive pathologically proven hemangiopericytoma (*arrowheads*) invading the right ethmoid air cells. (*From* Mafee MF, Valvassori GE, Becker M. Imaging of the head and neck. Stuttgart (Germany): Thieme; 2004. p. 263; with permission.) (*C*) Lateral DSA image from a follow-up right carotid injection in the same patient (*A*) demonstrates prominent feeding arteries and intense tumor blush (*arrowhead*) consistent with a hemangiopericytoma. (*B* and *C from* Mafee MF, Valvassori GE, Becker M. Imaging of the head and neck. Stuttgart (Germany): Thieme; 2004. p. 262; with permission.)

delayed equilibrium phase (>20–30-minute delay) versus the persisting homogeneous enhancement of orbital cavernous hemangiomas.

Because orbital veins are susceptible to venous pressures as a result of the absence of valves, type 2 distensible venous malformations and combined type 1 and type 2 distensible venous-lymphatic malformations may be identified using prone or Valsalva-induced expansion on additional CT and/or MR imaging (see Figs. 11–13) [2,3], providing a valuable technique to differentiate these lesions from orbital cavernous hemangiomas. Multiphase dynamic contrast CT and/or MR imaging remains the best approach to differentiate a subset of simulating type 1 venous-lymphatic and type 2 nondistensible venous malformations that demonstrate delayed enhancement patterns but do not expand using prone or Valsalva induction. In the past, color Doppler ultrasound and conventional DSA and/or venography have also been used in the diagnosis of distensible venous malformations as described [72,76].

Orbital lymphomas and pseudotumors may also morphologically mimic orbital cavernous hemangiomas on noncontrast or single-phase contrast CT and/

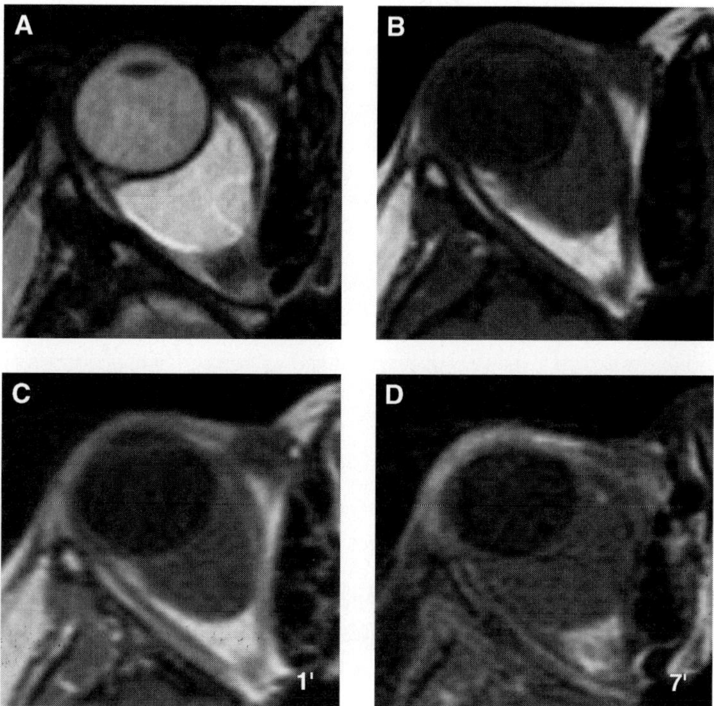


Fig. 18. Venous-lymphatic malformation (lymphangioma). Axial T2-weighted (TR/TE: 4200/99 ms) (*A*), axial T1-weighted (TR/TE: 500/14 ms) (*B*), axial T1-weighted (TR/TE: 500/14 ms) post–Gd-DTPA contrast (*C*), and axial T1-weighted (TR/TE: 400/9 ms) post–Gd-DTPA contrast fat-suppressed (*D*) MR images demonstrate a well-defined and homogeneous intraconal lesion simulating an orbital cavernous hemangioma, but more compatible with a venous-lymphatic malformation in an 8-year-old girl. The lesion shows absent or delayed vascular flow with no evidence of contrast enhancement in the early arterial/early venous phase (1 min in *C*) and late venous phase (7 min in *D*).

or MR imaging. Because these lesions are hypovascular, a delayed contrast enhancement pattern can occur similar to venous-lymphatic and venous malformations. Multiphase dynamic contrast CT and/or MR imaging again facilitates the differentiation of these lesions from orbital cavernous hemangiomas, which uniquely exhibit a persistent homogeneous enhancement pattern throughout the delayed equilibrium phases without washout.

### *Treatment*

Surgical treatment of orbital cavernous hemangiomas is mandated when clinical symptoms progress beyond exophthalmos as described, especially in cases of optic nerve compression. The most common approach is the lateral zygomatic-frontal orbitotomy or modified Krönlein procedure, because cavernous hemangiomas are predisposed to form in the lateral intraconal space. Despite the occasional complication of lateral rectus palsy, the modified lateral approach allows the greatest visualization or surgical exploration of the intraconal space and is a safer alternative to the transcranial approach [15,87]. Deeper lesions involving the orbital apex or within the optic canal require a transcranial (orbitocranial) approach with deroofing of the optic canal [13,16]. The transcranial approach is also indicated for lesions superior and medial to the optic nerve because it provides a superior exposure and cosmetic result but with increased morbidity. A less common anterior or transconjunctival approach is used mostly for extraconal lesions [35,88,89]. Dissection from the surrounding soft tissues is assisted by the well-encapsulated and isolated nature of orbital cavernous hemangiomas as opposed to orbital venous-lymphatic malformations, which are similar in appearance, but arborize into adjacent tissues [37]. En bloc removal of orbital cavernous hemangiomas is preferred when possible to limit residual and/or recurrent tissue and intra-

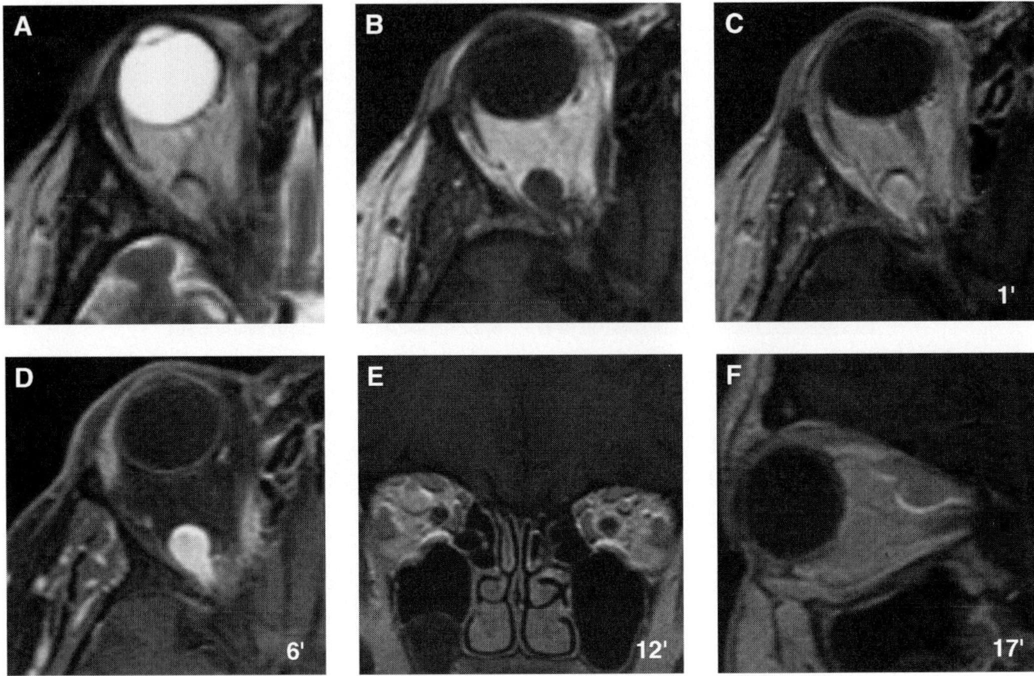


Fig. 19. Venous malformation (orbital varix). Using multiphase dynamic contrast 1.5-T MR imaging, axial T2-weighted (TR/TE: 5000/105 ms) (*A*), axial T1-weighted (TR/TE: 450/14 ms) (*B*), axial T1-weighted (TR/TE: 450/14 ms) post–Gd-DTPA contrast (*C*), axial T1-weighted (TR/TE: 600/9 ms) post–Gd-DTPA contrast fat-suppressed (*D*), coronal T1-weighted (TR/TE: 500/20 ms) post–Gd-DTPA contrast (*E*), and sagittal T1-weighted (TR/TE: 400/13 ms) post–Gd-DTPA contrast (*F*) MR images demonstrate a small well-defined and homogeneous intraconal lesion simulating an orbital cavernous hemangioma but more compatible with a venous malformation. The lesion shows homogeneous enhancement in the early arterial/early venous phase (1 min in *C*) and late venous phase (6 min in *D*) with persisting enhancement in the delayed equilibrium phases (12 min in *E*; 17 min in *F*). *E*, Lesion appears symmetric in position to the contralateral left superior ophthalmic vein.

operative hemorrhage [23], which is more problematic in deep lesions involving the orbital apex (Fig. 20). Although intraoperative bleeding from these vascular lesions may be more than expected, active arterial bleeding is unusual with hemostasis, and exsanguination is easily achieved because of their low-flow state [14,20].

Endovascular embolization techniques have been described for several high-flow vascular malformations and vascular tumors of the orbit secondary to promising advances in the field of interventional neuroradiology [85,90–92]. Excellent outcomes have been the standard with posttraumatic carotid cavernous fistulas, intracranial high-flow AVMs, and aneurysms [1]. However, treatment with embolization alone of low-flow vascular malformations, similar to orbital cavernous hemangiomas, is improbable because of the inaccessibility of small feeding arteries and multiple collateral pathways available for recanalization. Nevertheless, embolization of an intraosseous cavernous hemangioma has been reported prior to surgical resection using Gelfoam (Pharmacia and Upjohn Co., Kalamazoo, Missouri) material for homeostasis and cyanoacrylic for superselectively occluding the proximal feeding arteries. In select cases, presurgical embolization can decrease the arterial supply to the lesion, facilitating resection by reducing intraoperative time and blood loss. Conversely, because the end point of embolization is no longer complete vascular occlusion, surgery may reduce the complications of embolization, such as stroke, retinal ischemia, and vision loss [85]. In exceptional cases in which both embolization and surgery may be unsuccessful in treating symptomatic lesions because of inaccessibility or intraoperative blood loss, stereotactic radiosurgery has been reported to be successful

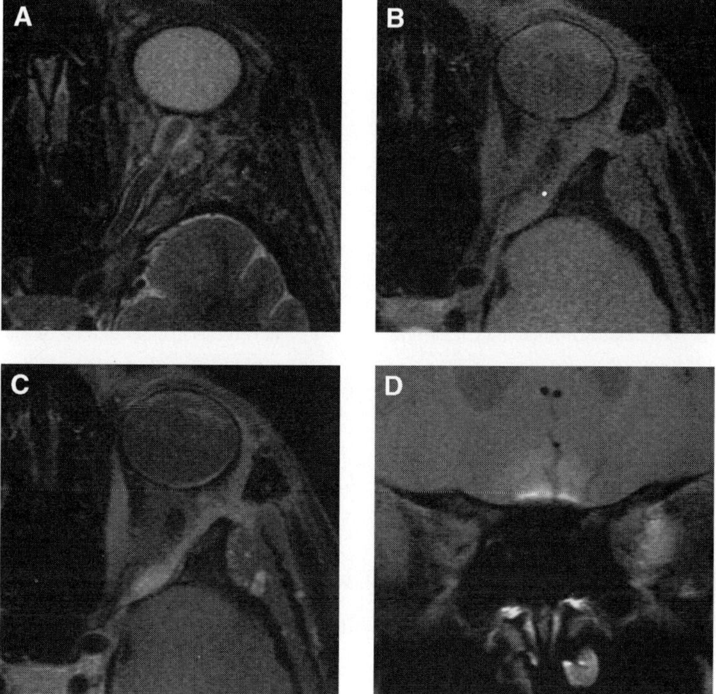


Fig. 20. Residual orbital cavernous hemangioma. Using single-phase contrast 3-T MR imaging, axial T2-weighted (TR/TE: 5300/108 ms) (*A*), axial T1-weighted (TR/TE: 500/22 ms) fat-suppressed (*B*), axial T1-weighted (TR/TE: 500/22 ms) post–Gd-DTPA contrast fat-suppressed (*C*), and coronal T1-weighted (TR/TE: 566/22 ms) post–Gd-DTPA contrast fat-suppressed (*D*) MR images demonstrate a small contrast-enhancing lesion (*C*, *D*) in the left orbital apex consistent with a residual cavernous hemangioma after surgical resection.

in treating cavernous hemangiomas involving the orbit and cavernous sinus [93].

## Summary

The histopathologic and diagnostic imaging characteristics of orbital cavernous hemangioma are compatible with its classification as a type 3 low-flow AVM. Orbital cavernous hemangiomas can be diagnosed with specific CT and/or MR imaging findings, especially using multiphase dynamic contrast scanning, allowing differentiation from simulating vascular malformations, vascular tumors, and other orbital tumors.

## Acknowledgments

The authors wish to thank the Departments of Radiology and Ophthalmology at the University of Illinois at Chicago Hospital, for great assistance in preparing this manuscript, specifically Dr. Galdino Valvassori, Dr. Deepak Edwards, Dr. Nikhil Balakrishnan, Yassir Aich, and Aura Smith. This work was approved by the Institutional Review Board of the University of Illinois at Chicago.

## References

[1] Tan WS, Wilbur AC, Mafee MF. The role of the neuroradiologist in vascular disorders involving the orbit. Radiol Clin N Am 1987;25(4):849–61.

[2] Rootman J. Vascular malformations of the orbit: hemodynamic concepts. Orbit 2003;22(2):103–20.

[3] Bilaniuk LT. Orbital vascular lesions. Role of imaging. Radiol Clin N Am 1999;37(1):169–83.

[4] Harris GJ. Orbital vascular malformations: a consensus statement on terminology and its clinical implications. Orbital Society. Am J Ophthalmol 1999;127(4): 453–5.

[5] Moss HM. Expanding lesions of the orbit. A clinical study of 230 consecutive cases. Am J Ophthalmol 1962;54:761–70.

[6] Reese AB. Tumors of the eye. Hagerstown (MD): Harper and Row; 1976.
[7] Kopelow SM, Foos RY, Straatsma BR, et al. Cavernous hemangioma of the orbit. Int Ophthalmol Clin 1971;11(3):113–24.
[8] Shields JA, Bakewell B, Augsburger JJ, et al. Classification and incidence of space-occupying lesions of the orbit. A survey of 645 biopsies. Arch Ophthalmol 1984;102(11):1606–11.
[9] Harris GJ, Jakobiec FA. Cavernous hemangioma of the orbit: a clinicopathologic analysis of sixty-six cases. In: Jakobiec FA, editor. Ocular and adnexal tumors. Birmingham: Aesculapius Publishing Co.; 1978. p. 741–81.
[10] Kennedy RE. An evaluation of 820 orbital cases. Trans Am Ophthalmol Soc 1984;82:134–57.
[11] Gunalp I, Gunduz K. Vascular tumors of the orbit. Doc Ophthalmol 1995;89(4):337–45.
[12] Harris GJ, Jakobiec FA. Cavernous hemangioma of the orbit. J Neurosurg 1979;51(2):219–28.
[13] McNab AA, Wright JE. Cavernous haemangiomas of the orbit. Aust NZ J Ophthalmol 1989;17(4):337–45.
[14] Ruchman MC, Flanagan J. Cavernous hemangiomas of the orbit. Ophthalmology 1983;90(11):1328–36.
[15] Mafee MF, Putterman A, Valvassori GE, et al. Orbital space-occupying lesions: role of computed tomography and magnetic resonance imaging. An analysis of 145 cases. Radiol Clin N Am 1987;25(3):529–59.
[16] Costa e Silva I, Symon L. Cavernous hemangioma of the optic canal. Report of two cases. J Neurosurg 1984; 60(4):838–41.
[17] Brown GC, Shields JA. Amaurosis fugax secondary to presumed cavernous hemangioma of the orbit. Ann Ophthalmol 1981;13(10):1205–9.
[18] Bradbury PG, Levy IS, McDonald WI. Transient uniocular visual loss on deviation of the eye in association with intraorbital tumours. J Neurol Neurosurg Psychiatry 1987;50(5):615–9.
[19] Orcutt JC, Tucker WM, Mills RP, et al. Gaze-evoked amaurosis. Ophthalmology 1987;94(3):213–8.
[20] Yamasaki T, Handa H, Yamashita J, et al. Intracranial and orbital cavernous angiomas. A review of 30 cases. J Neurosurg 1986;64(2):197–208.
[21] Acciarri N, Padovani R, Giulioni M, et al. Intracranial and orbital cavernous angiomas: a review of 74 surgical cases. Br J Neurosurg 1993;7(5):529–39.
[22] Zenobii M, Galzio RJ, Lucantoni D, et al. Spontaneous intraorbital hemorrhage caused by cavernous angioma of the orbit. J Neurosurg Sci 1984;28(1):37–40.
[23] Thorn-Kany M, Arrue P, Delisle MB, et al. Cavernous hemangiomas of the orbit: MR imaging. J Neuroradiol 1999;26(2):79–86.
[24] Gross HJ, Roth AM. Intraosseous hemangioma of the orbital roof. Am J Ophthalmol 1978;86(4):565–9.
[25] Colombo F, Cursiefen C, Hofmann-Rummelt C, et al. Primary intraosseous cavernous hemangioma of the orbit. Am J Ophthalmol 2001;131(1):151–2.
[26] Slem G, Ilcayto R. Hemangioma of the lacrimal gland in an adult. Ann Ophthalmol 1972;4(1):77–8.
[27] Wolin MJ, Holds JB, Anderson RL, et al. Multiple orbital tumors were cavernous hemangiomas. Ann Ophthalmol 1990;22(11):426–8.
[28] Ohbayashi M, Tomita K, Agawa S, et al. Multiple cavernous hemangiomas of the orbits. Surg Neurol 1988; 29(1):32–4.
[29] Fries PD, Char DH. Bilateral orbital cavernous haemangiomas. Br J Ophthalmol 1988;72(11):871–3.
[30] Sullivan TJ, Aylward GW, Wright JE, et al. Bilateral multiple cavernous haemangiomas of the orbit. Br J Ophthalmol 1992;76(10):627–9.
[31] Shields JA, Hogan RN, Shields CL, et al. Bilateral cavernous haemangiomas of the orbit. Br J Ophthalmol 2000;84(8):928.
[32] Johnson TE, Nasr AM, Nalbandian RM, et al. Enchondromatosis and hemangioma (Maffucci's syndrome) with orbital involvement. Am J Ophthalmol 1990; 110(2):153–9.
[33] McCannel CA, Hoenig J, Umlas J, et al. Orbital lesions in the blue rubber bleb nevus syndrome. Ophthalmology 1996;103(6):933–6.
[34] Chang EL, Rubin PA. Bilateral multifocal hemangiomas of the orbit in the blue rubber bleb nevus syndrome. Ophthalmology 2002;109(3):537–41.
[35] Scheuerle AF, Steiner HH, Kolling G, et al. Treatment and long-term outcome of patients with orbital cavernomas. Am J Ophthalmol 2004;138(2):237–44.
[36] Orcutt JC, Wulc AE, Mills RP, et al. Asymptomatic orbital cavernous hemangiomas. Ophthalmology 1991; 98(8):1257–60.
[37] Selva D, Strianese D, Bonavolonta G, et al. Orbital venous-lymphatic malformations (lymphangiomas) mimicking cavernous hemangiomas. Am J Ophthalmol 2001;131(3):364–70.
[38] Hood CI. Cavernous hemangioma of the orbit. A consideration of pathogenesis with an illustrative case. Arch Ophthalmol 1970;83(1):49–53.
[39] Mulliken JB, Glowacki J. Hemangiomas and vascular malformations in infants and children: a classification based on endothelial characteristics. Plast Reconstr Surg 1982;69(3):412–22.
[40] Mulliken JB, Young AE. Vascular birthmarks: hemangiomas and malformations. Philadelphia: WB Saunders; 1988.
[41] Wybar KC. A study of the choroidal circulation of the eye in man. J Anat 1954;88(1):94–8.
[42] Witschel H, Font RL. Hemangioma of the choroid. A clinicopathologic study of 71 cases and a review of the literature. Surv Ophthalmol 1976;20(6):415–31.
[43] Garner A. Cavernous hemangioma of the orbit. A consideration of its origin and development. Orbit 1988; 7:149–56.
[44] Zauberman H, Feinsod M. Orbital hemangioma growth during pregnancy. Acta Ophthalmol (Copenh) 1970; 48(5):929–33.
[45] Di Tommaso L, Scarpellini F, Salvi F, et al. Progesterone receptor expression in orbital cavernous hemangiomas. Virchows Arch 2000;436(3):284–8.
[46] Bilaniuk LT, Rapoport RJ. Magnetic resonance imag-

ing of the orbit. Top Magn Reson Imaging 1994;6(3): 167–81.

[47] Mafee MF, Miller MT, Tan W, et al. Dynamic computed tomography and its application to ophthalmology. Radiol Clin N Am 1987;25(4):715–31.

[48] Mafee MF, Valvassori GE, Becker M. Imaging of the head and neck. Stuttgart (Germany): Thieme; 2004.

[49] Hill JH, Mafee MF, Chow JM, et al. Dynamic computerized tomography in the assessment of hemangioma. Am J Otolaryngol 1985;6(1):23–8.

[50] Hill JH, Mafee MF, Lygizos NA, et al. Dynamic computed tomography. Its use in the assessment of vascular malformations and angiofibroma. Arch Otolaryngol 1985;111(1):62–5.

[51] Wilms G, Raat H, Dom R, et al. Orbital cavernous hemangioma: findings on sequential Gd-enhanced MRI. J Comput Assist Tomogr 1995;19(4):548–51.

[52] Ohtsuka K, Hashimoto M, Akiba H. Serial dynamic magnetic resonance imaging of orbital cavernous hemangioma. Am J Ophthalmol 1997;123(3):396–8.

[53] Freeny PC, Marks WM. Hepatic hemangioma: dynamic bolus CT. AJR Am J Roentgenol 1986;147(4): 711–9.

[54] van Leeuwen MS, Noordzij J, Feldberg MA, et al. Focal liver lesions: characterization with triphasic spiral CT. Radiology 1996;201(2):327–36.

[55] Gyldensted C, Lester J, Fledelius H. Computed tomography of orbital lesions. A radiological study of 144 cases. Neuroradiology 1977;13(3):141–50.

[56] Davis KR, Hesselink JR, Dallow RL, et al. CT and ultrasound in the diagnosis of cavernous hemangioma and lymphangioma of the orbit. J Comput Tomogr 1980;4(2):98–104.

[57] Savoiardo M, Strada L, Passerini A. Cavernous hemangiomas of the orbit: value of CT, angiography, and phlebography. AJNR Am J Neuroradiol 1983;4(3): 741–4.

[58] Wende S, Aulich A, Nover A, et al. Computed tomography or orbital lesions. A cooperative study of 210 cases. Neuroradiology 1977;13(3):123–34.

[59] Forbes GS, Sheedy II PF, Waller RR. Orbital tumors evaluated by computed tomography. Radiology 1980; 136(1):101–11.

[60] Sullivan JA, Harms SE. Surface-coil MR imaging of orbital neoplasms. AJNR Am J Neuroradiol 1986; 7(1):29–34.

[61] Hamm B, Fischer E, Taupitz M. Differentiation of hepatic hemangiomas from metastases by dynamic contrast-enhanced MR imaging. J Comput Assist Tomogr 1990;14(2):205–16.

[62] Whitney WS, Herfkens RJ, Jeffrey RB, et al. Dynamic breath-hold multiplanar spoiled gradient-recalled MR imaging with gadolinium enhancement for differentiating hepatic hemangiomas from malignancies at 1.5 T. Radiology 1993;189(3):863–70.

[63] Quillin SP, Atilla S, Brown JJ, et al. Characterization of focal hepatic masses by dynamic contrast-enhanced MR imaging: findings in 311 lesions. Magn Reson Imaging 1997;15(3):275–85.

[64] Bilaniuk LT, Atlas SW, Zimmerman RA. Magnetic resonance imaging of the orbit. Radiol Clin N Am 1987;25(3):509–28.

[65] Fries PD, Char DH, Norman D. MR imaging of orbital cavernous hemangioma. J Comput Assist Tomogr 1987;11(3):418–21.

[66] Ossoinig KC, Keenan TP, Bigar F. Cavernous hemangioma of the orbit. A differential diagnosis in clinical echography. Bibl Ophthalmol 1975;83:236–44.

[67] Sutherland GR. The contribution of echography in the diagnosis of proptosis. Br J Radiol 1978;51(602):116–21.

[68] Coleman DJ, Jack RL, Franzen LA. High resolution B-scan ultrasonography of the orbit. II. Hemangiomas of the orbit. Arch Ophthalmol 1972;88(4):368–74.

[69] Sklar EL, Quencer RM, Byrne SF, et al. Correlative study of the computed tomographic, ultrasonographic, and pathological characteristics of cavernous versus capillary hemangiomas of the orbit. J Clin Neuro-ophthalmol 1986;6(1):14–21.

[70] Jain R, Sawhney S, Berry M. Real-time sonography of orbital tumours, colour Doppler characterization: initial experience. Acta Ophthalmol Suppl 1992;204: 46–9.

[71] Aburn NS, Sergott RC. Orbital colour Doppler imaging. Eye 1993;7(Pt 5):639–47.

[72] Lieb WE. Color Doppler imaging of the eye and orbit. Radiol Clin N Am 1998;36(6):1059–71.

[73] Hatton MP, Remulla HD, Tolentino MJ, et al. Clinical applications of color Doppler imaging in the management of orbital lesions. Ophthal Plast Reconstr Surg 2002;18(6):462–5.

[74] Wolff-Korman PG, Kormann BA, Hasenfratz GC, et al. Duplex and color Doppler ultrasound in the differential diagnosis of choroidal tumors. Acta Ophthalmol Suppl 1992;204:66–70.

[75] Flaharty PM, Lieb WE, Sergott RC, et al. Color Doppler imaging. A new noninvasive technique to diagnose and monitor carotid cavernous sinus fistulas. Arch Ophthalmol 1991;109(4):522–6.

[76] Berges O. Colour Doppler flow imaging of the orbital veins. Acta Ophthalmol Suppl 1992;204:55–8.

[77] Deol AK, Terry JE, Seibert DA, et al. Hemangioma of the apical orbit diagnosed by radionuclide imaging. Optom Vis Sci 1994;71(1):57–9.

[78] Ki WW, Shin JW, Won KS, et al. Diagnosis of orbital cavernous hemangioma with Tc-99m RBC SPECT. Clin Nucl Med 1997;22(8):546–9.

[79] Murata Y, Yamada I, Umehara I, et al. Perfusion and blood-pool scintigraphy in the evaluation of head and neck hemangiomas. J Nucl Med 1997;38(6):882–5.

[80] Gdal-On M, Gelfand YA, Israel O. Tc-99m labeled red blood cells scintigraphy: a diagnostic method for orbital cavernous hemangioma. Eur J Ophthalmol 1999; 9(2):125–9.

[81] Sayit E, Durak I, Capakaya G, et al. The role of Tc-99m RBC scintigraphy in the differential diagnosis of orbital cavernous hemangioma. Ann Nucl Med 2001;15(2):149–51.

[82] Aron-Rosa D, Doyon D, Dassonville J. Angiography

in vascular malformations of the orbit. Mod Probl Ophthalmol 1975;14:146–55.
[83] Dilenge D. Arteriography in angiomas of the orbit. Radiology 1974;113(2):355–61.
[84] Numaguchi Y, Kishikawa T, Ikeda J, et al. Prolonged injection angiography for diagnosing intracranial neoplasms. Radiology 1980;136(2):387–93.
[85] Rootman J, Kao SC, Graeb DA. Multidisciplinary approaches to complicated vascular lesions of the orbit. Ophthalmology 1992;99(9):1440–6.
[86] Lloyd GA. Pathological veins in the orbit. Br J Radiol 1974;47(561):570–8.
[87] Arai H, Sato K, Katsuta T, et al. Lateral approach to intraorbital lesions: anatomic and surgical considerations. Neurosurgery 1996;39(6):1157–62.
[88] Acciarri N, Giulioni M, Padovani R, et al. Orbital cavernous angiomas: surgical experience on a series of 13 cases. J Neurosurg Sci 1995;39(4):203–9.
[89] Missori P, Tarantino R, Delfini R, et al. Surgical management of orbital cavernous angiomas: prognosis for visual function after removal. Neurosurgery 1994; 35(1):34–8.
[90] Kennedy RE. Arterial embolization of orbital hemangiomas. Trans Am Ophthalmol Soc 1978;76:266–77.
[91] Howard GM, Jakobiec FA, Michelsen WJ. Orbital arteriovenous malformation with secondary capillary angiomatosis treated by embolization with silastic liquid. Ophthalmology 1983;90(9):1136–9.
[92] Takahashi Y, Terasaki M, Maruiwa H, et al. Orbital hemangiopericytoma—case report. Neurol Med Chir (Tokyo) 1997;37(9):688–91.
[93] Thompson TP, Lunsford LD, Flickinger JC. Radiosurgery for hemangiomas of the cavernous sinus and orbit: technical case report. Neurosurgery 2000;47(3): 778–83.

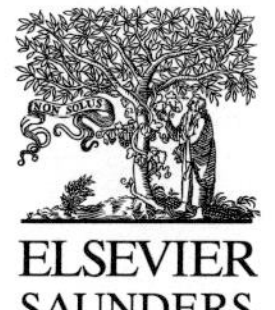

ELSEVIER
SAUNDERS

Neuroimag Clin N Am 15 (2005) 159 – 174

NEUROIMAGING
CLINICS OF
NORTH AMERICA

# Orbital Schwannoma and Neurofibroma: Role of Imaging

Rashmi Kapur, MD[a], Mahmood F. Mafee, MD[b], Reema Lamba, BSE[b], Deepak P. Edward, MD[a,*]

[a]*Department of Ophthalmology and Visual Sciences, University of Illinois at Chicago, MC 648, 1855 West Taylor Street, Chicago, IL 60612, USA*

[b]*Department of Radiology, University of Illinois at Chicago, 1740 West Taylor Street, MC 931, Chicago 60612, IL, USA*

Schwannomas, also known as neurilemmomas, are benign peripheral nerve sheath tumors that present as slowly progressing, well-defined, unilateral orbital masses. The tumor cells are purely Schwann cell in origin and constitute 1% of all orbital tumors [1,2]. Although it is conceivable that schwannomas can arise from the optic nerve meningeal sheath because of the trigeminal nerve innervation of this sheath, this tumor more commonly arises from the peripheral nerves in the orbit [1]. Because schwannomas are encapsulated noninvasive tumors, it is important to differentiate these tumors from other masses with a similar presentation. In this review, we discuss the role of radiologic imaging and its correlation to histopathologic evaluation to differentiate schwannomas from other orbital tumors with a similar clinical presentation. We also elaborate on specific differences between neurofibromas and schwannomas, which share many radiologic features.

This study was supported in part by a National Eye Institute Core Grant for Vision Research (EY01792), Bethesda, Maryland, and an unrestricted grant from Research to Prevent Blindness, Inc., New York, New York. It was also supported by a gift from Doris Semmler.

* Corresponding author.

*E-mail address:* deepedwa@uic.edu (D.P. Edward).

## Anatomic considerations

To understand the growth pattern and location of schwannomas, a basic understanding of the anatomic distribution of orbital nerves is necessary. Such an understanding helps in identifying the location and possible extension of schwannomas on CT and MR imaging. The ophthalmic nerve is the smallest division of the trigeminal nerve (Fig. 1A). It passes through the lateral wall of the cavernous sinus enclosed in a dural sheath. Just before it enters into the superior orbital fissure and the orbit, it divides into the frontal, lacrimal, and nasociliary branches (see Fig. 1A). The lacrimal nerve passes above the annular tendon, lateral to the frontal and trochlear nerves, in the superior orbital fissure (see Fig. 1B). It then courses forward along the upper border of the lateral rectus to reach the lacrimal gland (see Fig. 1) [3]. The frontal nerve, after its course through the superior orbital fissure, also passes above the annular tendon between the lacrimal and trochlear nerves (see Fig. 1B). Near the orbital margin, it divides into the supraorbital and supratrochlear branches (see Fig. 1A and B). The supraorbital nerve passes above the levator aponeurosis to leave the orbit at the supraorbital notch, whereas the supratrochlear nerve courses above the trochlea to ascend over the orbital margin (see Fig. 1B). These sensory nerves supply the upper eyelid, conjunctiva, and skin of the forehead [3]. Schwannomas more commonly arise from these sensory nerves, specifically the supraorbital,

1052-5149/05/$ – see front matter 
doi:10.1016/j.nic.2005.02.004

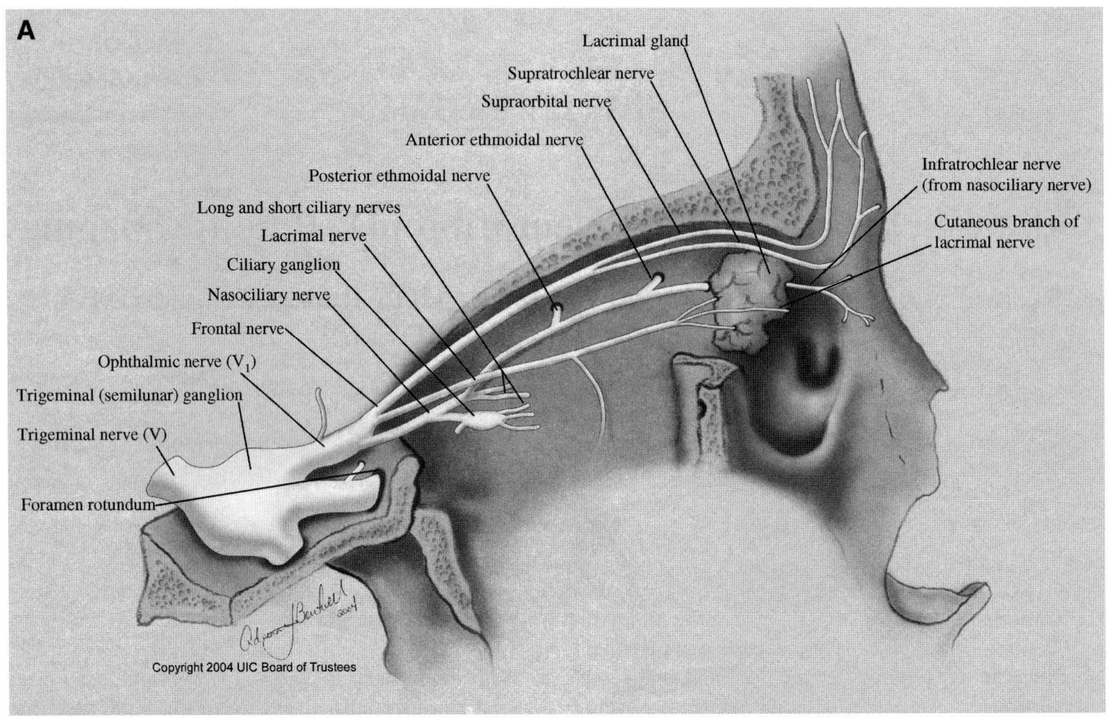


Fig. 1. (*A*) Sagittal section shows the course of the branches of the trigeminal nerve in the orbit and their bony anatomic relations. (*B*) Cranial view shows the intraorbital course of the orbital nerves and their relation to the extraocular muscles. (*C*) Cranial view shows the intraorbital course of the orbital nerves and their relation to the optic nerve. (Illustrations by Adrienne J. Boutwell and Lisa J. Birmingham © University of Illinois at Chicago Board of Trustees 2002; with permission.) (*D*) Axial T1W MR image obtained on a 3-T MR imaging system shows the supraorbital nerve (medial branch [*double white arrows*]), supraorbital nerve (lateral branch [*double white arrowheads*]), supratrochlear nerve (*black arrow*), frontal nerve (*white arrowhead*), nasociliary nerve (*black arrowhead*), and superior ophthalmic vein (*double black arrowheads*). (*E*) Coronal T1W MR image obtained on a 1.5-T MR imaging system shows the following: (1) superior oblique muscle; (2) superior rectus muscle; (3) lateral rectus muscle; (4) inferior rectus muscle; (5) medial rectus muscle; (6) presumed posterior ciliary artery and or ciliary ganglion; (7) nasociliary nerve; (8) supratrochlear nerve; (9) levator palpebral superioris; (10) frontal nerve; (11) lacrimal nerve, artery, and vein; (12) intermuscular septum; (13) presumed posterior ciliary artery; (14) oculomotor nerve (inferior ramus); and (15) medial orbital vein or inferior muscular artery. E, ethmoid sinus; L, lacrimal gland; MA, maxillary antrum; O, optic nerve; *single arrowhead*, superior ophthalmic vein; *arrowheads*, lateral collateral veins; *hollow curved arrow*, infraorbital nerve.

supratrochlear, and lacrimal nerves, and thus are usually outside the orbital muscle cone [4].

The nasociliary nerve is the only division of the ophthalmic nerve to pass through the superior orbital fissure within the annular tendon (see Fig. 1C) [3]. It is thus not uncommon to see schwannomas presenting as an intraconal mass [5]. The nasociliary nerve turns medially and follows in close relation to the ophthalmic artery to course above the optic nerve and below the superior rectus. The nerve then branches out into the sensory root of the ciliary ganglion and the long ciliary nerves, both of which course toward the globe in close relation to the optic nerve (see Fig. 1C) [3]. Because of this proximity to the optic nerve, schwannomas often result in compressive optic neuropathy, which is usually reversible on removal [6]. The other branches of the nasociliary nerve include the posterior ethmoidal nerve, infratrochlear nerve, and anterior ethmoidal nerve (see Fig. 1C) [3]. The divisions of the ophthalmic nerve and orbital motor nerves can be visualized on high-resolution MR imaging performed in 1.5-T and, in particular, 3-T MR systems (see Fig. 1D and E).

Rarely, schwannomas develop from one of the motor nerves, such as the oculomotor, trochlear, and

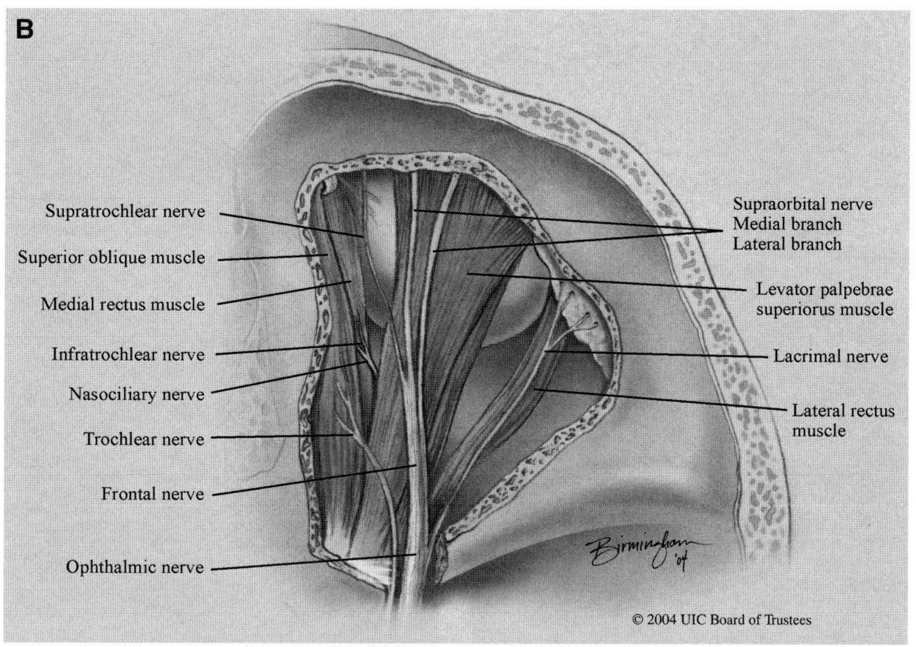


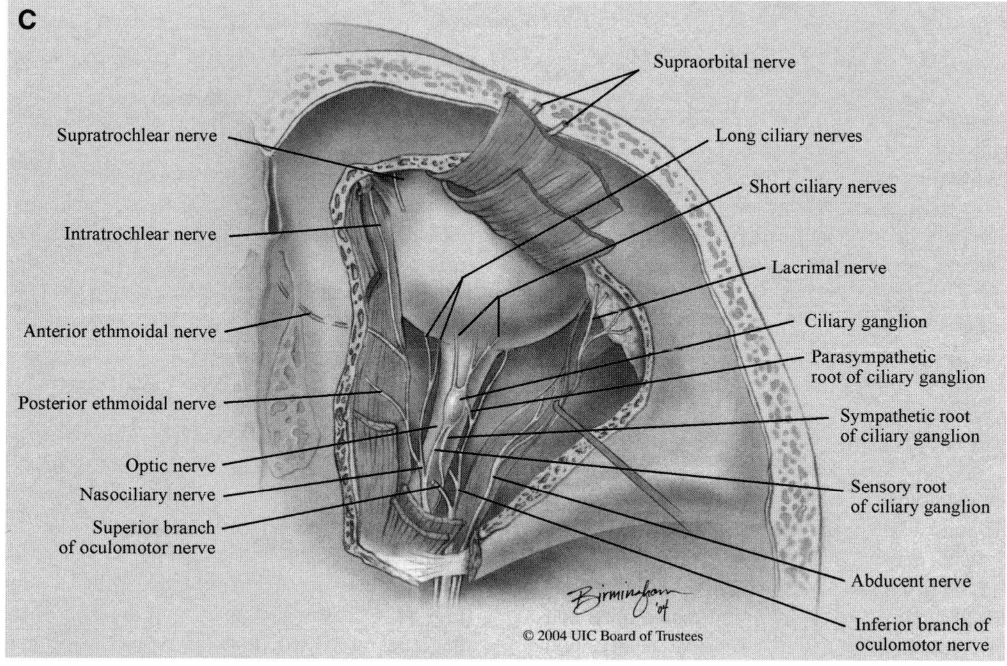


Fig. 1 (*continued*).

abducent nerves (see Fig. 1C) [7]. The oculomotor nerve divides into its superior and inferior branches at the anterior end of the cavernous sinus. These branches then separately enter the superior orbital fissure within the annular tendon (see Fig. 1C). The superior division turns medially above the optic nerve and courses behind the nasociliary nerve to supply the superior rectus and levator palpebral superioris. The inferior division immediately divides into branches for the medial and inferior recti and

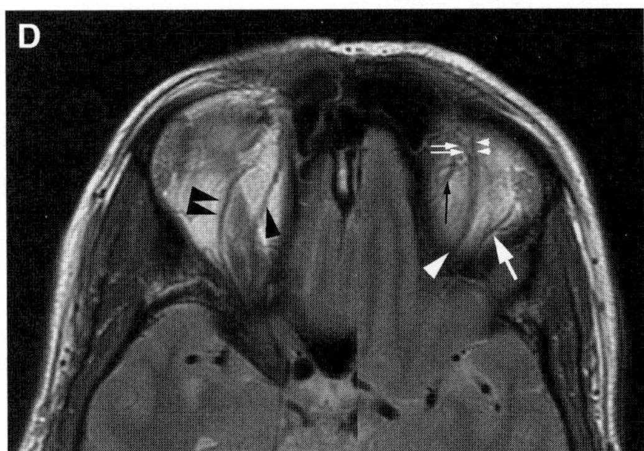


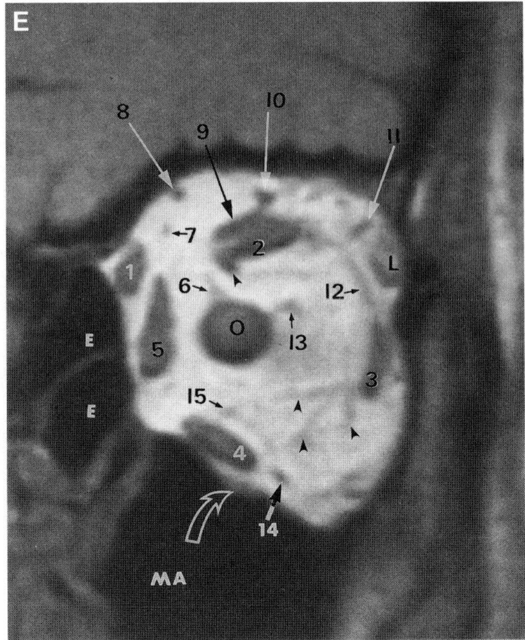


Fig. 1 (*continued*).

the inferior oblique (see Fig. 1C) [3]. The trochlear nerve, however, follows an extraconal course; therefore, schwannomas derived from motor nerve sheaths may also have an extraconal location (see Fig. 1B). Because of the course of these motor and sensory nerves, schwannomas can rarely grow along the nerve sheath to extend to the cavernous sinus (Fig. 2) [8].

## Clinical features

Schwannomas are usually seen in young to middle-aged adults and rarely in children [1]. There is no racial or sexual predilection. The most common presentation is painless insidious proptosis [1]. Intraconal tumors can lead to compressive optic neuropathy, resulting in decreased visual acuity, constricted fields, and a relative afferent pupillary defect [9,10]. When these tumors enlarge, they may also lead to limitation of extraocular motion and cause diplopia and strabismus [1,9,10]. Rarely, schwannomas may present with numbness in the distribution of the trigeminal nerve or with pain, or they may mimic the symptoms of sinusitis [10,11]. Von Recklinghausen neurofibromatosis (NF) is seen in 2% to 18% of cases [12].

On examination, an orbital mass may be palpable or visible [9]. Because masses more commonly arise from the supraorbital and supratrochlear branches, the patient may present with hypophthalmos with mild exophthalmos (2–4 mm) [1]. On fundus examination, there may be papilledema or optic atrophy with accompanying choroidal or retinal striae and an induced hyperopia because of compressive effects of the tumor [1,10,11,13].

## Histopathologic findings of schwannoma

On gross examination, schwannomas are smooth well-encapsulated masses with tan to yellow coloration, and they are fluctuant and friable on palpation (Fig. 3). Occasionally, there may be foci of hemorrhage or, rarely, calcification, or the lesion may undergo cystic degeneration (cystic schwannomas) [1].

Histologically, two patterns have been described, Antoni A and Antoni B (Fig. 4A and B). Antoni type A areas consist of well-differentiated spindle cells with ovoid nuclei and fine chromatin stippling. These cells demonstrate a fascicular arrangement with a background of fibrillary cell processes. The nuclei palisade to create picket fence type structures with interdigitating cytoplasmic processes, forming a pat-

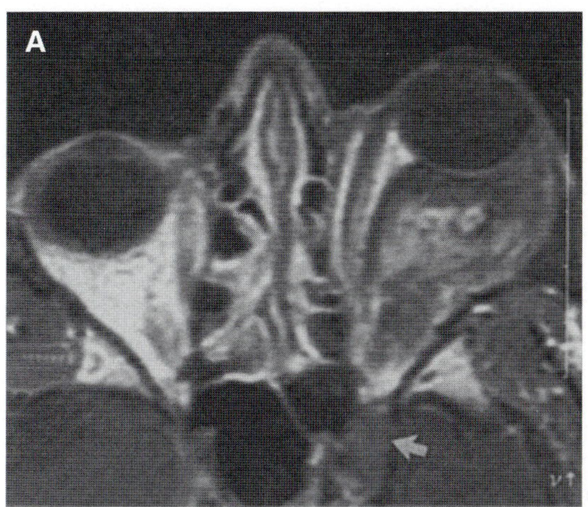


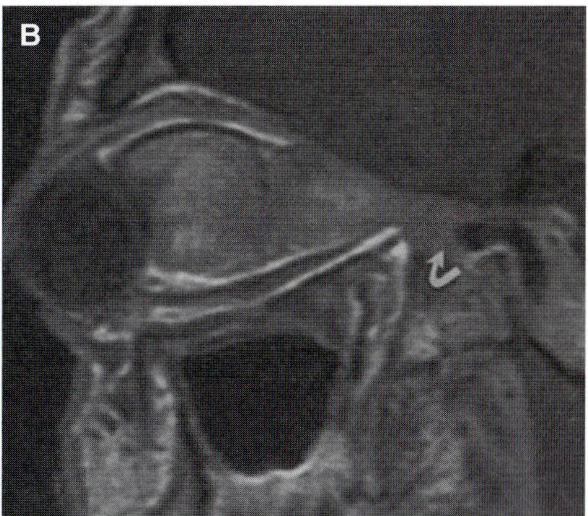


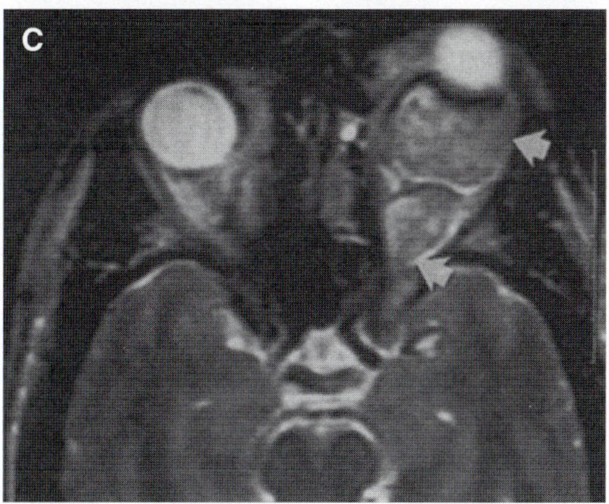


Fig. 2. (*A*) Axial postcontrast T1W MR image of a neurofibroma demonstrates heterogenous enhancement with displacement of the optic nerve. Note the extension into the anterior cavernous sinus (*arrow*) indicating that the mass is not arising from the optic nerve. (*B*) Sagittal postcontrast T1W MR image of the neurofibroma in *A* shows the tumor extension into the cavernous sinus (*arrow*). (*C*) Axial T2W MR image of neurofibroma in *A* and *B* shows the large retrobulbar intraconal neurofibroma (*arrows*). (*From* Carroll GS, Haik BG, Fleming JC, et al. Peripheral nerve tumors of the orbit. Radiol Clin N Am 1999;37(1):199.)

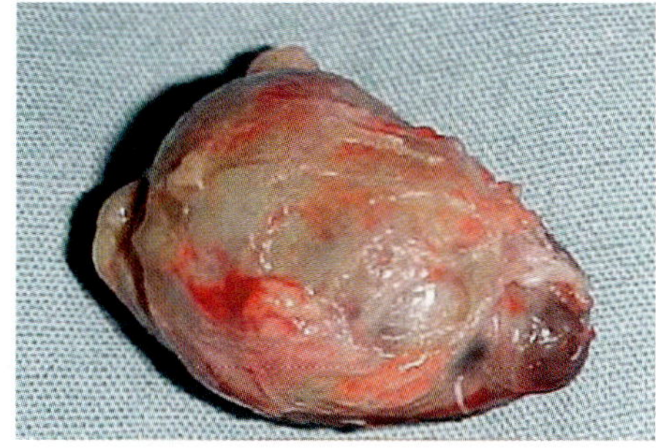

Fig. 3. Gross specimen of schwannoma. Note the smooth encapsulated mass with areas of yellow coloration.

tern known as Verocay bodies (see Fig. 4A) [14]. In Antoni type B areas, bipolar and multipolar cells are suspended in a loose myxoid matrix (see Fig. 4B). These cells may undergo secondary lipidization, adding a yellow hue to the gross coloration. The consistency of the tumor mass is dependent on which of these histologic patterns predominates, being more soft and cystic in tumors with a predominance of the Antoni B pattern. These tumors are moderately vascular and contain capillaries with thickened basement membranes [1]. Antoni B type areas are more vascular than Antoni A type areas, accounting for different signals on MR imaging enhancement with gadolinium injection [15]. There may also be perivascular lymphocytic cuffing [10].

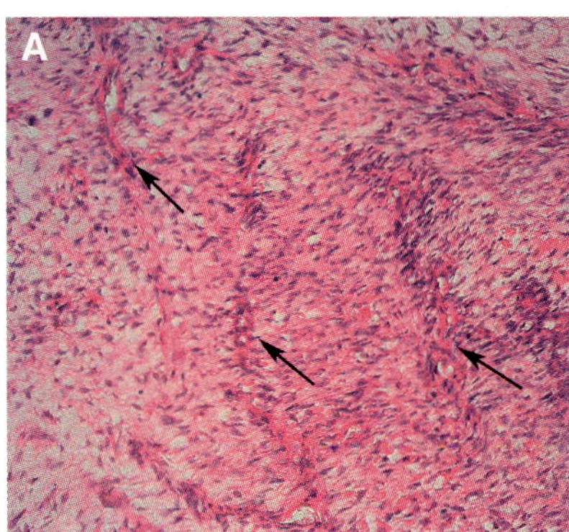


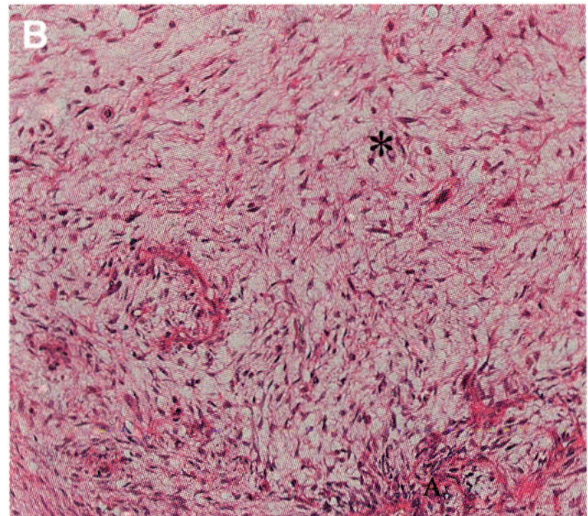


Fig. 4. (*A*) Schwannoma: Antoni A pattern. Note the picket fence arrangement of spindle-shaped cells (*arrows*). (*B*) Schwannoma: Antoni B pattern. Note the spindle-shaped cells in the looser myxoid tissue (*) (hematoxylin–eosin, original magnification ×20).

As these lesions age, they become more hypocellular, with a predominance of collagen producing the variant known as the ancient schwannoma. Areas of hypercellularity with nuclear pleomorphism and hyperchromatism may be seen surrounded by fibrosis with focal hyalinization [1,16]. Therefore, ancient schwannomas may not significantly enhance with contrast on CT or MR imaging because of decreased vascularity [16].

As a result of their neural crest origin, schwannomas demonstrate positive immunolabeling for S-100. On electron microscopy, the basement membrane may contain "long-spacing" collagen and banded areas, forming what are known as Luse bodies [1].

## Ancillary studies

Ancillary studies, such as ultrasound of the orbit, can sometimes be helpful to the clinician. On B-scan ultrasound, these tumors appear as encapsulated solid lesions containing cystic areas with well-demarcated borders and fairly high reflectivity [5,9,17]. An A-scan may demonstrate echographic findings of medium to high reflectivity representative of Antoni type A areas and areas of low reflectivity representative of Antoni type B pattern [5,17].

## CT and MR Imaging

On CT, schwannomas appear as smooth, ovoid, solitary, orbital retrobulbar masses, most commonly in the superior orbit with the long axis in the direction of the nerve, which is generally the anteroposterior direction [4,9]. The lesion can be seen in the extraconal or intraconal space (Figs. 5 and 6). Rarely, it may present as an intramuscular mass, however [18].

The tumor mass is usually isodense or slightly hyperdense when compared with the brain, and after injection of intravenous contrast medium, it often demonstrates homogeneous or heterogenous moderate to marked contrast enhancement (Figs. 5–7) [4,9]. The optic nerve may be displaced by the tumor mass, and the tumor mass may extend intracranially through the superior orbital fissure (see Fig. 2) [4]. Bony changes, such as widening of the superior orbital fissure, may be noted depending on tumor extent [9]. Also general or focal expansion of the orbit may

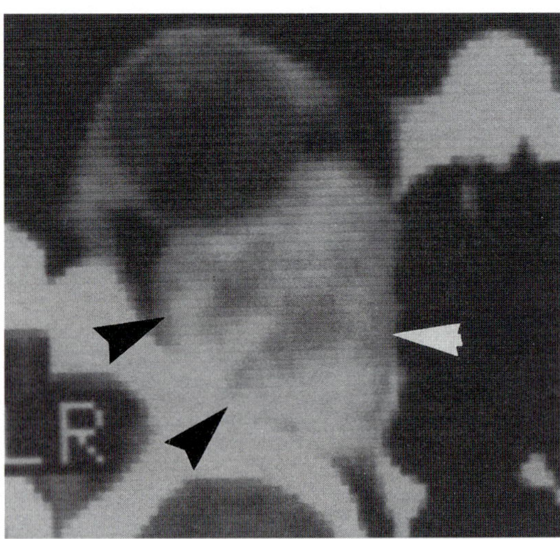


Fig. 5. Orbital schwannoma. Enhanced axial CT scan shows a well-defined enhancing intraconal mass compatible with a schwannoma (*arrowheads*).

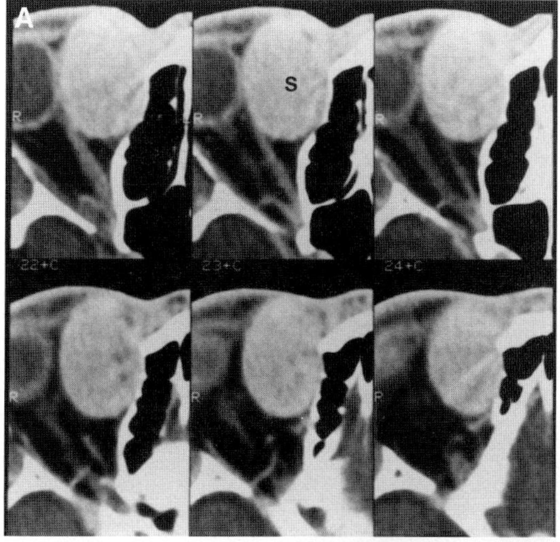


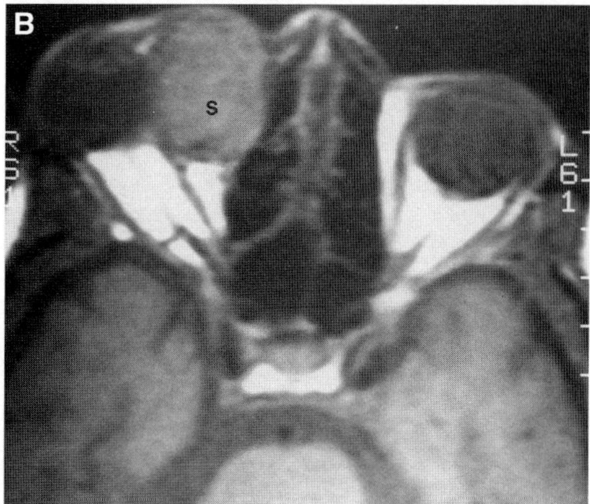


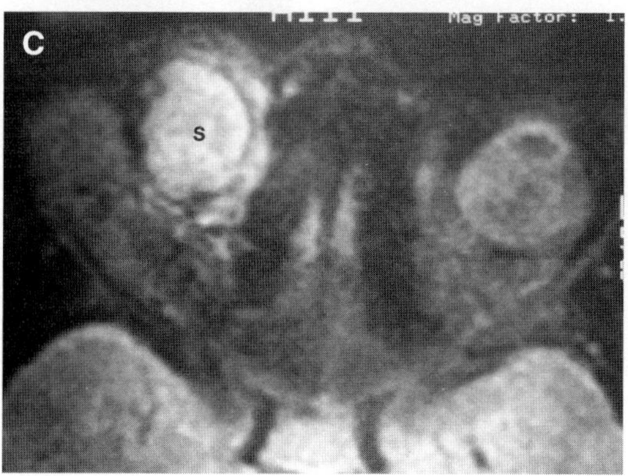


Fig. 6. Orbital schwannoma. (*A*) Enhanced serial CT scans of a schwannoma (S) show the well-defined extraconal tumor. Axial T1W (*B*) and T2W (*C*) MR images of the same patient show extraconal schwannoma (S).

be noted, although general enlargement is noted more often with intraconal tumors (see Fig. 5). Bony erosion may also be seen and is more common with tumors that have some extraconal extent [9].

MR imaging demonstrates the tumor as a well-circumscribed ovoid mass located in the extraconal or intraconal space (see Figs. 2, 6B, and 6C). It is most commonly seen in the superior orbit and is isointense with respect to the extraocular muscle and cerebral gray matter on T1-weighted (T1W) images and hyperintense on T2-weighted (T2W) images (see Fig. 7) [12]. In Antoni B areas, there is greater signal intensity on T2W images when compared with the more cellular Antoni A portion [15]. There may also be evidence of cavitary change on T2W images, which has been shown to indicate a predominance of Antoni B pattern when histopathologically examined [12]. With gadolinium infusion, there is increased enhancement in Antoni B type myxoid areas when compared with the more cellular Antoni A type areas (Fig. 7) [15]. However, this may not alwalys be the case.

## Cystic schwannomas

Schwannomas may undergo cavitary change, which on appears as a cystic mass with straw-colored fluid on gross pathologic examination. The cyst wall is composed of Antoni type A and B areas with minimal collagen [19]. Cystic schwannomas may appear as a homogeneous hypodense mass that does not enhance after contrast injection on CT because of their cystic nature. MR imaging can show the tumor as a well-defined lesion surrounded by a hypointense capsule [19]. The differential diagnosis

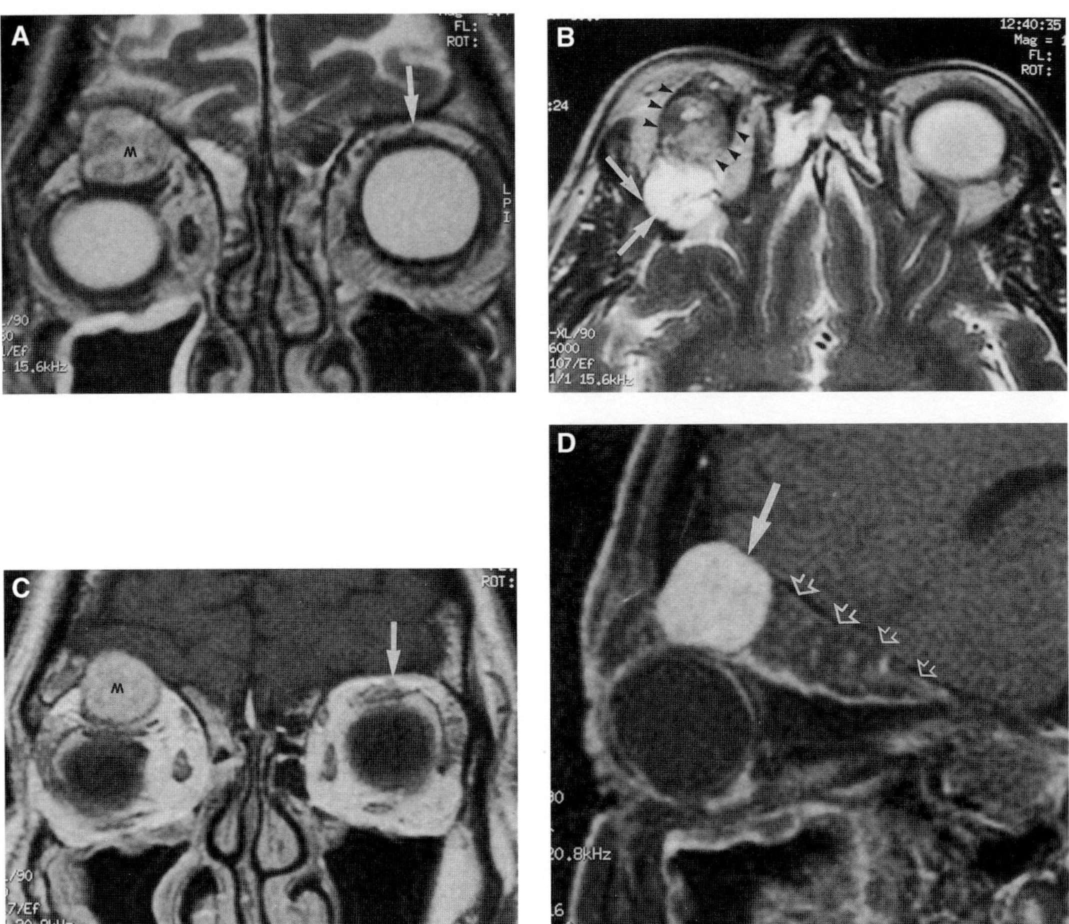


Fig. 7. Orbital frontal nerve schwannoma. (*A*) Coronal T2W MR image shows a mass (M) compatible with schwannoma. Note the normal left frontal nerve (*arrow*). Note fossa formation at the roof of the right orbit, which is indicative of a long-standing process. (*B*) Axial T2W MR image. Note the heterogenous signal intensity of this schwannoma, being markedly hyperintense posteriorly (*solid arrows*) and moderately hyperintense anteriorly (*black arrowheads*). (*C*) Enhanced axial T1W coronal MR image. Note the marked enhancement of the mass (M). The arrow points to the normal frontal nerve. (*D*) Enhanced sagittal T1W MR image. Note the marked enhancement of anterior portion of this schwannoma (*straight arrow*) and minimal enhancement of its posterior portion (*hollow arrows*). (Courtesy of Jan Lotz, MD, and Kobus Brits, MD, Cape Town, South Africa.)

includes cavernous hemangioma, dermoid cyst, hydatid cysts, mucocele, pyocele, lacrimal duct cyst, meningoencephalocele, epidermal inclusion cysts, hematic cyst, cholesterol granuloma, and lymphangioma [19–21].

## Malignant peripheral nerve sheath tumors

Malignant transformation of schwannomas is rare but has been previously reported [22]. It is thus important to understand the features of malignant peripheral nerve sheath tumors and to differentiate them from schwannomas, especially because of their common association with NF. These aggressive lesions consist of highly pleomorphic spindle cells with numerous mitotic figures and areas of myxoid tumor matrix. Peripheral palisading of nuclei may be present. The different patterns seen include malignant plexiform, alveolar-organoid, pseudoglandular, epithelioid, and neurotubular. Necrosis and heterotopic elements, such as bone and muscle, may be present, and these may be visible on CT and MR imaging. Immunostaining for S-100 may also be positive [1].

On CT, a poorly circumscribed mass with irregular margins can be seen, usually in the superior orbit, and there may be associated bony destruction [17]. MR imaging demonstrates a homogeneous signal on T1W, with small cystic areas on T2W. On gadolinium injection, diffuse enhancement with focal peripheral enhancement may be seen [23].

## Neurofibroma

Neurofibroma, especially the localized variant, is one of the more common differential diagnoses of orbital schwannomas (see Fig. 8). Both conditions can be seen in association with von Recklinghausen NF (Fig. 9). There are certain features that may help to differentiate between the two lesions, however. Unlike schwannomas, which are encapsulated, localized neurofibromas, although circumscribed, are not encapsulated. In addition, plexiform and diffuse schwannomas may present as massive overgrowths of the lids infiltrating the orbit along fascial planes. Through compressive effects on surrounding tissues, localized neurofibromas can, however, acquire a pseudocapsule. Histopathologically, these tumors consist of localized proliferations of endoneural fibroblasts and Schwann cells arranged into fascicles surrounded by an Alcian blue–positive myxoid matrix (Fig. 10A). The axonal component of neurofibromas, which is absent in schwannomas, can be demonstrated clearly with the Bodian stain. Similar to schwannomas, however, these tumors show positive immunostaining for S-100 antigen [1].

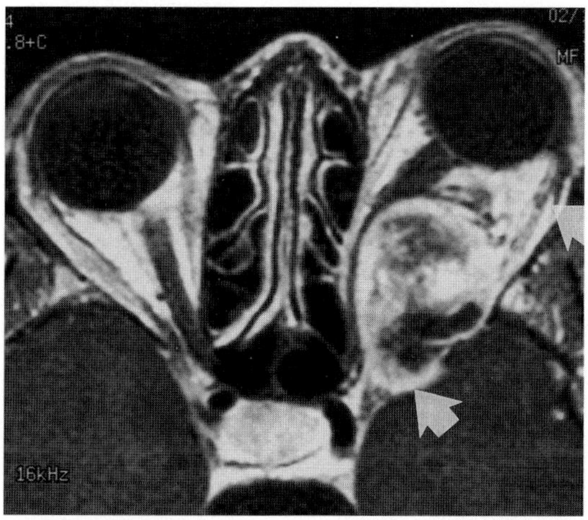

Fig. 8. Orbital neurofibroma. Axial enhanced T1W MR image shows a heterogenously enhancing neurofibroma (*arrows*).

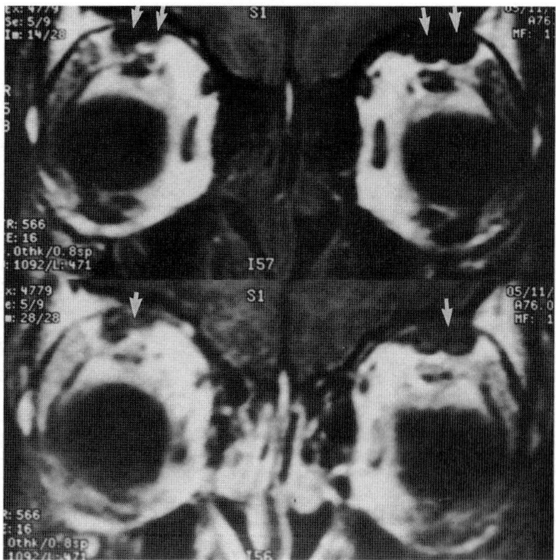

Fig. 9. Orbital frontal nerve neurofibroma in a patient with NF type 1. Coronal MR images show bilateral presumed frontal nerve neurofibromas (*arrows*).

On imaging, localized neurofibromas may appear similar to schwannomas, especially because both have a predilection for being extraconal masses in the superior orbit (Fig. 11) [15]. Often, the diagnosis can only be made on histopathologic examination. The CT density of the tumor mass is similar to that of the brain, and there is moderate to marked enhancement after intravenous contrast injection, as seen in schwannomas [9]. Some differences that have been noted, however, include slight irregularities of the borders of the lesion on CT because of the lack of true encapsulation [1]. Also of note, several case series have shown that widening of the superior orbital fissure is more commonly seen with schwannomas [8,9,24]. On MR imaging, neurofibromas show homogeneous or heterogenous isointense to slightly hyperintense signal when compared with extraocular muscle on the T1W images (Fig. 11A), homogeneous or heterogenous hyperintense signal on the T2W images, and moderate to marked heterogenous enhancement with contrast (see Figs. 8, 11B, and 11C). The myxoid matrix surrounding the areas of Schwann cell proliferation demonstrates greater enhancement [15].

## Differential diagnosis

The differential diagnosis of schwannoma includes neurofibroma (Fig. 7), hemangiopericytoma, fibrous

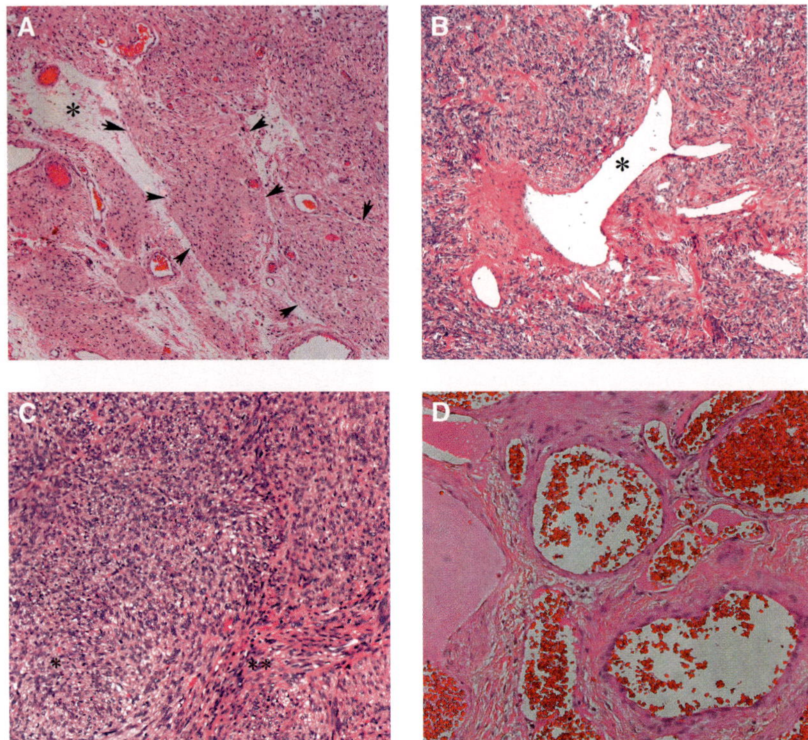


Fig. 10. (*A*) Plexiform neurofibroma. The microphotograph demonstrates bundles (*arrowheads*) of proliferating Schwann cells and endoneural fibroblasts separated by a myxoid matrix (*) (hematoxylin–eosin, original magnification ×10). (*B*) Hemangiopericytoma. The tumor displays a prominent vascular pattern of sinusoidal spaces (staghorn pattern) (*) surrounded by solid areas composed of ovoid to spindle-shaped cells (hematoxylin–eosin, original magnification ×10). (*C*) Fibrous histiocytoma. The tumor shows a characteristic storiform pattern. There is a mixture of fibroblast (**) and histiocyte-like (*) cells (hematoxylin–eosin, original magnification ×20). (*D*) Cavernous hemangioma. The microphotograph demonstrates large cavernous spaces lined by endothelial cells and filled with red blood cells. Note the dense fibrosis of the interstitial trabeculae separating the cavernous channels (hematoxylin–eosin, original magnification ×20).

histiocytoma, cavernous hemangioma, meningioma, leiomyoma, neuroblastoma, rhabdomyosarcoma, malignant peripheral nerve sheath tumors, optic nerve glioma, orbital lymphomas, and isolated metastasis (Table 1). Being able to differentiate between these lesions is especially important, because a number of them are associated with NF.

## Hemangiopericytoma

Hemangiopericytomas are vascular tumors that arise from the capillary pericytes and are seen mostly in middle-aged women [25]. Larger tumors may present with optic nerve and extraocular dysfunction [1]. Because of their vascular origin, these tumors have a different appearance from schwannomas on histopathologic examination. They may have one of three patterns; a prominent vascular pattern with sinusoidal and staghorn vessels lined by oval to spindle-shaped endothelial cells, a more solid pattern in which the vascularity may be minimal, or a combination of these two patterns (see Fig. 10B) [1]. Unlike schwannomas, the tumor matrix in hemangiopericytomas stains positively with reticulin [1].

On CT, hemangiopericytomas may also present as superior orbital masses. Their margins may be less distinct, however, because of their tendency to invade adjacent tissue. Bony erosion may be present. Also, because of their vascular nature, these tumors may show marked enhancement with contrast [4,15]. On MR imaging, these tumors are isointense to slightly hyperintense with respect to extraocular muscle on T1W images and show variable but predominantly increased signal on T2W images. With

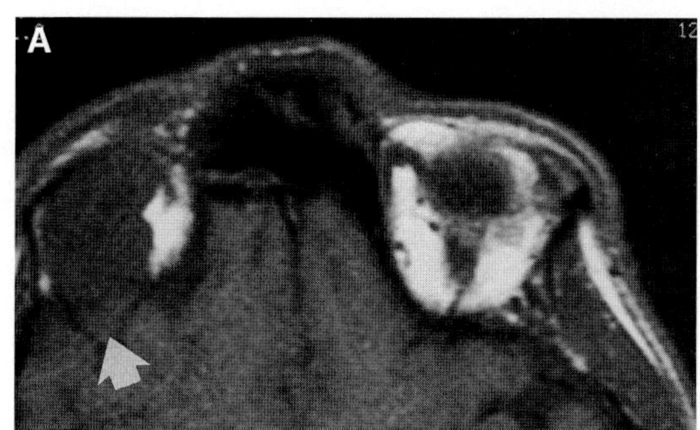


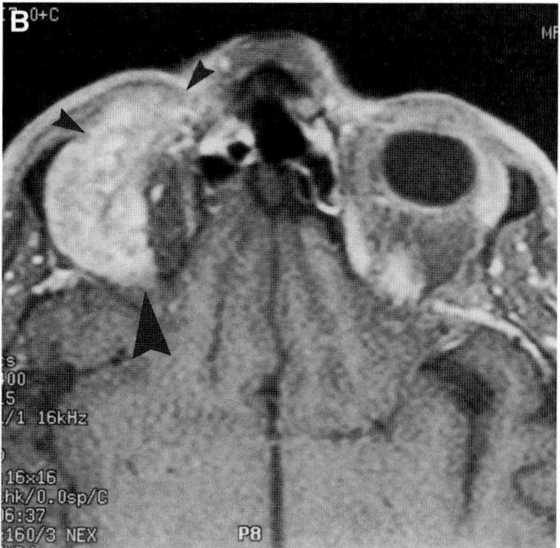


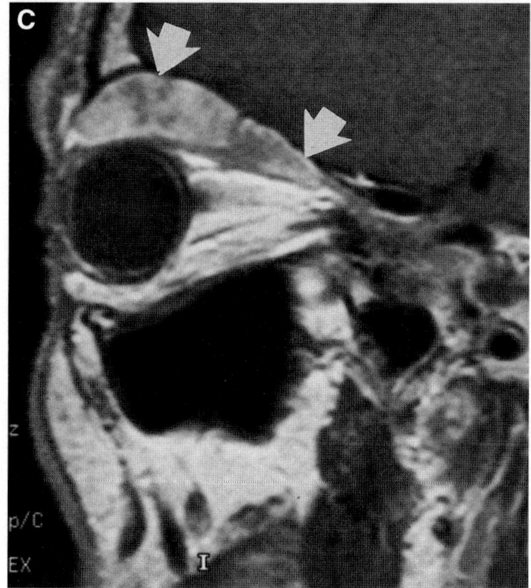


Fig. 11. Frontal nerve neurofibroma. Axial T1W (*A*), axial enhanced fat suppression T1W (*B*), and sagittal enhanced T1W (*C*) MR images show a neurofibroma (*A, arrow; B, arrowheads*) arising from the right frontal nerve. The sagittal enhanced T1W MR image in *C* shows a frontal nerve schwannoma (*arrows*). Note that unlike the orbital neurofibroma in Fig. 10, this neurofibroma appears homogeneous in pre- and postcontrast T1W MR images. (*From* Mafee MF, Valvassori GE, Becker M, editors. Imaging of the head and neck. 2nd edition. Stuttgart (Germany): Thieme; 2004. p. 266; with permission.)

gadolinium, these masses show moderate to marked diffuse contrast enhancement [15]. With increased vascularity, hemangiopericytomas display marked enhancement with gadolinium on MR imaging [1]. The best way to differentiate them from schwannomas is through carotid angiography. Hemangiopericytomas show an early florid blush, whereas schwannomas show a slight to moderate late vascular blush [4,10].

## Fibrous histiocytoma and solitary fibrous tumor of the orbit

Fibrous histiocytomas and solitary fibrous tumors of the orbit may be difficult to differentiate from schwannomas. Larger tumors can present with optic nerve and extraocular dysfunction [1]. The term "fibrous histiocytoma" denotes the biphasic cell population, which consists of spindle-shaped

Table 1
Radiologic and pathologic features of other differential diagnoses of orbital schwannomas

| Lesion | CT | MR image | Pathology | Other differentiating features |
|---|---|---|---|---|
| Rhabdomyosarcoma | Intraconal or extraconal mass. May be very bulky. Still well delineated. Isodense to muscle. Moderate to marked contrast enhancement. Bony erosion seen in large lesions. May infiltrate surrounding tissues [14]. | Hypointense to muscle on T1W and hyperintense to muscle on T2W. Moderate to marked enhancement on enhanced T1W MR image. | Embryonal, alveolar, and pleomorphic patterns. Embryonal form: fascicles of spindle-shaped cells and strap cells. Nuclei may palisade. Alveolar form: more frequently seen in the inferior orbit and in association with an extraocular muscle. Cells arranged along connective tissue trabeculae. Pleomophic form: multinucleated strap cells with abundant eosinophilic cytoplasm [14]. | May present with rapidly progressive proptosis and/or may be present at birth. Can be mistaken with capillary hemangioma or venolymphatic malformation. Seen in children or young adults [24]. |
| Optic nerve glioma | Marked, diffuse tortuous enlargement of the optic nerve with characteristic fusiform appearance due to kinking and buckling [4]. Unlike schwannomas, lesion can extend from the apex into the optic cananl [9]. May often even show expansion of optic canal [15]. May show areas of lucencies from cystic changes [28]. Mild to moderate contrast enhancement [4]. | T1W: isointense signal to muscle T2W: variable, If tumor is fusiform, homogenous high signal intensity. If tumor is lobulated, more heterogenous signal. May show a peripheral hyperintense area surrounding a hypointense core in tumors with arachnoid hyperplasia. Variable enhancement with contrast [15]. | Well-differentiated spindle- shaped cells with elongated nuclei and delicate processes arranged in a parallel or intertwining pattern [1]. May demonstrate Rosenthal fibers, which are eosinophilic structures that represent areas of degeneration in the astrocytes. There may also be arachnoid hyperplasia [17]. | Associated with NF-1. Clinical features: disproportion between advanced visual loss and low degrees of proptosis (2–4 mm) [1]. Seen under age of 20 [24] |
| Meningioma | Well-defined tubular thickening of the optic nerve [28]. Unlike schwannomas, lesion can extend from the apex into the optic canal [9]. Calcification of lesion is common [4]. Moderate to | Uniform thickening or globular appearance of the intraorbital segment of the optic nerve [28]. T1W: variable signal, mostly iso- to hypointense to brain T2W: variable signal, isointense | Whorls and sheets of meningothelial cells. Variable amounts of fibrous and vascular tissue. May contain psammoma bodies-concentric layers of calcification [29]. | Associated with NF. Clinical features: Disproportion between advanced visual loss and low degrees of proptosis (2–4 mm) [1]. Seen in adults [24]. |

| | | | | |
|---|---|---|---|---|
| | marked contrast enhancement [4]. Central lucent areas can be seen after contrast agent and may show the optic nerve with calcification (ie, "railroad sign") [15,28]. | to hyperintense to brain If calcification is present within tumor, low signal intensities are seen on T1W and T2W. Marked enhancement with contrast [15]. | | Carotid angiography: multiple tumor vessels and a late blush [10]. |
| Orbital lymphoma | Homogenous masses that mold themselves to surrounding structures with no bony destruction. High density when compared to brain. Mild to moderate enhancement with contrast [30]. | T1W: Isointense to hyperintense to muscle [15]. T2W: hyperintense signal to muscle [15]. Mild to moderate enhancement with contrast. | Predominantly a B-cell tumor. All patterns of B-cell lymphoma may be seen. Monotonous B cells with hyperchromatic nucleoli and scant cytoplasm. Increased nuclear: cytoplasmic ratio and mitotic figures [29]. | 53% of patients develop systemic lymphoma [31]. Extraorbital disease is present in 19% of patients at the time of ophthalmic presentation [32]. |
| Neuroblastoma | Large, irregular poorly circumscribed orbital mass with associated bony destruction and periosteal reaction. Hyperostosis may be present [17,33]. | Intense enhancement with gadolinium infusion [34]. | Small hypochromatic cells with scant cytoplasm and delicate eosinophilic processes forming a fibrillary background. Nuclei are hyperchromatic and display peripheral palisading. Areas of necrosis may be present [1,17]. Positive immunostaining for S-100, neuron-specific enolase, and neurofilament [1,14]. | Seen more commonly in children. If it is a metastatic neuroblastoma, increased urinary secretion of vanilyllmandelic acid [33]. |
| Leiomyoma | Smooth, circumscribed lesion [1]. Moderate to marked enhancement with contrast [17]. | T1W: Hypointense to muscle T2W: Hyperintense to muscle with moderate to marked contrast enhancement. | Fascicles of elongated spindle cells with lateral nuclear palisading in a fibrillary background of thin actin filaments. Nuclei are ovoid or cigar shaped. Chromatin stippling more marked than that seen in schwannomas. More intense eosinophilic cytoplasm. Immunohistochemistry-S100 negative. Muscle actin and desmin positive [1]. | Adolescence and early adult life [24]. |

collagen-producing fibroblasts and lipid-containing multinucleated histiocytes. Microscopically, these tumors show a "storiform," twisted, cartwheel pattern of tumor cells that are S-100–negative with absence of nuclear palisading (see Fig. 10C) [1]. In contrast, solitary fibrous tumors of the orbit consist of spindle-shaped cells dispersed in a background of collagen bands and can be seen in variable pathologic patterns [26]. Fibrous histiocytomas and solitary fibrous tumors of the orbit can both show positive immunostaining for CD34 and vimentin [1,26]. Therefore, it is also difficult to differentiate fibrous histiocytomas from solitary fibrous tumors of the orbit.

Similarly, on radiologic imaging, it may be difficult to differentiate between fibrous histiocytomas and solitary fibrous tumors of the orbit. Similar to schwannomas, fibrous histiocytomas are most commonly seen in the superior orbit. Fibrous histiocytomas arise in the orbital fat, however [1]. On CT imaging, a well-circumscribed tumor with marked enhancement can be seen [4]. Solitary fibrous tumors of the orbit may also show similar CT density, with marked enhancement with contrast on CT [26]. Malignant and long-standing variants of both tumors may have surrounding bony erosion, however [17, 26]. On MR imaging, these lesions show a heterogenous isointense signal with respect to the extraocular muscles on T1W images [17,27]. Some of the areas that are hypointense in T1W images of fibrous histiocytomas may remain hypointense on T2W images. On T2W MR images, these masses appear hyperintense or isointense to brain. With gadolinium, both lesions demonstrate moderate heterogenous enhancement [17,27].

## Cavernous hemangioma

Cavernous hemangiomas are benign, encapsulated, slowly progressive vascular tumors seen in the

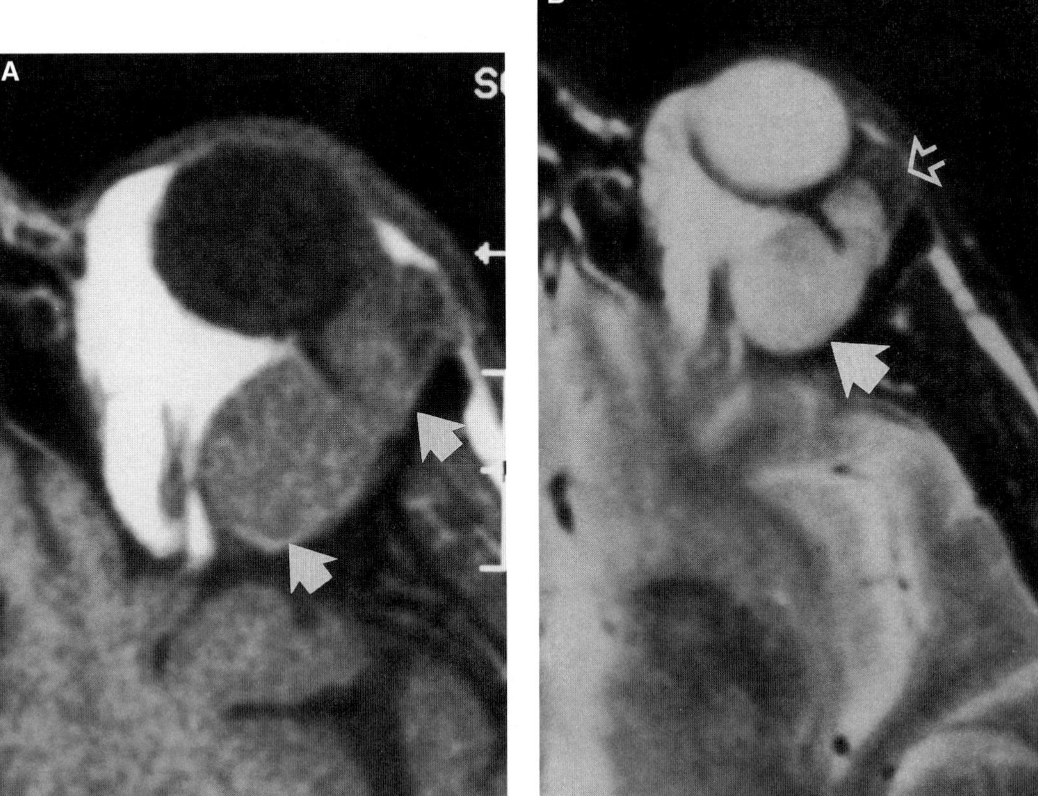


Fig. 12. Schwannoma arising from lacrimal nerve. Axial T1W (*A*), T2W (*B*), and enhanced fat suppression (*C*) MR images show a large orbital schwannoma (*arrows*). Note the anterior displacement of the lacrimal gland (*hollow arrow* in *B*).

second to fourth decades of life. Histopathologically, these tumors are composed of large, endothelium-lined, venous spaces with fibrous septae in between (see Fig. 10D) [15]. On CT, these lesions appear as well-defined, ovoid, lobulated, frequently intraconal masses, often in the temporal quadrant. These benign tumors tend to be of increased density, however, with variable contrast enhancement, because there is slow intratumor circulation. This is better appreciated by means of a CT dynamic study. Orbital bone expansion and rarely calcification of these lesions may also be seen [4]. On MR imaging, these lesions seem to have a homogeneous isointense to slightly hyperintense signal with respect to the extraocular muscles on T1W images and homogeneously high signal intensity on T2W images. With gadolinium infusion, these vascular lesions demonstrate heterogenous moderate enhancement (see article by Ansari et al elsewhere in this issue) [15].

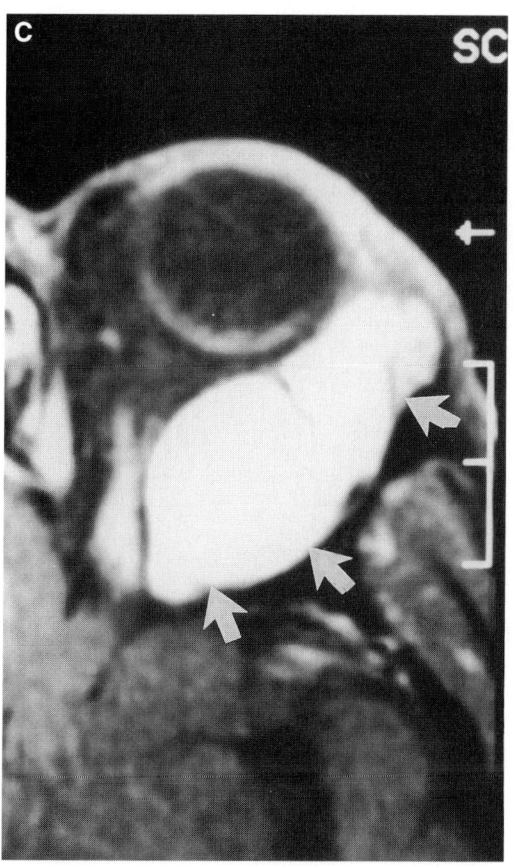


Fig. 12 (*continued*).

## Course

It may take many years for schwannomas to recur; even on recurrence, these tumors have low malignant potential [1]. Malignant transformation is rare but has been reported [22]. Recurrent tumors may be hypercellular without frank pleomorphism but with increased mitotic figures. These are probably more aggressive tumors that are still benign in nature. These tumors should be managed more aggressively, however [1].

## Management

Because schwannomas are well-circumscribed encapsulated masses, treatment consists of total excision. Because of the friable nature of the lesion, however, excision may not be as trivial. Because the tumor is derived from Schwann cells and thus is typically located along the periphery of the nerve, the mass can be stripped away from the nerve with minimal damage to the nerve [1]. The surgical approach is dependent on tumor location and extent and may require a combined orbitotomy and craniotomy [10].

## Summary

Schwannomas are well-circumscribed ovoid masses that most commonly present in the superior orbit. Although it may be difficult to differentiate these benign masses from other orbital tumors on radiologic imaging, the CT and, in particular, the MR imaging characteristics can sometimes point to the diagnosis of a nerve sheath tumor (Figs. 7, 9, 11, and 12). A definitive diagnosis can be made through correlation with histopathologic findings, however. In most cases, schwannomas have low malignant potential, and with total excision, recurrence is rare.

## Acknowledgments

The authors thank Dr. Geeta Vemuganti and Drs. Jan Lotz and Kobus Britz of Cape Town, South Africa for their assistance in the development of this article. This work was approved by the Institutional Review Board of the University of Illinois at Chicago.

## References


[1] Albert DM, Jakobiec FA. Principles and practice of ophthalmology. 2nd edition. Philadelphia: WB Saunders; 2000.

[2] Shields JA, Shields CL, Scartozzi R. Survey of 1264 patients with orbital tumors and simulating lesions: the 2002 Montgomery Lecture, part 1. Ophthalmology 2004;111:997–1008.

[3] Bron AJ, Tripathi RC, Tripathi BJ, editors. Innervation and nerves of the orbit. In: Wolff's anatomy of the eye and orbit. 8th edition. London: Chapman and Hall; 1997. p. 178–210.

[4] Mafee MF, Putterman A, Vavassori GE, et al. Orbital space-occupying lesions: role of computed tomography and magnetic resonance imaging. An analysis of 145 cases. Radiol Clin N Am 1987;25(3):529–59.

[5] Byrne BM, van Heuven WAJ, Lawton AW. Echographic characteristics of benign orbital schwannomas (neurilemomas). Am J Ophthalmol 1988;106:194–8.

[6] Allman MI, Frayer WC, Hedges TR. Orbital neurilemoma. Ann Ophthalmol 1977;9(11):1409–13.

[7] Shen WC, Yang DY, Ho WL, et al. Neurilemmoma of the oculomotor nerve presenting as an orbital mass: MR findings. AJNR Am J Neuroradiol 1993;14(5): 1253–4.

[8] Shields JA, Kapustiak J, Arbizo V, et al. Orbital neurilemoma with extension through the superior orbital fissure. Arch Ophthalmol 1986;104:871–3.

[9] Dervin JE, Beaconsfield M, Wright JE, et al. CT findings in orbital tumours of nerve sheath origin. Clin Radiol 1989;40(5):475–9.

[10] Rootman J, Goldberg C, Robertson W. Primary orbital schwannomas. Br J Ophthalmol 1982;66:194–204.

[11] Cockerham KP, Cockerham GC, Stutzman R, et al. The clinical spectrum of schwannomas presenting with visual dysfunction: a clinicopathologic study of three cases. Surv Ophthalmol 1999;44(3):226–34.

[12] Gunduz K, Shields CL, Gunalp I, et al. Orbital schwannoma: correlation of magnetic resonance imaging and pathology findings. Graefes Arch Clin Exp Ophthalmol 2003;241:593–7.

[13] Mohan H, Sen DK. Orbital neurilemmomas presenting as retrobulbar neuritis. Br J Ophthalmol 1970;54: 206–7.

[14] Spencer WH. Ophthalmic pathology: an atlas and textbook. 4th edition. Philadelphia: WB Saunders; 1996.

[15] DePotter P, Shields JA, Shields CL. MRI of the eye and orbit. Philadelphia: JB Lippincott; 1995.

[16] Khwarg SI, Lucarelli MJ, Lemke BN, et al. Ancient schwannoma of the orbit. Arch Ophthalmol 1999; 117(2):262–4.

[17] Shields JA. Diagnosis and management of orbital tumors. Philadelphia: WB Saunders; 1989.

[18] Capps DH, Brodsky MC, Rice CD, et al. Orbital intramuscular schwannoma. Am J Ophthalmol 1990; 110:535–9.

[19] Lam DSC, Ng JSK, To KF, et al. Cystic schwannoma of the orbit. Eye 1997;11:798–800.

[20] Tsuzuki N, Katoh H, Ohnuki A, et al. Cystic schwannoma of the orbit: case report. Surg Neurol 2000; 54:385–7.

[21] Mafee MF. The orbit. In: Mafee MF, Valvassori GE, Becker M, editors. Imaging of the head and neck. 2nd edition. Stuttgart (Germany): Thieme; 2004. p. 196–204.

[22] Schatz H. Benign orbital neurilemoma: sarcomatous transformation in von Recklinghausen's disease. Arch Ophthalmol 1971;86:268–73.

[23] Briscoe D, Mahmood S, O'Donovan DG, et al. Malignant peripheral nerve sheath tumor in the orbit of a child with acute proptosis. Arch Ophthalmol 2002;120:653–5.

[24] Cantore G, Chiapetta P, Raco A, et al. Orbital schwannomas: report of nine cases and review of the literature. Neurosurgery 1986;19:583–8.

[25] Kumar V, Abbas AK, Fausto N. Robbins and Cotran pathologic basis of disease. 7th edition. Philadelphia: Elsevier; 1999.

[26] Krishnakumar S, Subramanian N, Mohan ER, et al. Solitary fibrous tumor of the orbit: a clinicopathologic study of six cases with review of the literature. Surv Ophthalmol 2003;48:544–54.

[27] Romer M, Bode B, Schuknecht B, et al. Solitary fibrous tumor of the orbitã two cases and a review of the literature. Eur Arch Otorhinolaryngol 2005;262: 81–8.

[28] Azar-Kia B, Naheedy MH, Elias DA, et al. Optic nerve tumors: role of magnetic resonance imaging and computed tomography. Radiol Clin N Am 1987;25(3): 561–81.

[29] Yanoff M, Duker JS. Ophthalmology. London: Mosby; 1999.

[30] Flanders AE, Espinosa GA, Markiwicz DA, et al. Orbital lymphoma role of CT and MRI. Radiol Clin N Am 1987;25(3):601–13.

[31] Jenkins C, Rose GE, Bunce C, et al. Histological features of ocular adnexal lymphoma (REAL classification) and their association with patient morbidity and survival. Br J Ophthalmol 2000;84:907–13.

[32] Jenkins C, Rose GE, Bunce C, et al. Clinical features associated with survival patients with lymphoma of the ocular adnexa. Eye 2003;17:809–20.

[33] Shields JA, Shields CL. Atlas of orbital tumors. Philadelphia: Lippincott Williams & Wilkins; 1999.

[34] Tamase A, Nakada M, Hasegawa M, et al. Recurrent intracranial esthesioneuroblastoma outside the initial field of radiation with progressive dural and intraorbital invasion. Acta Neurochir (Wien) 2004;146: 179–82.

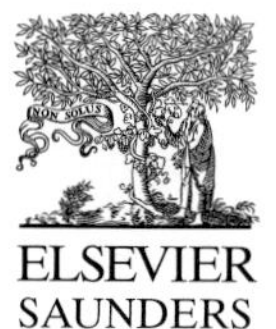

ELSEVIER
SAUNDERS

Neuroimag Clin N Am 15 (2005) 175 – 201

NEUROIMAGING
CLINICS OF
NORTH AMERICA

# The Optic Nerve: Radiologic, Clinical, and Pathologic Evaluation

Alfred L. Weber, MD[a,b,c,d,e,*], Paul Caruso, MD[a,b], Nelson R. Sabates, MD[c,f]

[a]Massachusetts Eye and Ear Infirmary, 243 Charles Street, Boston, MA 02114, USA
[b]Harvard Medical School, Boston, MA, USA
[c]University of Missouri at Kansas City Medical School, Kansas City, MO, USA
[d]King Faisal Hospital and Research Center, Riyadh, Saudi Arabia
[e]King Khaled Eye Hospital, Riyadh, Saudi Arabia
[f]Eye Foundation of Kansas City–Truman Medical Centers, Kansas City, MO, USA

The radiologic investigation of the optic nerve plays an integral part in the diagnostic evaluation of diverse lesions of the optic pathways including inflammatory diseases, vascular disorders and benign and malignant tumors [1]. These radiologic modalities consist principally of CT and MR imaging and, in vascular lesions, MR angiography and conventional angiography.

The selection of radiologic studies and their focus is based on the ophthalmologic examination. The ophthalmologist, after a careful history and evaluation of visual function, visual fields, pupillary abnormalities, and optic kinetic findings, can often determine the suspected location of lesions in the anterior or posterior visual pathways. Furthermore, inspection of the eye, including adnexal structures and funduscopy, provides additional information in the clinical assessment of these patients. With technical advances in the last few years, CT and MR imaging can detect lesions and determine their location and extent with high sensitivity and specificity.

* Corresponding author. Massachusetts Eye and Ear Infirmary, 243 Charles Street, Boston, MA 02114.

*E-mail address:* alweber1@aol.com (A.L. Weber).

## Methods of examination

### *CT*

CT usually plays a complementary role to MR imaging in the evaluation of the optic nerves but may be the first-line modality in patients unable to tolerate MR imaging (eg, patients who are clinically unstable and those who have pacemakers or non–MR-compatible aneurysm clips).

CT is important in assessing the optic canal and orbital apex, in evaluating the relation of inflammatory conditions such as pseudotumor or sinogenic orbital cellulitis to the orbit or optic nerve, and in evaluating meningiomas that may result in hyperostosis of the osseous orbit or mineralization along the nerve itself.

Multidetector CT scanners represent a further technical advance over conventional helical CT scanners. Multidetector scanners provide shorter acquisition times, decreased tube current load, and improved spatial resolution. The improvement in reformats with multidetector scanners essentially obviates the need for rescanning the patient in a second coronal plane [2].

At the Massachusetts Eye and Ear Infirmary, the authors use a multidetector scanner in helical mode to image the orbit and optic nerve with the patient in the supine position, in the axial plane, using 1-mm collimation, 120 to 140 kV, and 120 to 140 mA. The images are reconstructed in bone and soft tissue

1052-5149/05/$ – see front matter 
doi:10.1016/j.nic.2005.02.011

algorithms in 1.25-mm sections with 0.6-mm overlap and then reformatted in the coronal plane. CT oblique sagittal reformats may be advantageous in outlining the optic nerve, which courses at an angle of 30° to 40° off the midsagittal plane of the skull. Moreover, the enlarged optic nerve displays a tortuous, undulating course that is difficult to project in the axial plane. Iodinated contrast material is used in the evaluation of inflammatory diseases and tumors. CT demonstrates the bony structures, such as the sphenoid bone including the sphenoid sinus, the optic canals, and the sella turcica, to best advantage. Moreover, CT optimally demonstrates areas of calcification, which occur commonly in optic nerve sheath meningiomas.

## MR imaging

MR imaging is the modality of choice for imaging the optic nerves, chiasm, and postchiasmatic optic pathways. MR imaging distinguishes the meningeal, cerebrospinal fluid (CSF), and axonal portions of the optic nerve better than CT and without the use of ionizing radiant energy [3]. At the Massachusetts Eye and Ear Infirmary, the standard imaging protocol for the optic nerves includes 3-mm coronal short tau inverse recovery (STIR) images, 3-mm axial T1-weighted images, and, after administration of gadolinium, 3-mm axial fat-saturation T1-weighted images and coronal high-resolution non–fat-saturation T1-weighted images. STIR images are sensitive for detecting abnormal signal intensity of the optic nerve in neoplasia and in metabolic or demyelinating diseases such as multiple sclerosis. Normally, beyond 2 years of age, the central myelinated fibers of the optic nerve appear isointense to the frontal lobe white matter. The authors have found that the use of fat saturation may be advantageous to detect enhancement within the nerve in optic neuritides and in optic nerve tumors, but non–fat-saturated postgadolinium high-resolution T1-weighted MR images provide better resolution of the orbital apex and optic canal. Parasagittal images along the long axis of the nerve are sometimes used to complement the routine sequences, can depict the entire nerve along its often sinuous course, and may be of use in imaging optic nerve gliomas in which the nerve may become tortuous and kinked. Use of gadopentetate dimeglumine is important in the detection of the often coarse perineural enhancement that occurs in optic nerve meningiomas and that is seen variably in optic nerve gliomas.

For evaluation of chiasmatic lesions, a similar protocol is used and complemented with sagittal high-resolution T1- or T2-weighted images. A high-resolution heavily T2-weighted sequence (eg, CISS; Siemens, Erlangen, Germany) or 3D-Fiesta (General Electric, Milwaukee, Wisconsin) may be of further use in evaluating lesions that extrinsically compress the chiasm or postcanalicular optic pathways. For posterior visual pathway lesions, sagittal T1, axial T2, and fluid-attenuated inversion recovery sequences of the brain are routinely used with optional gadolinium enhancement.

### *Normal anatomy*

The orbital portion of the optic nerve courses obliquely posteriorly, superiorly, and medially from the optic disc to the optic canal. The total length of the optic nerve ranges from 45 to 50 mm. The intraocular portion is the shortest and measures 1 mm; the intraorbital portion, the longest, is 30 mm; the intracanalicular portion is 6 mm, and the intracranial portion is 10 to 16 mm [4]. The optic nerve measures approximately 4 to 6 mm in transverse diameter. The orbital segment of the optic nerve often describes a sinuous course. Histologically, the optic nerve consists of bundles of myelinated axons interspersed with connective tissue septae that contain blood vessels. The nerve is surrounded by three layers: (1) the dura, which extends from the intracranial dura forming a tough outer layer; (2) the arachnoid; and (3) the pia mater, which fuses to the outer surface of the nerve proper. The optic nerve passes through the optic canal, which measures approximately 4 to 9 mm in length and 4 to 6 mm in transverse diameter Within the optic canal, the optic nerve runs posteriorly and medially, forming an angle of approximately 35° with the midsagittal plane. The optic canal also contains the ophthalmic artery and branches of the sympathetic carotid plexus. Within the canal, the dura of the optic nerve and the periosteum of the bone are fused. The space between the pia mater and the arachnoid of the optic nerve communicates with the intracranial subarachnoid space and contains CSF. After leaving the optic canals, the optic nerves converge at the optic chiasm. The intracranial optic nerves extend posteriorly and medially and ascend at an angle of 45° to reach the chiasm. Above the intracranial segments of the optic nerves lie the frontal lobes of the brain, the olfactory tracts, and, usually, the anterior cerebral and anterior communicating arteries. The lateral aspect of the optic nerve is adjacent to the internal carotid artery as the vessel emerges from the cavernous sinus. Inferiorly, the posterior ethmoid and the sphenoid sinuses are adjacent to the optic nerves.

## Pathology of optic nerve tumors

The types of optic nerve tumors are listed in Box 1 and are discussed more fully in the text.

### *Primary optic nerve tumors*

#### *Optic nerve gliomas*

Optic nerve gliomas are uncommon tumors. They represent approximately 1.5% to 3.5% of all orbital tumors, 0.6% to 7.0% of all intracranial tumors, 1.7% to 7.0% of all gliomas, and 2% to 5% of gliomas in the pediatric age group [5,6]. Optic nerve gliomas outnumber meningiomas by a ratio of 4:1 and account for 66% of all optic nerve tumors. The peak incidence is between 2 and 8 years of age, with 75% manifesting in the first decade and 90% within the first 2 decades of life. Optic nerve gliomas, however, have been reported from birth to age 79 years [7,8]. There is a slight female preponderance. Patients who have involvement of the hypothalamus present at a younger age group, often younger than 6 years [5,9]. A common initial symptom is proptosis associated with decreased visual acuity [10,11]. The loss of visual acuity is more severe in postchiasmal tumors, notably when located in the optic tracts [12]. Other presenting signs and symptoms include nystagmus, strabismus, central or paracentral field defects, dyschromatopsia, and an afferent pupillary defect [6]. Lesions of the optic nerve are commonly associated with disc edema, which can be seen on funduscopy. If the edema persists, atrophy may ensue in approximately 6 to 8 weeks. Optic nerve gliomas grow slowly but may grow in spurts [13–15] or be dormant without any significant increase in size over many years. They may decrease in size or, in rare instances, regress completely [16–18]. Spontaneous regression of an optic nerve glioma in patients who have neurofibromatosis has been reported [19]. Because of this erratic growth, follow-up over many years is necessary [20–22]. There is a high association of optic nerve gliomas with neurofibromatosis type 1 (NF-1), which has varied from 12% to 37% [23]. The evidence of NF-1 may be subtle, such as the presence of Lish nodules of the iris or café au lait spots. The clinical presentation of optic pathway gliomas is earlier and more severe in sporadic tumors than in tumors associated with NF-1 [22].

Optic nerve glioma in the anterior visual pathway may be limited to the orbital optic nerve or extend into the intracranial cavity (Fig. 1). In an analysis of 63 cases by Yanoff and associates [24] in 1978, the orbital optic nerve was involved in 48%, the orbital and intracranial optic nerve in 24%, the intracranial optic nerve and chiasm in 10%, and chiasm in 5% of cases.

On pathologic examinations, optic nerve gliomas resemble juvenile pilocytic astrocytomas [25–28]. They are composed of elongated, spindle-shaped pilocytic astrocytes with absence of mitotic figures reflecting a benign histopathology. Oligodendroglial cells are also present in small numbers; if oligodendroglial cells are numerous, the tumor is designated as an oligodendroglioma.

Optic nerve gliomas grow slowly and are locally invasive with no tendency to malignant transforma-

**Box 1. Tumors of the optic nerve**

*Primary optic nerve tumors*
- Optic nerve glioma
  - Optic nerve glioma and neurofibromatosis
  - Malignant optic nerve glioma
- Optic nerve sheath meningioma
- Medulloepithelioma
- Ganglioglioma
- Hemangioblastoma
- Choristoma

*Secondary optic nerve tumors*
- Metastatic disease to optic nerves
  - Hematogenous
    - Breast
    - Lung
    - Gastrointestinal tract
  - Invasion of optic nerve from globe
    - Retinoblastoma
    - Uveal melanoma
  - Invasion from orbit
  - Extension from paranasal sinuses
    - Benign and malignant tumors
    - Mucoceles
    - Infection
  - Spread of tumor through the subarachnoid space
    - Meningeal carcinomatosis
    - Non-Hodgkin's lymphoma
    - Leukemia
    - Myeloma
  - Primary brain tumors
    - Glioblastoma multiforme
    - Primitive neuroectodermal tumor
    - Gliomatosis cerebri

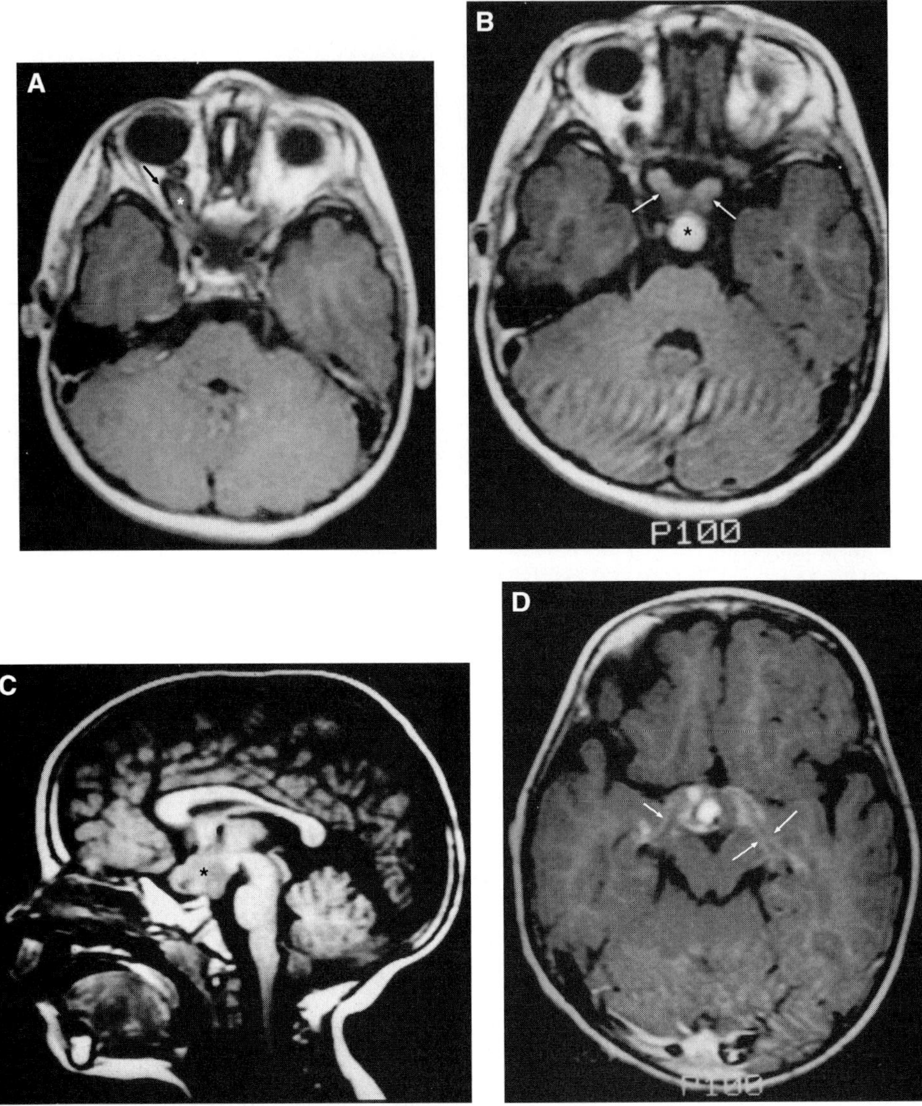


Fig. 1. Bilateral optic nerve gliomas with extension to the chiasm, hypothalamus, optic tracts, and optic radiation. (*A*) Axial T1-weighted image shows enlargement of the optic nerves. Note low-intensity layer around right optic nerve consistent with perineural gliosis (*arrow*). (*B*) Axial T1-weighted image demonstrates enlarged intracranial optic nerves (*arrows*) and chiasm (*asterisk*). (*C*) Lateral T1-weighted image visualizes tumor in the hypothalamus (*asterisk*). (*D*) Axial T1-weighted image after gadolinium introduction shows heterogeneous uptake of contrast material in the enlarged chiasm. Note linear extension of enhancing tumor into both optic tracts (*arrows*). (*E*) Axial T1-weighted image after gadolinium administration shows uptake of tumor in the geniculate bodies. (*F*) Axial FLAIR image illustrates high-signal-intensity tumor in both optic tracts.

tion. They cause fusiform enlargement of the optic nerve, which is completely invested by an intact and often thinned and stretched dura [27]. If they extend through the optic foramen, they often have a dumbbell-shaped configuration. On cut section, they are firm on palpation but may have soft areas of myxomatous consistency imparting a gelatinous appearance to the nerve [23]. Cystic degeneration within the tumor has been described [28]. Hemorrhage with hematoma formation and necrosis occurs infrequently in optic nerve gliomas but may lead to blindness and sudden proptosis [29–31]. The normal histologic architecture of the optic nerve is completely effaced from the tumor growth within the nerve. Cross-

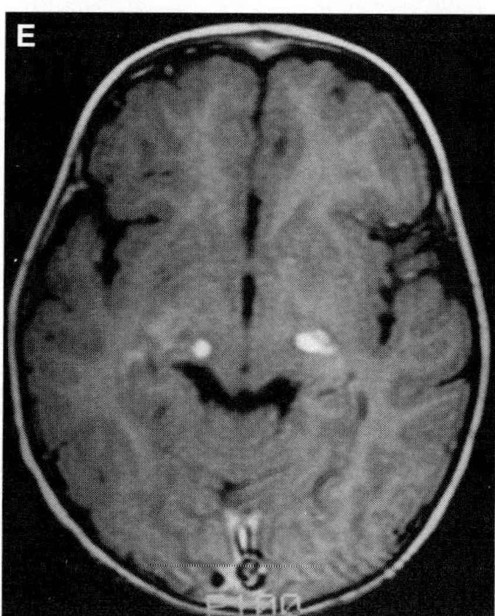


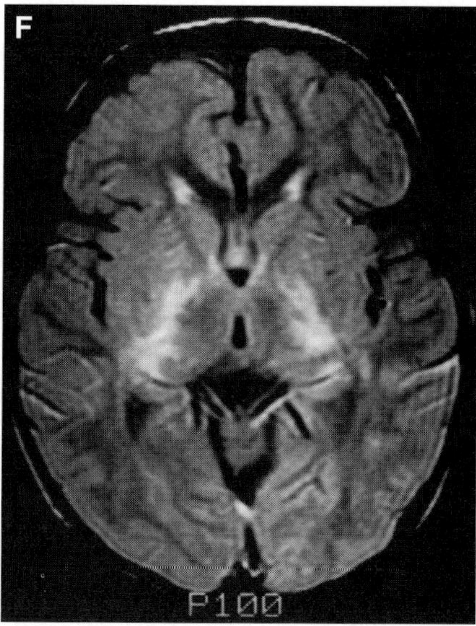


Fig. 1 (*continued*).

section of an excised optic nerve glioma reveals a layer of arachnoidal tissue of varying thickness surrounding the tumor, covered by a stretched intact dura. This thickened tissue is formed by proliferation of meningothelial cells and fibroblasts intermingled with astrocytes. The term perineural gliomatosis has been proposed by Stern and associates [27] for this admixture of perineural tissue (Fig. 1) [24]. The perineural gliomatosis may extend beyond the limits of the intraneural portion of the glioma, making assessment of tumor extension difficult [32]. On MR imaging, perineural gliomatosis is depicted as a low signal intensity on T1-weighted images and on T2-weighted images as an area of high signal intensity surrounding a central area of lesser signal intensity [33]. Some reports state that there is no gadolinium enhancement of the perineural arachnoidal hyperplasia [34]. If the arachnoidal gliomatosis is protuberant, an optic nerve meningioma may mistakenly be diagnosed [35,36].

Extension of optic nerve glioma to the globe with intraocular seeding has been described in a patient who has neurofibromatosis [37]. This phenomenon should be differentiated from gliomas that arise in the optic nerve head [38,39]. Seeding within the subarachnoid space cranially and in the spinal canal has been observed in a patient who has a suprasellar chiasmal pilocytic astrocytoma [40]. A related tumor is the ganglioneuroma, which has been reported in the optic nerves and chiasm [41].

The management of optic nerve gliomas is controversial, and reported statistics and results of treatment vary considerably among published reports [9,42–45]. Patients who have anterior visual pathway gliomas, particularly patients who have NF-1, should not be treated unless there is clear clinical or neuroimaging evidence of progression [6,46,47]. In 1969 Hoyt and Baghdassarian [48] reported that 75% of patients who had untreated gliomas had improved or stable visual acuity.

There is increased mortality with intracranial extension, especially with hypothalamic involvement. In recent years, surgery, through orbitotomy or a transcranial approach, has been performed for orbital or intracranial optic nerve gliomas after significant visual loss has developed in patients who have severe proptosis, a blind, painful eye, or for biopsy of a chiasmal tumor [43]. A rare occurrence of regrowth after resection of the optic nerve, referred to as phantom optic nerve, has been observed [49]. Radiotherapy has been reserved mainly for intracranial tumors, including chiasmatic gliomas [42,50]. After radiation therapy, visual improvement or stability and tumor regression have been observed in some cases [51]. Because of small sample sizes, short follow-up intervals, and inadequate radiologic demonstration of tumor extent before the availability of MR imaging, no firm conclusions can be drawn concerning outcome.

Chemotherapy is being tried, and preliminary data suggest some potential value [52,53]. Optic gliomas are considered true neoplasms. They may invade the leptomeninges, notably in patients who have NF-1.

Before the introduction of CT and MR imaging, conventional radiologic studies, consisting of optic

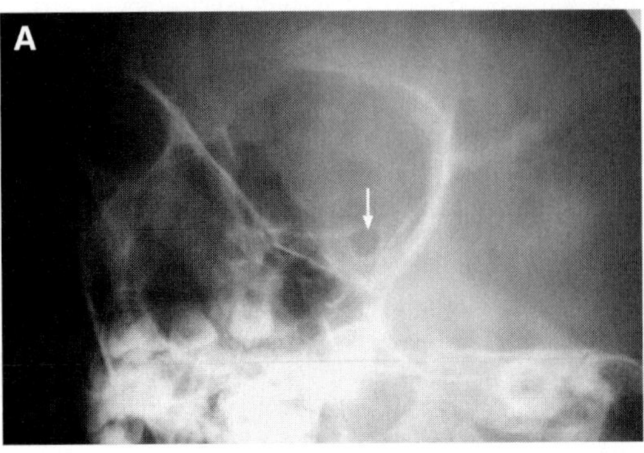


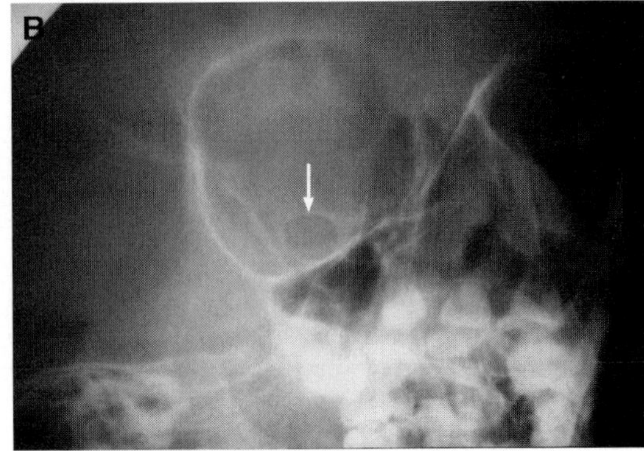


Fig. 2. Left optic nerve glioma. (*A*) Conventional optic foramen view shows normal right optic foramen (*arrow*). (*B*) Conventional optic foramen view illustrates enlarged left optic foramen with well-defined cortex.

foramen views, were obtained (Fig. 2). These studies showed concentric enlargement of the optic foramen in more than 50% of cases. The cortical margins are well preserved with no evidence of irregularity or sclerosis [54]. Not all optic nerve gliomas that extend through the optic canal cause enlargement of the foramen on radiologic studies, however. Extension to the chiasm with formation of a bulky mass may lead to enlargement and depression of the chiasmatic sulcus, flattening of the tuberculum sellae, undercutting of the anterior clinoid process, and thinning of the optic strut [55]. These radiologic findings reflect the slow growth of optic nerve gliomas. On basal CT sections with bone window setting, the entire length of the optic canal is visualized (Fig. 3B). On CT with soft tissue windows, intraorbital optic nerve gliomas are characterized by fusiform or sausage-shaped enlargement (Fig. 4) [55]. In a small percentage of cases, there may be marked fusiform to globular enlargement of the optic nerve glioma with almost complete obliteration of the intraconal orbital fat (Fig. 5A). Axial CT with bone window delineates the dimension of the enlarged bony optic canal (Fig. 5B). The tumor margins are smooth, and there is a sharp interface with the surrounding orbital fat. On CT, optic nerve gliomas are isodense with brain and show slight to moderate enhancement following the introduction of contrast material. CT, however, does not allow the separation of the individual optic nerve layers and CSF space. MR imaging provides optimal assessment of optic nerve gliomas [56–59]. There is enlargement of the optic nerve sheath complex with a configuration that may be tubular, fusiform, eccentric, or globular, with kinking and tortuosity noted in cases that have marked enlargement of the nerve (Fig. 5). On TI-weighted images, hypo- or isointensity of the

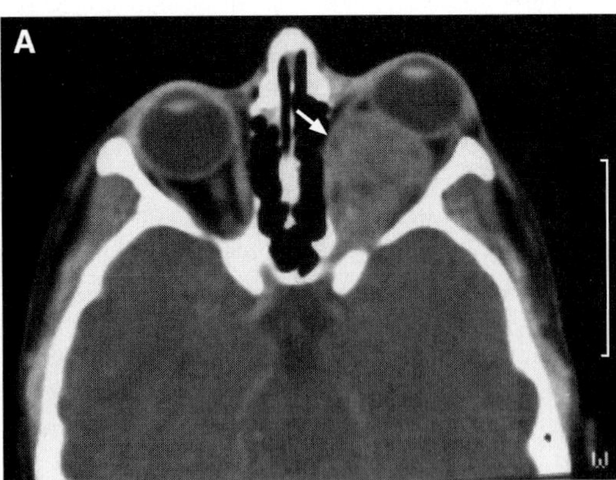


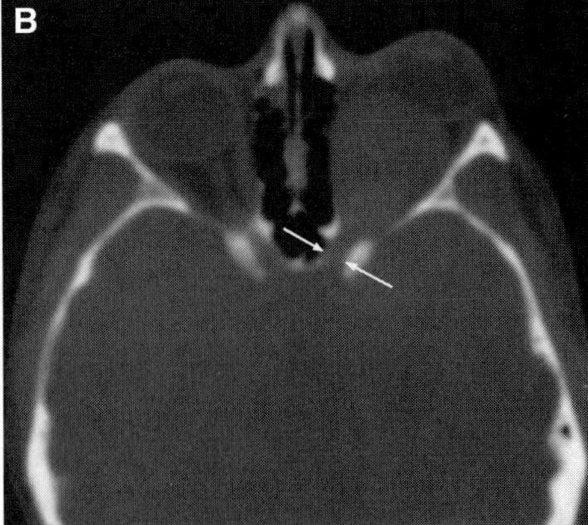


Fig. 3. Large left optic nerve glioma. (*A*) Axial CT study reveals a large, slightly heterogeneous mass within the orbital cavity. Note slight medial deviation of the lamina papyracea medially (*arrow*). (*B*) Axial scan through the orbits with bone window setting shows funnel-shaped enlargement of the left optic canal (*arrows*). Note normal right optic canal.

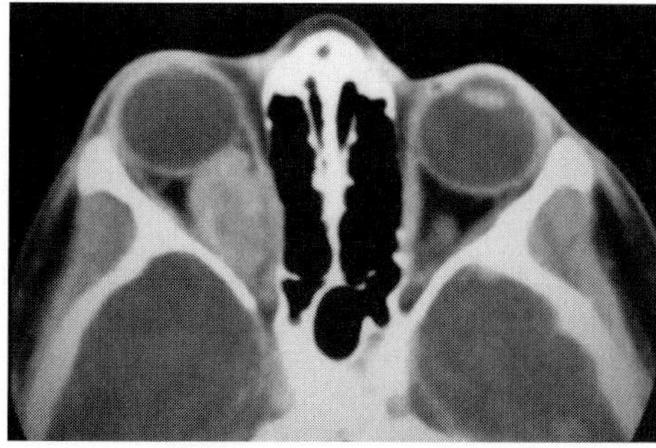

Fig. 4. Right optic nerve glioma. Axial CT study reveals a homogeneous spindle-shaped mass with well-defined margins consistent with an optic nerve glioma.

optic nerve glioma is present (Fig. 5A and B), whereas on the T-2 weighted images there is often increased signal intensity of the lesion (see Fig. 1F). The enhancement of optic nerve glioma on MR imaging can vary from no enhancement to slight to marked homogeneous or heterogeneous enhancement (Fig. 6). The more aggressive tumors reveal enhancement on MR imaging, whereas nonenhancement is more common in stationary glioma. Peripheral enhancement of optic nerve gliomas and chiasmatic gliomas may reflect extraneural growth of tumor within the subarachnoid space intermixed with gliomatous tissue contrasted against nonenhancing central tumor (see Fig. 1D). Extension of optic nerve gliomas to the chiasm through the optic canal produces a dumbbell-shaped configuration [55]. Optic nerve gliomas may be associated with dilatation of the subarachnoid space reflected by widening of the high-intensity CSF fluid on the T2-weighted images. This dilatation may be secondary to obstruction in the outflow of CSF or trapping of fluid by perineural gliomatosis.

Gliomas of the anterior visual pathway may be limited to one or both optic nerves or may extend posteriorly into the chiasm and, in advanced cases, to

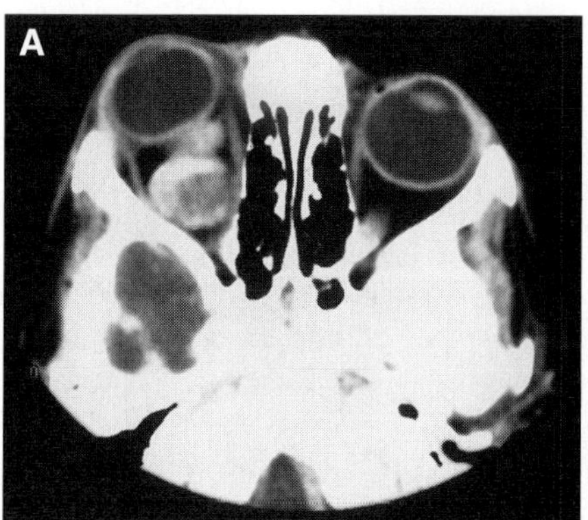


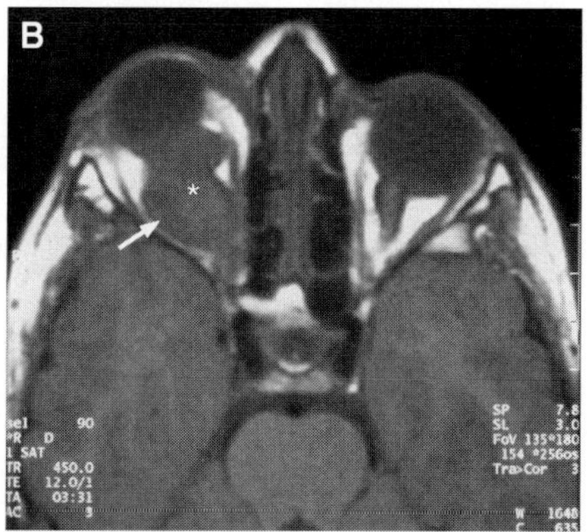


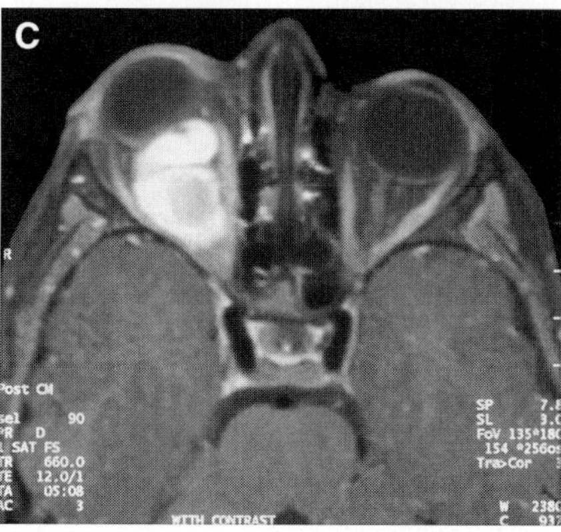


Fig. 5. Right optic nerve glioma with hamartomatous dysplasia in the cerebellum. (*A*) Axial CT section outlines a large heterogeneous glioma in the right orbit. Note proptosis of globe. (*B*) Axial T1-weighted image through the orbit shows a hypointense, tortuous, slightly heterogeneous optic nerve glioma (*asterisk*). There is a hypointense layer at the margin of the nerve (*arrow*) consistent with perineural gliosis interspersed with cerebrospinal fluid. (*C*) Axial T1-weighted image after gadolinium administration shows marked enhancement of the tumor.

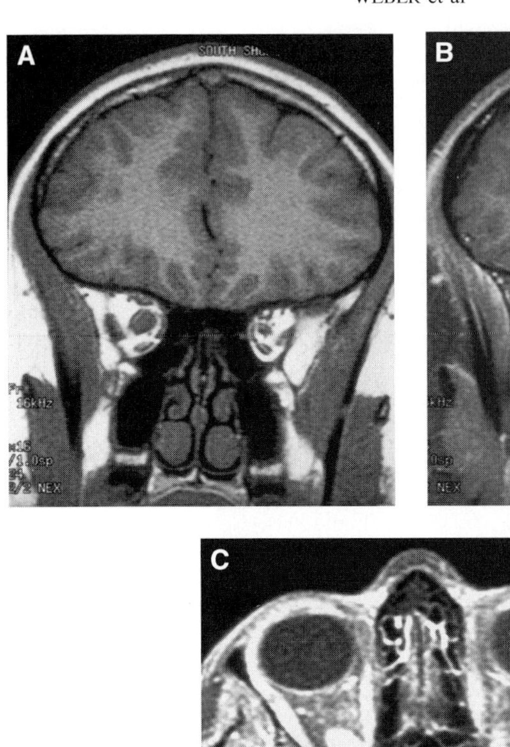


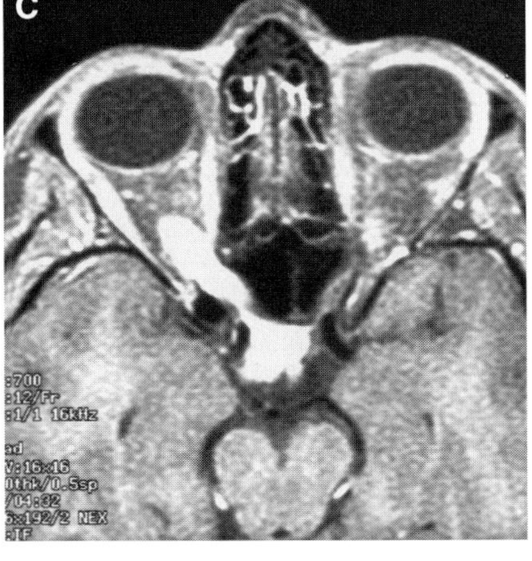


Fig. 6. Right optic nerve glioma extending to the chiasm and displaying marked homogeneous enhancement. (*A*) Right T1-weighted coronal image shows enlargement of the hypointense optic nerve. (*B*) T1-weighted image after gadolinium administration and fat suppression demonstrates marked homogeneous enhancement of the enlarged right optic nerve. (*C*) Axial T1-weighted image after gadolinium administration illustrates enhancement of the optic nerve and extension through the enlarged optic canal to the chiasm.

the optic tracts and least common optic radiation unilaterally or bilaterally (see Fig. 1) [55,60,61]. When angiography has been performed, no hypervascularity of optic nerve gliomas has been observed. Calcifications in optic nerve gliomas are not demonstrated but may occur following radiation therapy. Rarely, tumor may extend into the sphenoid sinus or sella turcica and have the appearance of an intrasellar or sphenoid sinus lesion [62]. Extension of gliomas into the postchiasmal pathway, including optic tracts and optic radiation, may form a large mass growing into the adjacent brain [55,60]. Associated enlargement of the sylvian, suprasellar arachnoid, and prepontine cisterns may be present. Large tumors in the suprasellar area may simulate other suprasellar tumors, but involvement of the intraorbital optic nerves can be helpful in the differential diagnosis of these suprasellar masses. Some of these tumors in the chiasm and hypothalamus are prone to necrosis with formation of irregular cystic areas (Fig. 7) [63].

### *Optic nerve glioma and neurofibromatosis*

Optic nerve glioma may occur in association with neurofibromatosis [46,64,65]. The incidence of optic nerve glioma in NF-1 has been reported to be approximately 15%, whereas approximately 12% to 37% of optic pathway gliomas have signs of NF-1

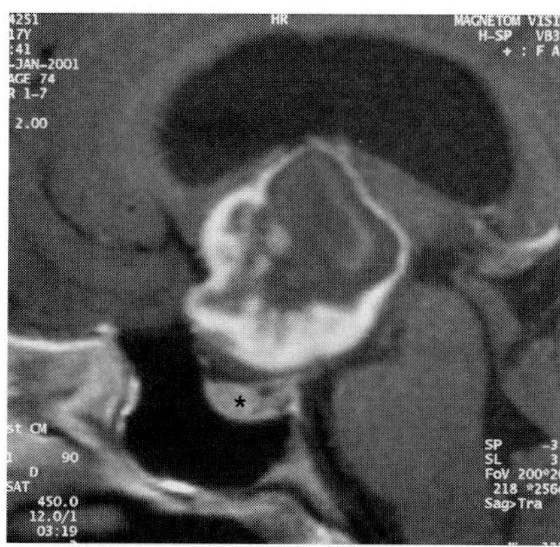

Fig. 7. Chiasmal and hypothalamic glioma with central necrosis. Lateral T1-weighted image after gadolinium introduction demonstrates central necrosis. The remaining tumor wall is irregular. Note dilatation of the lateral ventricles.

[66,67]. The condition is inherited in an autosomal dominant fashion. As in patients who do not have neurofibromatosis, the growth rate is variable, but involvement of both optic nerves is more common. Like patients who have optic nerve gliomas without NF-1, patients with NF-1 and gliomas have visual dysfunction including decreased visual acuity and visual field defects that can be related to tumor location by MR imaging [12]. (On MR imaging some optic nerve gliomas in patients who have NF-1 display dilatation of the subarachnoid space around the optic nerve or perineural, arachnoidal gliomatosis around the optic nerve glioma [34,58,59,68,69]. Optic nerve gliomas may extend posteriorly with involvement of the chiasm and optic tracts and adjacent anatomic areas, especially the hypothalamus, and extend less commonly to the optic radiation (see Fig. 1C) [69,70]. They rarely involve the optic radiation, but involvement of optic radiation may signal a more aggressive optic pathway glioma in patients who have NF-1. Patients who have NF-1 and optic gliomas are more likely to develop a second primary central nervous system (CNS) tumor, and long-term follow-up is advised [65,71,72]. A frequent finding is the association of hamartomatous lesions of the brain including cerebellum, brainstem, basal ganglia, thalamus, deep capsular and periventricular white matter, and corpus callosum in patients who have NF-1 [58,68,69,71]. These hamartomatous areas are reflected by increased signal intensity on the long T2-weighted images and proton density images. They exhibit no mass effect or edema and fail to enhance with gadolinium. A change in size (either an increase or decrease) has been observed. The benign nature of these hamartomatous lesions is further exemplified by their presence on MR imaging studies performed for a routine work-up in asymptomatic patients, for follow-up of NF-1 patients, or for evaluation of nonophthalmologic symptoms in patients who have NF-1. They display increased signal intensity on T2-weighted images and sporadically on TI-weighted images. A decrease in size and signal intensity has been reported over time. The hamartomatous lesions are composed of dysplastic glial tissue in the white matter of the various parts of the brain. A diagnostic problem occurs when the lesions are interspersed with tumor tissue. Enhancement of the lesion or change in size and configuration over a limited period supports a tumor etiology. Optic nerve gliomas in patients who have NF-1 have also been reported in patients who have tuberous sclerosis and von Hippel-Lindau disease [73,74].

*Malignant optic nerve glioma*

Malignant optic nerve glioma is a rare tumor of the optic pathway that is distinct from the benign optic nerve glioma of childhood [75–82]. It is more prevalent in males, and the peak incidence is between 40 and 50 years of age. The presenting symptoms include rapid loss of vision (most commonly bilateral) associated with dyschromatopsia, field defects, optic disc edema or atrophy, afferent pupillary defect, and orbital pain. The tumor is usually bilateral and predominantly involves the intracranial optic nerves and chiasm with secondary extension to the hypothalamus, optic tracts, and third ventricle. Tumor location limited to the intraorbital optic nerve is less common. Histologic examination of biopsy and necropsy material reveals anaplastic astrocytoma or glioblastoma multiforme. Primary neuroectodermal tumor also has been observed (Fig. 8) [77]. The overall mortality rate of this disease approaches 100%, with a mean survival of 9 months following initial diagnosis. Treatment by radiation therapy and chemotherapy thus far has not significantly altered the fatal outcome. The preferred imaging modality is MR imaging with gadolinium, because, in the early stages of the disease, only slight enlargement of the anterior optic pathway may be visible and is only illustrated with gadolinium enhancement. At this early stage, the tumor simulates an early inflammatory process including optic neuritis or sarcoid. Before MR imaging was available, the early diagnosis was often made by surgical intervention with a biopsy [80]. Further tumor growth leads to enlargement of the optic nerves and chiasm and involvement of the optic tracts, hypothalamus, and adjacent brain.

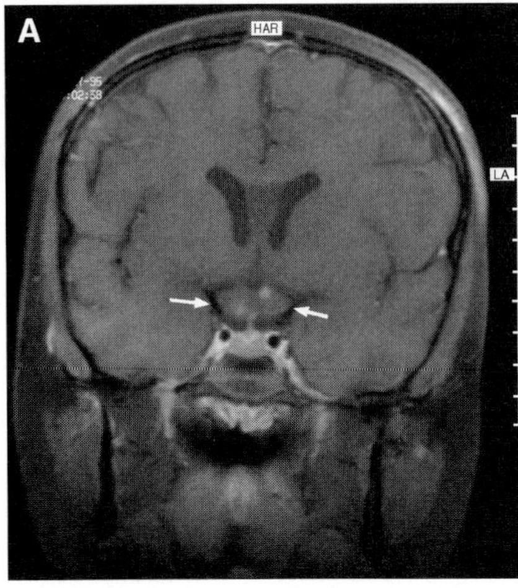

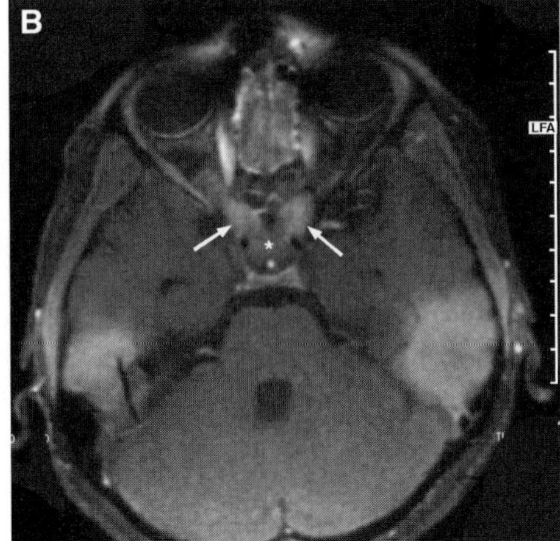

Fig. 8. Primary neuroectodermal tumor of the brain invading both intracranial optic nerves including the chiasm. (*A*) Coronal T1-weighted postgadolinium section through the chiasm defines an enlarged, partially enhancing chiasm (*arrows*). (*B*) Axial T1-weighted image after gadolinium introduction demonstrates diffuse enhancement of both enlarged intracranial optic nerves.

Metastases to the neural axis have been reported [78]. The extent of the tumor is delineated optimally with MR imaging [83]. The enhancement is variable and similar to the findings in aggressive malignant gliomas of the brain.

*Optic nerve sheath meningioma*

Meningiomas are classified as primary if they originate from the meninges of the orbital optic nerve and as secondary if they extend into the orbit from the meninges in the intracranial cavity, notably the sphenoid bone [23]. A less common third type arises from ectopic nests of meningothelial cells in the orbit. Optic nerve sheath meningioma represents less than 1% of all meningiomas [84] and constitutes approximately 3% to 5% of orbital tumors. The tumor occurs predominantly between the ages of 30 and 50 years but can occur at any age, including childhood [85]. The mean age of presentation of primary optic nerve sheath meningiomas is lower than that of intracranial meningiomas. There is a 3:1 female predominance.

Primary intraorbital meningiomas in children are more aggressive than similar tumors in adults. The

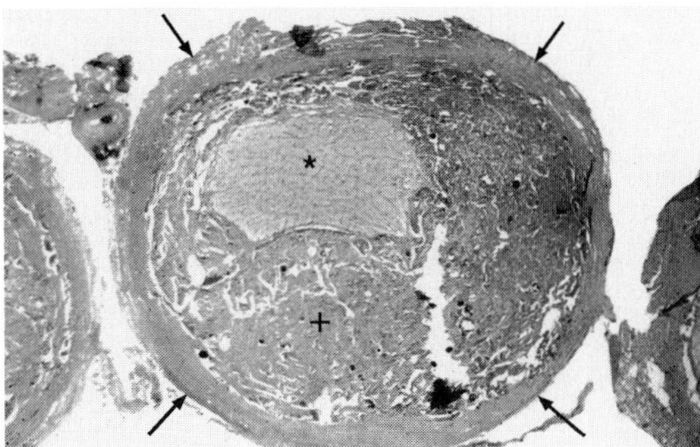

Fig. 9. Histopathologic cross-section through the optic nerve reveals the central normal axons of the optic nerve (*asterisk*) surrounded by thick layers of meningioma (*cross*). The outermost layer represents the dura (*arrows*).

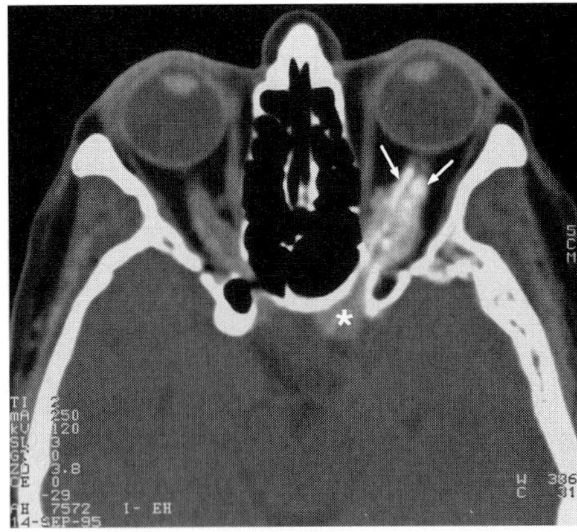

Fig. 10. Bilateral optic nerve sheath meningioma with speckled small calcifications on the left. Axial CT section through the orbits reveals diffuse thickening of both optic nerves with small tumor calcifications on the left (*arrows*). Note hypointense linear structure within the optic nerves. On the left there is a slight intracranial extension of the meningioma shown by a small enhancing mass at the cranial end of the optic canal (*asterisk*).

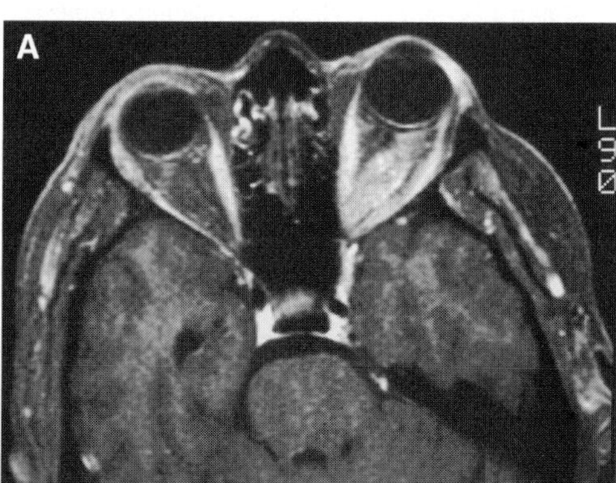


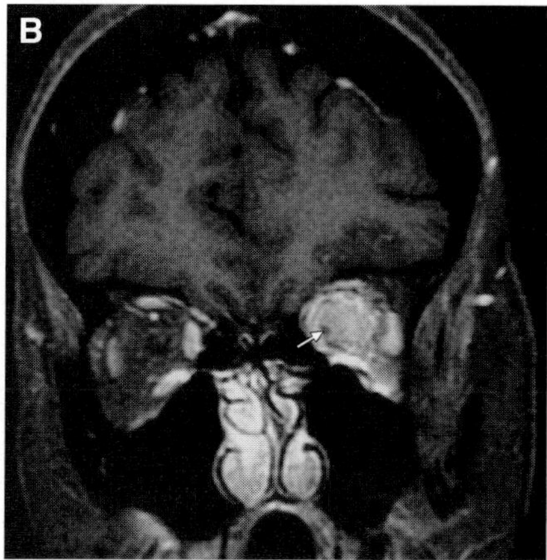


Fig. 11. Left optic nerve meningioma with fat suppression. (*A*) Axial and (*B*) coronal T1-weighted images after gadolinium introduction and fat suppression show an enhancing left optic nerve sheath meningioma. On the coronal image (*B*), there is a hypointense oval structure consistent with the optic nerve embedded within the meningioma (*arrow*).

most frequent symptoms are progressive loss of vision, slowly progressive axial proptosis, disc edema, pallor [86,87], and, uncommonly, enophthalmos [88]. Papilledema is present in the early stages and eventually proceeds to atrophy, reflected by a white, sharply delimited disk on funduscopy. Ophthalmologic examination demonstrates central scotoma with generalized constriction of the visual field or overall depression of the visual field. These findings become progressively worse, and eventually the patient may become blind. Optociliary shunt vessels are occasionally demonstrated in the papillary area on funduscopy. Optic nerve sheath meningiomas originate in the capsules of the arachnoid enveloping the optic nerve. The optic nerve usually is embedded in the tumor (Fig. 9). The tumors grow along the nerve and may penetrate the dura and expand into the adjacent orbital fat [22,89]. They are unilateral tumors, but bilateral optic nerve sheath meningiomas are seen occasionally, especially in patients who have NF-1 (Fig. 10) [90]. The histologic types are the same as in meningiomas encountered in the intracranial cavity. Growth may be circumferential along the optic nerve sheath, imparting a tubular configuration to the enlarged optic nerve. The tumor margins are often slightly irregular and lobulated with variable thickness. They show marked enhancement, and therefore fat suppression techniques should be used (Figs. 11 and 12). They may, however, grow eccentrically from the optic nerve sheath and cause asymmetrical

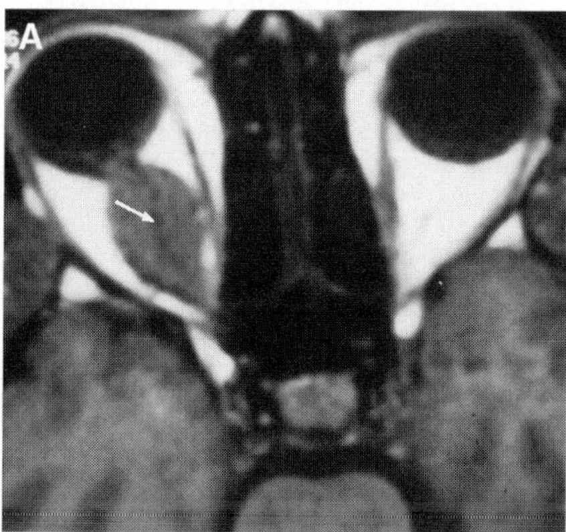


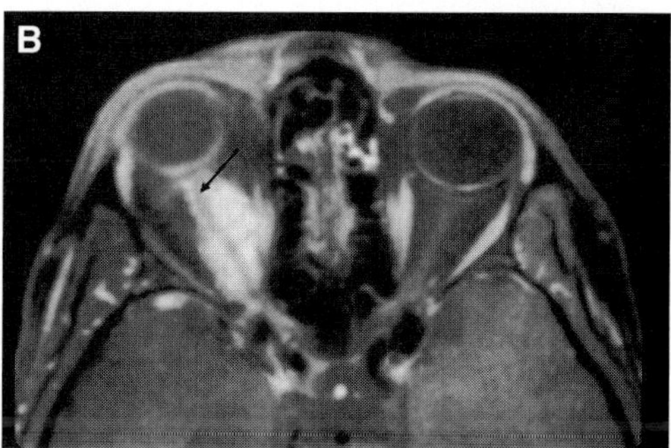


Fig. 12. Right optic nerve sheath meningioma. (*A*) Axial T1-weighted mage displays a spindle-shaped, hypointense meningioma arising from the right optic nerve sheath. Note hypointense nerve surrounded by tumor (*arrow*). (*B*) Axial T1-weighted image after gadolinium administration with fat suppression shows an asymmetric, moderate-sized, enhancing meningioma surrounding a low-signal-intensity optic nerve (*arrow*).

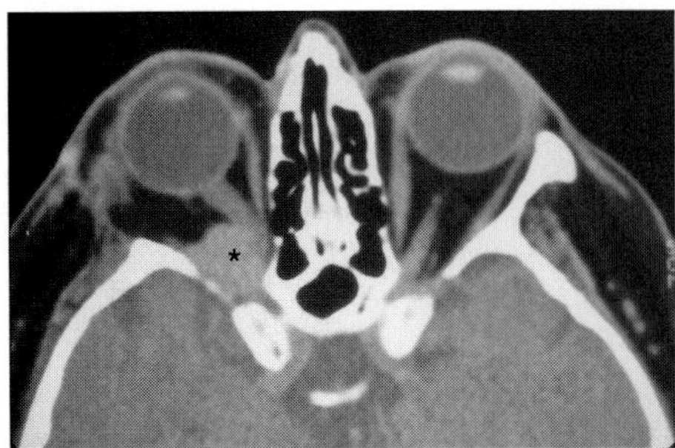

Fig. 13. Asymmetric meningioma in the apex of the left orbit. Axial CT scan through the orbits outlines an isodense meningioma (*asterisk*) in the apex of the orbit displacing the optic nerve medially.

enlargement of the entire or part of the optic nerve sheath (Fig. 13). If eccentric growth prevails, the optic nerve may be located at the margin of the tumor with concomitant displacement away from the tumor, often medially. In these circumstances, the optic nerve sheath meningioma may simulate a tumor within the orbit that has encroached on the optic nerve. Significant globular extrinsic growth is frequently encountered in the optic nerve near the globe. The dura is thinned because of spreading into the adjacent sclera. Optic nerve sheath meningiomas, in rare instances, may grow into the optic disc of the eye and adjacent choroid with tumor visible on funduscopy as a bulging mass at the disc [91]. They have been associated with cysts distal to the tumor [92]. Eventually the tumor may grow along the septae into the core of the optic nerve. A special group of meningiomas may be confined to the optic canal and most posterior portion of the orbital apex and defy early diagnosis [93,94]. They cause progressive loss of vision, and a diagnosis of optic neuritis is falsely made. On imaging studies with slices thicker than 3 mm, no mass is visible in the orbital apex or sellar/parasellar area. In such cases, thin sections (3 mm and less) in different projections by MR imaging with gadolinium enhancement are required. CT with thin slices may illustrate minor bone changes, notably sclerosis or alteration in size of the foramen; these changes have been observed in about 50% of cases [89,93].

Meningiomas tend to be hyperdense on CT studies, and 12.5% to 31% reveal globular, linear, or plaquelike calcifications (see Fig. 10) [89,95]. Contrast enhancement in optic nerve sheath meningioma is often intense surrounding the nonenhancing optic nerve within the tumor mass. On axial and coronal MR imaging studies, a lucent central cord is noted throughout the dense enhancing tumor (see Figs. 11 and 12). Optic nerve sheath meningiomas may extend from the orbital part of the sheath into the optic canal and cause enlargement and, occasionally, hyperostosis of the margin of the canal [89].

On MR imaging, optic nerve sheath meningiomas reveal low signal intensity on the TI-weighted (see Fig. 12A) and T2-weighted images [96]. MR imaging frequently fails to demonstrate small areas of calcification within the optic nerve sheath. Larger amounts of calcium are reflected by low signal intensity on the T1-weighted and T2-weighted images. There is frequently marked enhancement of the meningioma, similar to meningiomas in the intracranial cavity (see Figs. 11 and 12B). Extension into the optic canal and adjacent intracranial cavity is demonstrated optimally with gadolinium-enhanced MR imaging (see Figs. 10, 14, and 16)). Fat suppression techniques should be used to contrast the enhancing tumor against the darkened fatty tissue (see Fig. 11) [97]. Meningiomas that arise within the intracranial cavity, particularly from the tuberculum sellae, anterior clinoid processes, and lesser wing of sphenoid, may secondarily invade the optic nerve sheath in the optic canal and may further extend into the orbital apex. These lesions are well delineated on MR imaging with gadolinium enhancement using different projections, such as axial, coronal, and parasagittal (Fig. 15). Clinically, they cause marked compromise in vision, often without proptosis.

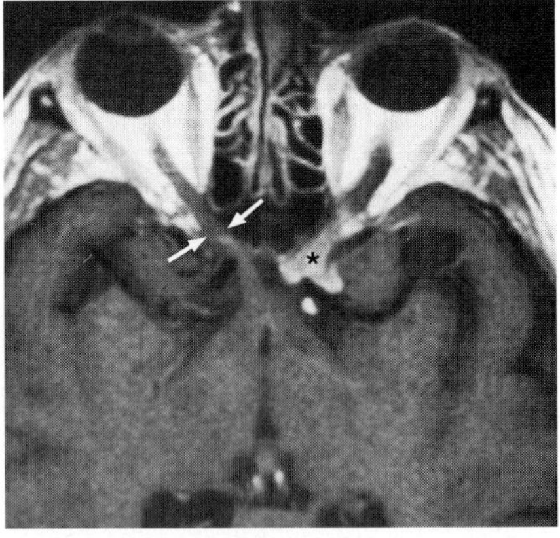

Fig. 14. Meningioma in the left optic canal and tuberculum sellae. Axial T1-weighted section after gadolinium administration shows a moderately enhancing meningioma in the left optic canal and adjacent tuberculum sellae (*asterisk*). Compare with normal right optic nerve in optic canal (*arrow*).

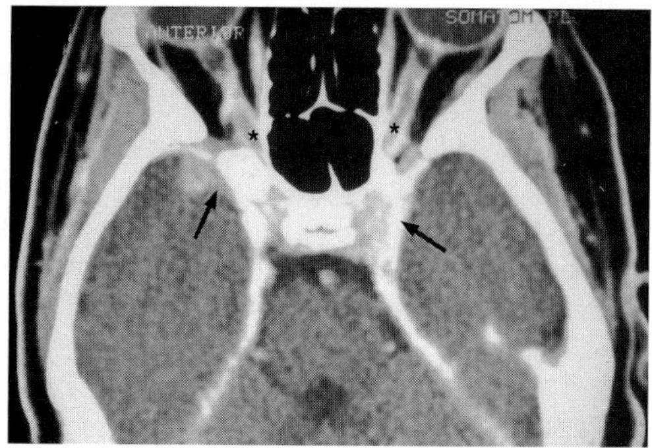

Fig. 15. Bilateral sphenoid wing meningioma extending into the left and right optic canals and apices of the left and right orbits. Axial CT section through the orbits defines an enhancing meningioma arising from the left and right sphenoid wings (*arrows*) with extension to the apices of both orbits and adjacent optic canals. The optic nerves reveal enhancement, possibly because of secondary invasion by the meningiomas.

The treatment of meningiomas depends on the clinical course over time, principally as they affect vision [98]. No treatment is indicated if the vision is stable or only slight deterioration is found on follow-up examinations. Treatment, however, is indicated, after serial follow-up examinations document a progressive decline in visual acuity and visual field defects or further enlargement of the tumor on imaging studies [1]. The treatment consists of fractionated stereotactic conformal radiotherapy, which seems most likely to preserve visual function. Visual improvement often is perceptible after 1 to 3 months of therapy [99,100].

*Medulloepithelioma*

Medulloepithelioma is a rare tumor composed of multilayered sheets of poorly differentiated neuroepithelial cells that are similar to embryonic retinal and ciliary epithelial cells [101,102]. The tumor has been categorized as teratoid and nonteratoid. In addition to the medullary cells, nonteratoid medulloepithelioma demonstrates tissue elements (eg, cartilage) that are not native to the tissue of origin. The tumor is irregular and reveals variable local aggressiveness, but distant metastases do not occur. Medulloepithelioma most commonly arises from the ciliary body region as a bulky, variable-sized mass but may occur in the optic nerve and disc. There is expansion of the dura of the nerve and occasionally invasion into the adjacent orbital fat after penetration through the dura.

*Melanocytoma*

Melanocytoma, a relatively uncommon, unilateral lesion, is a heavily pigmented tumor with an average size of 2 × 1 mm and shape. The tumor is located in the optic nerve head but may extend into the contiguous choroid and retina or, rarely, to the optic nerve near the lamina cribrosa [38,103]. The tumor also occurs in the ciliary body and the meninges of the intracranial cavity, chiefly the posterior fossa, and spine [104–106]. Melanocytoma is considered a variant of a nevus and is composed of large, round, pigmented melanocytes displaying benign features. There is a male predominance with an age range between 14 and 79 years. The mean age of onset is 50 years [104]. Approximately 37% to 50% of lesions occur in blacks, whereas less than 1% of melanomas occur in the black population. The tumor is stationary, but slow growth is observed in some cases [107]. Rarely, the tumor undergoes malignant transformation into a malignant melanoma [108,109]. On CT, the tumor appears as a small, enhancing mass showing slight extension to the optic nerve near the lamina cribrosa (Fig. 16). The signal intensities of melanocytoma on MR imaging are thought to display features similar to those of a melanoma (eg, high T1- and low T2-weighted signal intensities with enhancement) [110,111].

*Ganglioglioma*

Ganglioglioma is a rare tumor affecting the optic nerve and remaining anterior visual pathway [112].

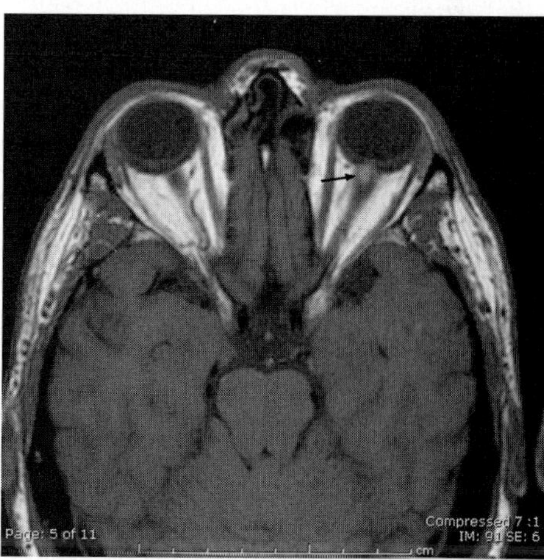

Fig. 16. Melanocytoma in the optic nerve head and adjacent optic nerve. Axial T1-weighted image shows a hyperdense lesion at the optic nerve head and adjacent optic nerve (*arrow*).

Eighty percent of these lesions occur during the first 3 decades of life. Histologic examination demonstrates a mass composed of neurons and glial cells characteristic of ganglioglioma [113]. The optic nerve shows diffuse enlargement similar to that observed in optic nerve glioma and meningioma [114]. The clinical and biologic behavior depends on the glial component. A case that had rapid growth secondary to proliferation of pilocytic glial cells and association with NF-1 has been described [115].

*Hemangioblastoma*

Hemangioblastomas occur predominantly in the cerebellum, spinal cord, and retina. They occur uncommonly in the orbit or the optic nerve [116–119]. Hemangioblastomas are highly vascularized tumors; the histologic origin is poorly defined. They are the most frequent manifestation of the von Hippel-Lindau disease but also occur as sporadic nonhereditary tumors [118]. Almost all the lesions are sharply demarcated from the adjacent nerve and, thus, potentially are resectable. They are more common in the prechiasmatic optic nerve and display marked enhancement (Fig. 17). The patients experience progressive loss of vision to the point of blindness.

*Choristoma*

Choristoma is an uncommon optic nerve lesion that is probably malformative and nonneoplastic in nature [120]. It usually causes progressive visual loss and optic atrophy. It is composed of adipose tissue and smooth muscle involving and often invading the optic nerve or chiasm [121] On T1-weighted MR imaging, a choristoma has high signal intensities generated by the fatty tissue intermixed with low signal intensities generated by the muscular tissue. Fat-suppression techniques provide further evidence of the presence of fat, an integral part of a choristoma [122,123]. Even if imaging studies are highly suggestive of the diagnosis, pathologic confirmation is required.

## Secondary optic nerve tumors

The optic nerve is involved by secondary optic nerve tumors more frequently than by primary optic nerve tumors [23,124]. Secondary malignant tumors from a variety of sources and routes of spread afflict the optic nerve (see Box 1). These tumors include

1. Hematogenous metastases [125]
2. Extension from ocular tumors
3. Compression or, rarely, invasion by tumor adjacent to the nerve in the orbital cavity
4. Extension of tumor from the sellar/parasellar area through the subarachnoid space [126]
5. Seeding of tumor within the subarachnoid space from sources outside the neural axis principally from carcinomas [125]
6. CNS tumors extending to the chiasm and optic nerves, including primary neuroectodermal tumors (see Fig. 8), glioblastomas [77], and gliomatosis cerebri [127]

Unlike orbital and choroidal metastases, which are relatively common, metastatic disease to the optic nerve from different sources, especially isolated in-

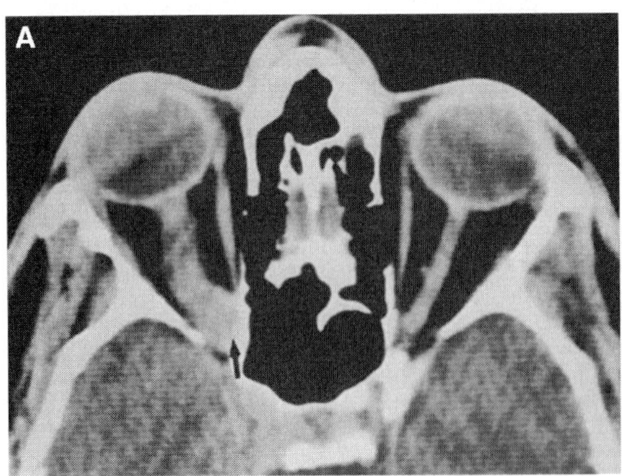


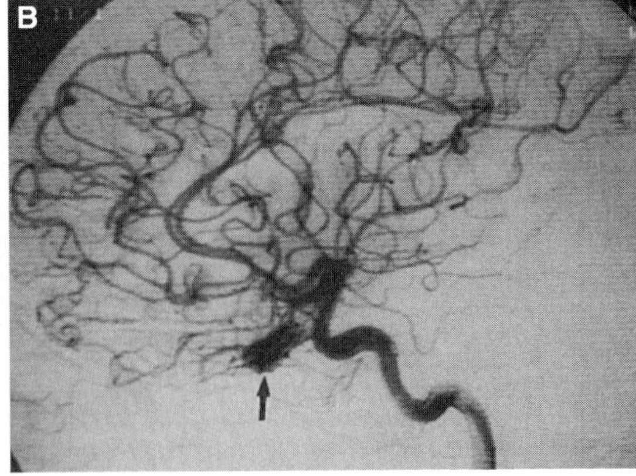


Fig. 17. Hemangioblastoma of the right optic nerve. (*A*) Contrast CT scan shows an enhancing optic nerve hemangioblastoma (*arrows*). (*B*) Lateral carotid angiogram reveals an intense tumor blush (*arrows*). (*From* Mafee MF, Goodwin J, Dorodi S. Optic nerve sheath meningiomas: role of MR imaging. Radiol Clin North Am 1999;37;55.)

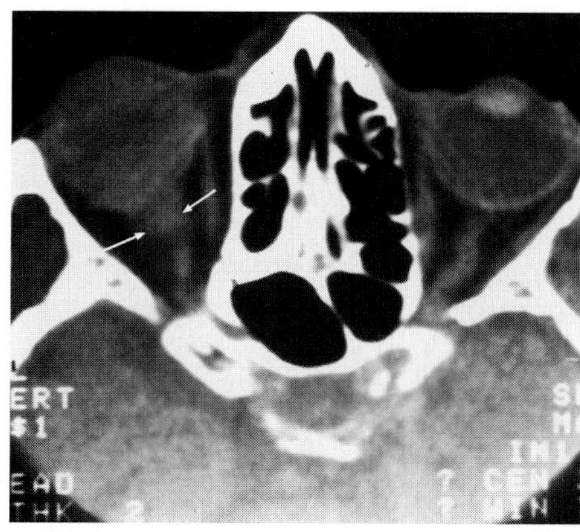

Fig. 18. Melanoma of the right globe extending into the optic nerve. Axial CT section through the midglobe shows expansion of the optic nerve near the optic disc (*arrows*).

volvement of the optic nerve with metastatic tumor, has been observed rarely [128–132]. A report from the Massachusetts Eye and Ear Infirmary and Massachusetts General Hospital described 205 cases of optic nerve malignancies between 1962 and 1987 [124]. Of these 205 cases, 36 (18%) were primary tumors of the optic nerves. The remaining cases were of secondary origin: 134 (79%) were intraocular tumors, 70 [41%] were intraocular melanoma, and 64 [38%] were retinoblastoma); 20 (12%) were metastases of solid tumors from distant sites; 8 (5%) were hematopoietic malignancies; and 6 (4%) were brain tumors. Among the solid metastatic tumors, carcinoma of the breast and lung were the most common sources. In a report by Ferry and Font [133] of 227 reported cases metastatic to the eye and orbit, only 3 cases (1.3%) involved the optic nerve or optic nerve sheath. In 1970 in a review by Ginsberg [129] of 115 previously reported cases (with the addition of two of his own cases), the optic nerve involvement was as follows: choroidal metastases with optic nerve invasion (39%), direct blood born implantation (33%), meningeal carcinomatosis (20%), and extraocular metastases (8%). Among these 117 cases, the sources of the metastases were as follows: breast carcinoma (33%), lung carcinoma (11%), stomach (6%), pancreas (3%), melanoma primary site unknown (2%), uterus (2%), and ovary (2%). Secondary optic nerve involvement can also occur from metastases in the bony part of the optic canal, as has been documented in metastatic prostate carcinoma and metastatic neuroblastoma [134].

Most patients who have optic nerve metastases present with progressive loss of vision with a poor prognosis. In patients who have retinal or optic nerve metastases, the median survival is approximately 9 months after the onset of visual symptoms but is slightly longer when the primary lesion is a breast carcinoma [130]. Most patients who have optic nerve metastases have other systemic metastases at the time they present with ocular involvement. Metastatic disease, notably from prostate carcinoma, has also been reported to involve the optic canal with secondary compression of the optic nerves [135].

Treatment options for metastases to the eye, including metastases to the optic nerve, include observation, radiotherapy to the eyes and optic nerves with visual-saving potential, and enucleation for pain control.

Primary ocular tumors are the most common source of secondary optic nerve tumors [23]. It has been suggested that increased intraocular pressure predisposes the optic nerves to involvement by intraocular tumors. Retinoblastoma and melanoma are the most common intraocular tumors with extension to the optic nerve (Figs. 18 and 19) [136,137].

Retinoblastoma has a predisposition to optic nerve invasion [138,139]. In 240 cases published by Christmas et al [124], 64 (26.7%) invaded the optic nerve, and 14 of the 64 tumors extended beyond the lamina cribrosa. Factors leading to an increased incidence of optic nerve involvement are seeding into the vitreous and necrotic undifferentiated tumors. Optic nerve invasion, along with cases showing penetration of the coats of the eye and choroidal invasion, is associated with a poorer prognosis.

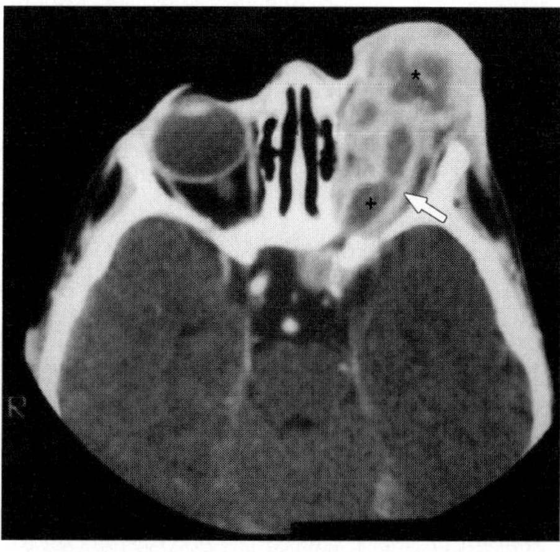

Fig. 19. Retinoblastoma invading the left optic nerve. Axial CT scan demonstrates a proptotic globe (*asterisk*) showing marked increase in density secondary to tumor. There is extension of tumor along the optic nerve, which is thickened and displays marginal enhancement (*arrow*) with a lucent central bandlike core (*asterisk*). Note tumor in the optic canal (*arrows*).

Uveal melanoma invasion of the optic nerve is usually limited to the portion anterior to the lamina cribrosa and occurs in 0.3% to 8% of cases. Involvement beyond the lamina cribrosa of the juxtapapillary type of melanoma has been reported to occur in 62% of cases [140]. Posterior spread may occur to the orbital optic nerve, prechiasmatic optic nerve, chiasm, and brain [136,137,141].

Acute leukemia of the optic nerve is encountered most commonly in acute lymphoblastic leukemia but has also been reported in acute myeloblastic leukemia and adult leukemia. Several reports state the incidence to be 13% to 16% [142,143]. The ophthalmoscopic findings consist of papilledema and optic disc pallor associated with variable loss of visual acuity. On imaging studies, notably MR imaging, there may be diffuse enlargement of the optic nerve sheath complex reflecting invasion of the meninges or the optic nerve, with a variable degree of enhancement [144,145].

Lymphoma involves the CNS, including the optic nerve, either as a primary (most common) or as a secondary tumor [146–148]. Secondary disease more often involves the meningeal, perivascular, and spinal epidural areas. Optic nerve extension occurs most often in longstanding or recurrent systemic lymphoma. Non-Hodgkin's lymphoma is the most common histopathologic type; rarely, Hodgkin's lymphoma involves the optic nerve. Non-Hodgkin's lymphoma involves ocular tissues either as a primary tumor or as secondary metastasis from systemic disease [146,147]. Diagnosis is based on the identification of malignant cells in the eye by biopsy. Primary intraocular lymphoma cells have been identified in the optic nerve and also in the ciliary body, iris, and choroid of a small number of patients by histopathology or radiographically [144]. Diffuse enlargement of the optic nerve sheath complex is best illustrated on MR imaging [149–152]. If the lymphoma envelops the optic nerve, a meningioma may be suspected [153].

Multiple myeloma has been reported to involve the optic nerve and causes multiple other findings in the eye in addition to cranial nerve findings [154].

Meningeal carcinomatosis is the consequence of diffuse metastatic disease to the meninges of the brain and spinal cord. The source of the original tumor includes a variety of lesions, such as various carcinomas, non-Hodgkin's and Hodgkin's lymphomas, melanoma, and multiple myeloma. In a series by Little et al [155], the optic nerve was affected in 4 of 29 patients (20%). Other cranial nerves are often affected in addition to the optic nerve [156]. Intracranial germinomas often disseminate by the ventricular and subarachnoid pathways; seeding to the perioptic arachnoid space is unusual but has been reported in one case [157]. Visual loss occurs in approximately one third of patients who have meningeal carcinomatosis, first afflicting one eye followed by extension to the other eye. Blindness may eventually ensue. Because of the close proximity of the posterior ethmoid air cells and sphenoid sinus, pathologic processes have easy access to the optic canals and optic nerves [158]. Pathologies, notably lesions arising within the posterior ethmoid cells and sphenoid sinus [159,160], including bacterial inflammatory diseases [161], granulomatous and fungus infections [162,163], mucoceles [164,165], benign tumors such as osteomas, fibrous dysplasia [166], and malignancies may involve the optic nerves. Among 42 cases of sphenoid sinus carcinoma, 5 revealed optic nerve and chiasmal invasion [159]. Nasopharyngeal carcinoma may invade the orbital apex including the optic canal and cause cranial nerve deficits and visual impairment [167,168]. Malignant teratoma of the optic nerve has also been described [169].

The preferred imaging studies include MR imaging with conventional and inversion recovery sequences and gadolinium enhancement with fat suppression in different planes, as previously discussed. They range from a negative study with diffuse infiltrations causing only minimal thickening of the optic nerve to moderate enlargement of the optic nerve sheath complex. There is a variable amount of enhancement after introduction of contrast material in a nerve sheath complex that may be enlarged or appear of normal caliber (Fig. 20). The metastasis may be situated in the chiasm and extend into the intracranial optic nerves (Fig. 21). The MR imaging findings are not specific and may simulate optic neuritis [132]. They should be interpreted in corre-

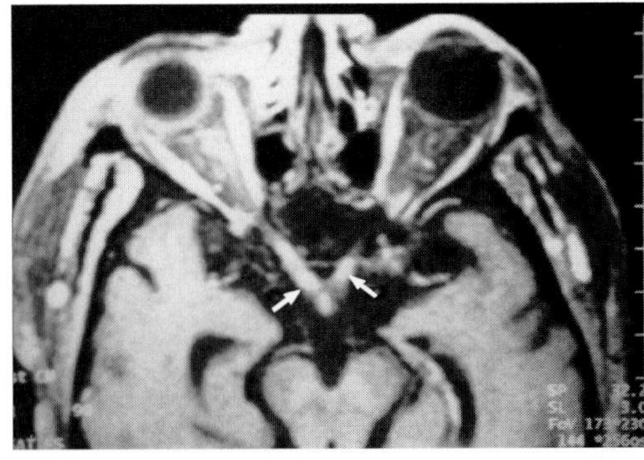

Fig. 20. Metastases from breast carcinoma to both optic nerves. Axial T1-weighted MR scan after gadolinium injection reveals enhancement of both optic nerves (*arrows*).

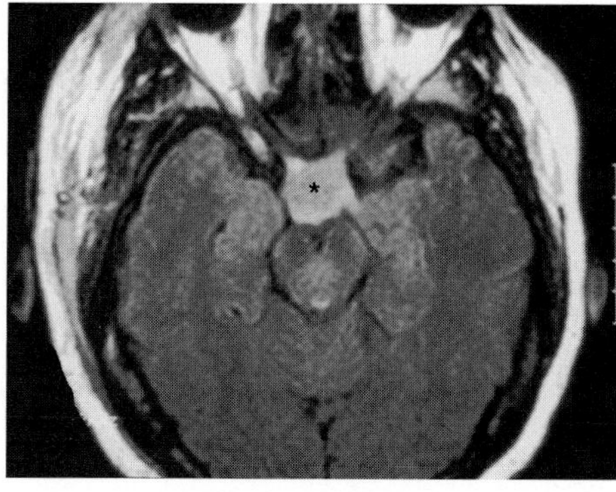

Fig. 21. Metastases from breast carcinoma to chiasm and slight invasion of adjacent intracranial optic nerves. Axial proton density image shows increased signal intensity of the enlarged chiasm and origin of optic nerves consistent with tumor (*asterisk*).

lation with the clinical findings and the patient's history, especially the presence of a primary malignant tumor. CT is indicated for assessment of bony structures, especially the optic canal. Often the history is pivotal in the evaluation, because patients who have metastatic disease to the eye and optic nerves often complain of vision loss and pain or have other known metastatic disease. If there is no known primary tumor elsewhere—as occurs in 20% of cases—a meningioma or optic neuritis may mistakenly be considered [132,170].

**Box 2. Inflammatory and other lesions of the optic nerve**

*Inflammatory lesions*

- Optic neuritis
- Optic nerve sarcoid
- Radiation-induced optic neuritis
- Optic nerve tuberculoma

*Miscellaneous lesions*

- Arachnoid cyst
- Dilation of the subarachnoid space of the optic nerve sheath
  - Hydrocephalus
  - Pseudotumor cerebri
  - Idiopathic
  - Neurofibromatosis 1
  - Optic nerve hypoplasia

*Inflammation*

Inflammatory (and miscellaneous) lesions of the optic nerve are listed in Box 2 and are described more fully in the following sections.

*Optic neuritis*

Optic neuritis is a common disease entity that afflicts younger patients; the mean age of onset is 29 to 30 years. It is the initial manifestation in 15% to 20% of patients who have multiple sclerosis, and approximately 35% to 40% of patients who have multiple sclerosis develop optic neuritis in the course of the disease [171,172]. The disease is rare in children, in whom the risk for development of multiple sclerosis is low. Optic neuritis may be symptomatic or asymptomatic. The disease is characterized by loss of vision, ipsilateral eye pain, and dyschromatopsia [173]. The initial attack is unilateral in 70% and bilateral in 30% of adult patients. Loss of vision may occur very rapidly (within days) or chronically within a period of 1 to 2 weeks. A variant of optic neuritis occurs in a small number of patients in whom a chronic, progressive, demyelinating optic neuropathy is characterized by slowly progressive visual loss without remission. CT scanning in optic neuritis reveals slight enlargement and contrast enhancement of the optic nerves. These features, however, are nonspecific [174] MR imaging is more sensitive for imaging multifocal plaques in the optic nerve, chiasm [175], or white matter [176]. MR imaging abnormalities are characterized by slight enlargement of the optic nerve complex and by increased signal intensities on the T2-weighted images along with enhancement after gadolinium introduction (Figs. 22 and 23) [177]. These imaging findings have been demon-

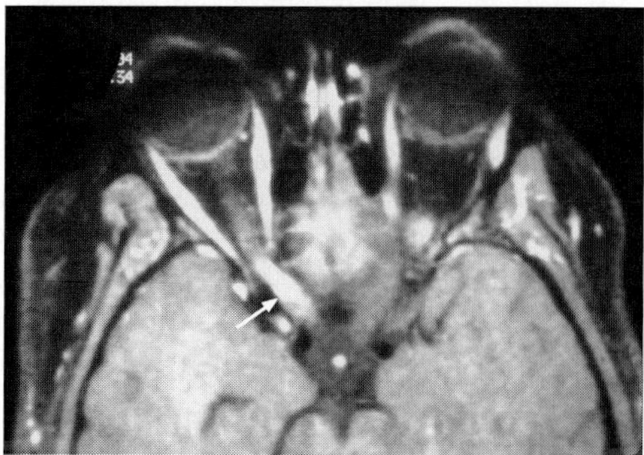

Fig. 22. Optic neuritis of the right optic nerve. Axial enhanced T1-weighted image shows enhancement of optic canal segment of the right optic nerve with no enlargement (*arrow*).

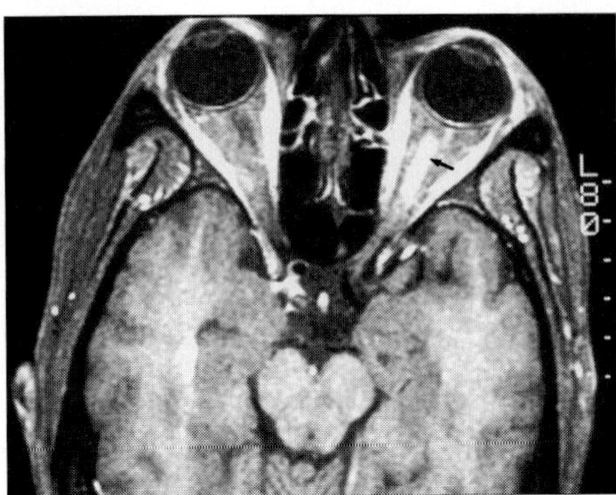

Fig. 23. Optic neuritis of the left optic nerve. Axial fat-suppressed MR scan shows enhancement of the mid segment of the left optic nerve (*arrow*).

strated in 56% to 72% of adult patients who have isolated optic neuritis and in 90% to 98% of patients who have clinically definitive active multiple sclerosis [178]. The increased signal intensity on T2-weighted images is the result of inflammation and dilatation of the optic nerve sheath together with enhancement of the optic nerve sheath following introduction of gadolinium [179]. Rarely, there may be moderate marked enlargement of the optic nerve mimicking an optic nerve glioma or meningioma [180]. The diagnostic yield is increased when inversion recovery sequences are used and possibly with the addition of a surface coil. The demonstration of increased signal intensity of the optic nerve and chiasm, however, is nonspecific and does not allow a definitive diagnosis of multiple sclerosis. The site and the longitudinal extent of the lesion vary. Lesions may be located anterior near the optic nerve head, throughout the entire orbital optic nerve, intracanalicularly, and in intracranial portions of the optic nerve. A single lesion or several discontinuous lesions may be present within the respective optic nerves. The retrobulbar segment is most commonly involved. The differential diagnosis of unilateral optic neuritis includes ischemic optic neuropathy, syphilis, HIV-associated optic neuropathies, collagen vascular disease, amyopathic dermatomyositis, and viral infections (Fig. 24).

### *Optic nerve sarcoid*

Sarcoidosis is a granulomatous disease with a worldwide distribution. It involves many organ systems [181] and affects the central nervous system including the visual pathway in 5% of cases. Sarcoid may involve the uveal tract (the most common location) and the optic nerve sheath [182] with associated involvement of the intracranial optic nerves and chiasm [183]. The orbital fat is less commonly infiltrated, but the lacrimal glands are frequently involved [184–187]. The optic nerves may be the first and only manifestation of sarcoidosis [188–190]. In a reported case, sarcoid developed in the orbital apex followed by involvement of the opposite optic nerve. Several discontinuous lesions may be present within the respective optic nerves and chiasm [191,192]. The diagnosis of sarcoid is strongly suggested if other clinical findings are documented, especially a positive chest radiograph. On imaging studies, the optic nerve is diffusely enlarged [193,194]. The configuration of the nerve may be smooth, tubular, or slightly lobulated or may be eccentrically enlarged [182,185]. On MR imaging, marked enhancement of the sarcoid granulomata usually occurs following the introduction of gadolinium (Fig. 25) [195]. If the lesion is confined to the optic nerve, however, the MR imaging features are not specific, and other lesions, principally optic neuritis and ischemic optic neuropathy, must be considered [192]. In some cases, optic nerve sarcoidosis may resemble a meningioma or glioma, particularly if marked thickening of the optic nerve sheath has developed [196].

### *Radiation-induced optic neuritis*

Radiation given to the orbits, paranasal sinuses, nasopharynx, brain, and sella may include the anterior visual pathway. The damage to the optic nerve and chiasm depends on the total amount of radiation and fractionation during treatment [197,198]. The average time for acute radiation optic neuropathy to occur ranges from approximately 6 months to 2 years, with an average of 18 months after treatment

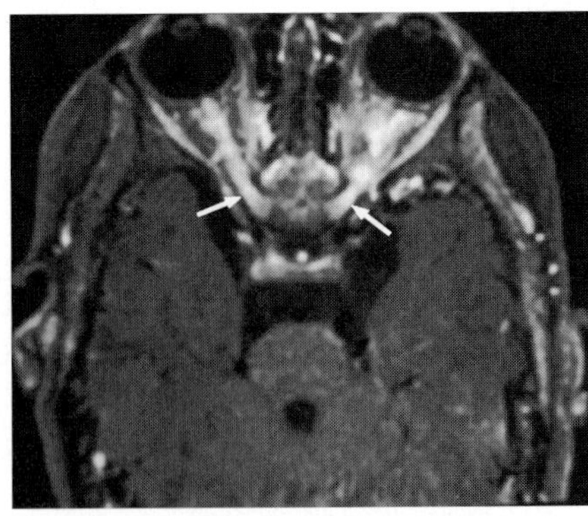

Fig. 24. Viral optic neuritis in a child aged 2 years. Axial T1-weighted scan after gadolinium introduction shows enhancement of both optic nerves (*arrows*).

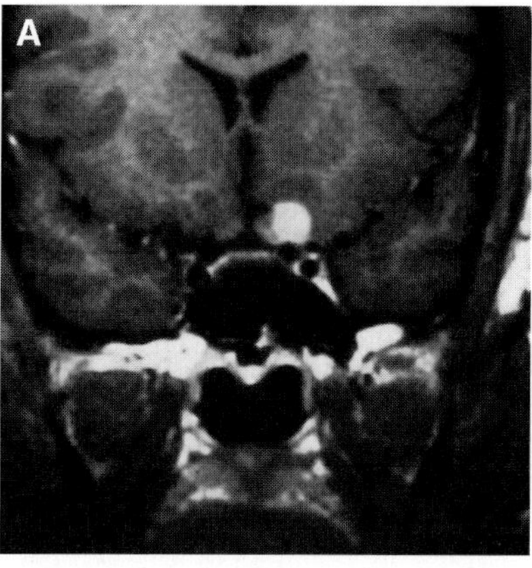


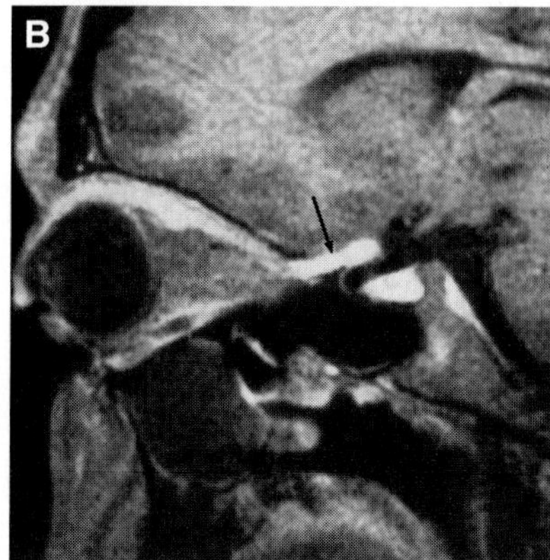


Fig. 25. Sarcoid of the left optic nerve. (*A*) Coronal contrast MR scan demonstrates homogeneous enhancement of the slightly enlarged left intracranial optic nerve. (*B*) Sagittal view demonstrates the enhancing intracranial segment of the optic nerve (*arrow*).

with a total dose of 50 Gy or a single dose of greater than 10 Gy [199]. Visual loss may result from lesions of the optic nerve disk, retrobulbar segment of the optic nerve, optic chiasm, or retrochiasmatic pathways. The second eye may show clinical manifestations of optic neuropathy many months after the diagnosis of the first involved eye. Spontaneous improvement in visual function may rarely occur. Treatment has been disappointing, but if visual dysfunction is detected early, hyperbaric oxygen might be beneficial. On MR imaging, there is enhancement of the optic nerve or chiasm associated with swelling, and, in some cases, necrosis may ensue (Fig. 26) [200]. The acute inflammatory stage is followed years later by atrophy nerve structures. The enhancement of the optic nerve probably is based on increased permeability of the blood–brain barrier.

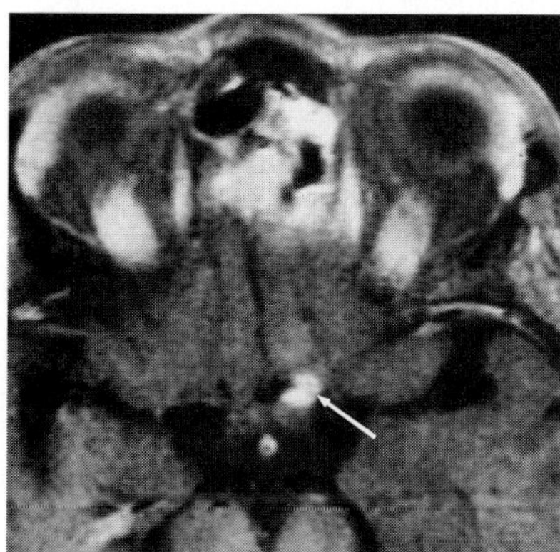

Fig. 26. Optic neuritis after radiation for undifferentiated carcinoma of the sinuses. Localized enhancement of the left optic nerve near the origin of the chiasm (*arrow*).

MR imaging findings may antedate visual loss in chiasmal radiation injury [201,202]. In addition to the radiation-induced changes to the optic pathway, these patients may have disc swelling, peripapillary exudates, hemorrhages, and subretinal fluid on funduscopy.

### *Optic nerve tuberculoma*

Involvement of the optic nerve and chiasm by tuberculous inflammatory disease with exudate is common, but tuberculomas in the optic nerve sheath are rare [203–207]. Most optic chiasmatic tuberculomas occur as a late complication of tuberculous optic chiasmatic meningitis. They may manifest as a mass and simulate a glioma. The imaging features on CT and MR imaging are not specific, and commonly a biopsy with a culture is indicated for the final diagnosis.

## Miscellaneous lesions

### *Arachnoid cyst*

Arachnoid cysts of the optic nerve sheath are uncommon [208,209]. In most cases, the cause is unknown, but a patient who had a perioptic cyst distal to a meningioma has been reported [92]. These cysts extend along the intraorbital optic nerve sheath and appear as fusiform dilatation of the subarachnoid space [203–213]. The MR imaging findings are the same as reported in arachnoid cysts of the intracranial cavity, including low T1- and high T2-weighted signal intensities with no enhancement after gadolin-

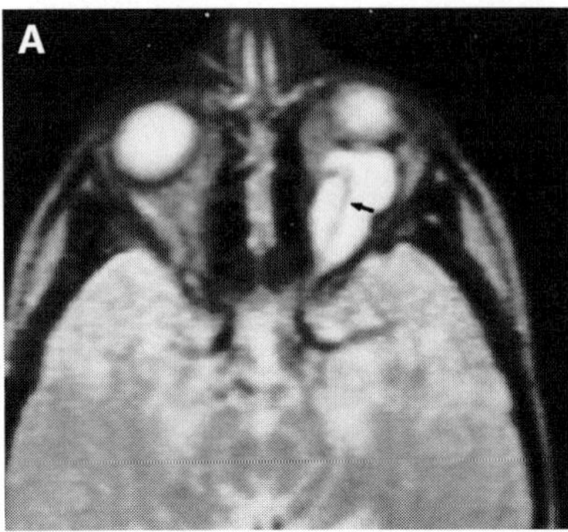


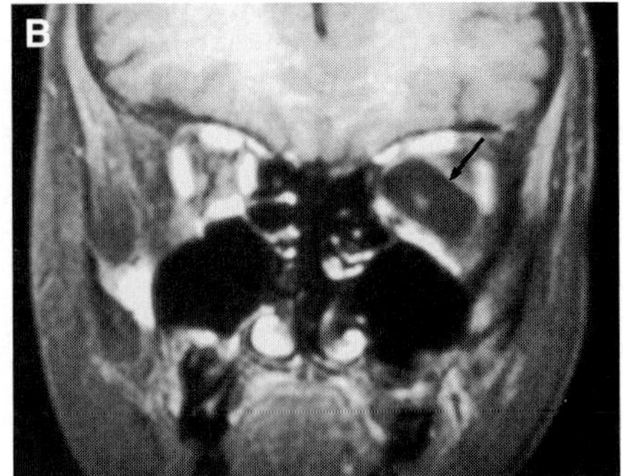


Fig. 27. Arachnoid cyst of the left optic nerve sheath. (*A*) Axial T2-weighted image through the optic nerves shows a high-signal-intensity arachnoid cyst enveloping the optic nerve. Faint structure with low signal intensity represents the partially visualized optic nerve (*arrows*). (*B*) Coronal T1-weighted image after gadolinium administration shows the low-signal-intensity arachnoid cyst (*arrow*). Note the low-signal-intensity central structure representing the optic nerve.

ium introduction. In the authors' case material, they encountered a chiasmatic glioma with an arachnoid cyst (Fig. 27).

*Dilatation of subarachnoid space of optic nerve sheath*

Optic nerve sheath dilatation is encountered in hydrocephalus, pseudotumor cerebri, neurofibromatosis [214,215], idiopathic optic nerve hydrops, and in patients who have unknown etiologies. MR imaging displays the typical findings of CSF fluid in the dilated subarachnoid space with low T1- and high T2-signal intensities.

*Optic nerve hypoplasia*

Congenital optic nerve hypoplasia is a common unilateral or bilateral abnormality of the eye. The underlying pathology is a reduction in the retinal ganglion cells and their nerve fibers. It is a clinical diagnosis and is characterized by early-onset strabismus, poor vision, nystagmus, and diminished pupillary light reflex. On funduscopic examination, the optic nerve head is small in diameter; there is disc pallor and abnormal termination of the retinal pigment epithelial cells. Optic nerve hypoplasia, also known as septo-optic dysplasia, is associated with a wide range of neurologic and endocrine disorders, including absent septum pellucidum, hypoplasia of the corpus callosum, various pituitary abnormalities, and arachnoid cyst (optimally evaluated with MR imaging) [216,217]. On MR imaging of the optic nerves, the cross-sectional area is diminished in diameter to less than 2.9 mm [218,219]. Brodsky [220] distinguished five categories of optic nerve hypoplasia: (1) isolated optic nerve hypoplasia; (2) absence of septum pellucidum; (3) posterior pituitary ectopia; (4) hemispheric migration abnormalities; and (5) intrauterine perinatal hemispheric injuries.

## Summary

Optic nerve lesions encompass a wide spectrum of different disease entities, including inflammatory diseases, primary and secondary benign and malignant tumors, and miscellaneous abnormalities. CT and MR imaging with optional administration of contrast material are the modalities used in the diagnostic assessment. The most common primary optic nerve tumor is the optic nerve glioma, followed by the optic nerve meningioma. Optic nerve gliomas occur predominantly in children and reveal slow growth with erratic unpredictable growth spurts; malignant transformation is rare. Up to 70% of cases are associated with NF-1, with display of hamartomas in the brain and associated other lesions. Perioptic gliomatosis occurs, in some cases surrounding or enveloping the optic nerve glioma. Perineural gliomatosis is characterized by increased signal intensities on T2-weighted images. Optic nerve glioma most commonly involves the orbital optic nerves (in 46% of cases) and the orbital and intracranial optic nerve combined (in 25% of cases). On MR imaging, an optic nerve glioma exhibits low T1 and high T2 signal intensities. The enhancement varies from no enhancement to marked homogeneous enhancement to heterogeneous enhancement. Observation of the tumor with no treatment is justified because of the stationary behavior or slow intermittent growth of these tumors. More aggressive tumors that cause visual deterioration are treated with surgery, irradiation, and chemotherapy. Optic nerve sheath meningiomas, shown by symmetric or asymmetric thickening of the nerve, occur most commonly in middle-aged women and display slow growth with gradual progressive deterioration in vision. About 12% of optic nerve sheath meningiomas contain calcium % and demonstrate marked enhancement. They may be confined to the orbit but can extend intracranially through the optic canal. Intracranial meningiomas may invade the optic nerve sheath from the sphenoid bone. Secondary optic nerve tumors are more common than primary optic nerve tumors. The most common source for optic nerve extension is the globe: 25% to 30% of retinoblastomas and less than 5% of uveal melanomas invade the nerve.

Metastases from distant sources are less common; breast and lung the most common sources, followed by the gastrointestinal tract. Meningeal carcinomatosis, including leukemia and lymphoma, is another source of secondary optic nerve tumors. A diverse group of lesions, including inflammatory diseases, mucoceles, and tumors arising in the posterior ethmoid sinuses and sphenoid sinus, can extend into the optic canal and cause visual impairment and blindness.

Optic nerve neuritis has various causes but is commonly associated with multiple sclerosis (in 35% to 40% of cases). Slight enlargement to swelling of the optic nerve is seen with enhancement. Other areas in the visual pathway (eg, the chiasm) may also be involved. Sarcoid involves the CNS, including the optic pathway, in about 5% of cases. Isolated involvement of the optic nerve is less common than involvement of the optic nerve with other parts of the anterior visual pathway, including the chiasm. Sarcoid granulomas cause enlargement of the optic nerve or chiasm and are associated with marked enhancement. Radiation-induced optic neuritis is suggested if the patient complains of vision loss after previous radiation that included the anterior visual pathway in the radiation field.

Benign tumors and choristomas are uncommon in the optic nerve. They include ganglioglioma, hemangioblastoma, medulloepithelioma, and melanoblastoma. The choristoma displays fatty tissue around the optic nerve, suggesting the diagnosis in a patient who has visual impairment. Melanoblastoma is located in the optic nerve head showing high T1- and low T2-signal intensities based on the large amount of pigment within the lesion. Dilatation of the surrounding perioptic subarachnoid space or cyst formation is occasionally demonstrated. On MR imaging, this dilatation reflected by typical signal intensities of CSF in the dilated spaces. Optic nerve hypoplasia is common and is demonstrated by MR imaging along with the frequently associated anomalies of the brain.

## References

[1] Miller NR. Primary tumours of the optic nerve and its sheath. Eye 2004;18(11):1026–37.

[2] McCollough C, Zink F. Performance evaluation of a multi-slice CT system. Med Phys 1999;26:2223–30.

[3] Hendrix LE, Kneeland JB, Haughton VM, et al. MR imaging of optic nerve lesions: value of gadopentetate dimeglumine and fat suppression technique. AJNR Am J Neuroradiol 1990;11:749–54.

[4] Rootman J. Diseases of the orbit: a multidisciplinary approach. London: JB Lippincott; 1988. p. 281–5.

[5] Dutton JJ. Gliomas of the anterior visual pathway. Surv Ophthalmol 1994;38:427–57.

[6] Thompson CR, Lessell S. Anterior visual pathway gliomas. Int Ophthalmol Clin 1997;37(4):261–79.

[7] Lertchavanakul A, Baimai C, Siwanuwatn R, et al. Optic nerve glioma in infancy: a case report of the youngest patient in Thailand. J Med Assoc Thai 2001; 84(Suppl 1):137–41.

[8] Wulc AE, Bergin DJ, Barnes D, et al. Orbital optic nerve glioma in adult life. Arch Ophthalmol 1989; 107(7):1013–6.

[9] Jans AJ, Drundy R, Canaan A, et al. Optic pathway and hypothalamic/chiasmatic gliomas in children younger than age 5 years with a 6 year follow-up. Cancer 1995;75:1051–9.

[10] Cirak B. Optic nerve glioma. J Neurosurg Spine 2003;99(2):246–53.

[11] Ellsworth C, Alvord MD, Loftsen S. Gliomas of the optic nerve or chiasm. Neurosurg 1988;68:85–98.

[12] Balcer LJ, Liu GT, Heller G, et al. Visual loss in children with neurofibromatosis type 1 and optic pathway gliomas: relation to tumor location by magnetic resonance imaging. Am J Ophthalmol 2001; 131(4):442–5.

[13] Borit A, Richardson Jr EP. The biological and clinical behaviour of pilocytic astrocytomas of the optic pathways. Brain 1982;105:161–87.

[14] Condon JR, Rose FC. Optic nerve glioma. Br J Ophthalmol 1967;51:703–6.

[15] Thiagalingam S, Flaherty M, Billson F, et al. Neurofibromatosis type 1 and optic pathway gliomas: follow-up of 54 patients. Ophthalmology 2004;111(3): 568–77.

[16] Parazzini C, Triulzi F, Bianchini E, et al. Spontaneous involution of optic pathway lesions in neurofibromatosis type 1: serial contrast MR evaluation. AJNR Am J Neuroradiol 1995;16(8):1711–8.

[17] Parsa CF, Hoyt CS, Lesser RL, et al. Spontaneous regression of optic gliomas: thirteen cases documented by serial neuroimaging. Arch Ophthalmol 2001; 119(4):516–29.

[18] Yoshikawa G, Nagata K, Kawamoto S, et al. Remarkable regression of optic glioma in an infant. Case illustration. J Neurosurg 2003;98(5):1134.

[19] Brzowski AE, Bazan C, Mumma JV, et al. Spontaneous regression of optic glioma in a patient with neurofibronatosis. Neurology 1992;42:679–81.

[20] Alvord J, Lofton S. Gliomas of the optic nerve or chiasm. Outcome by patients' age, tumor site, and treatment. J Neurosurg 1988;68(1):85–98.

[21] Listernik R, Charrow J, Greenwald M, et al. Natural history of optic pathway tumors in children with neurofibromatosis type 1: a longitudinal study. J Pediatr 1994;125:63–6.

[22] Listernik R, Louis DN, Packer RJ, et al. Optic pathway gliomas in children with neurofibromatosis type 1. Ann Neurol 1997;41(2):143–9.

[23] Spencer WH. Optic nerve. In: Spencer WH, editor. Ophthalmic pathology, vol. 3. Philadelphia: WB Saunders; 1996. p. 513–622.

[24] Davis RL, Zimmerman LE. Juvenile pilocytic astrocytoma of the optic nerve: clinico-pathologic study of sixty three cases. In: Jakobiec FA, editor. Ocular and adnexal tumors. Birmingham: Yanoff Aesculapius; 1978. p. 685–707.

[25] Bilgric S, Erbengi A, Tinaztepe B. Optic glioma of childhood: clinical histopathological, and histochemical observations. Br J Ophthalmol 1989;73:832–7.

[26] Robertson AC, Brewin TB. Pilocytic astrocytoma. Clin Radiol 1980;31:471–2.

[27] Stern J, Jakobiec FA, Housepian EM. The architecture of optic nerve gliomas with and without neurofibromatosis. Arch Ophthalmol 1980;98:505–11.

[28] Wilson WB, Finkel RS, McCleary L, et al. Large cystic glioma. Neurology 1990;40:1898–2000.

[29] Applegate LJ, Pribram FW. Hematoma of optic nerve glioma: a cause of sudden proptosis. J Clin Neuroophthalmol 1989;9:15–9.

[30] Charles NC, Nelson L, Brookner AR, et al. Pilocytic astrocytoma of the optic nerve with hemorrhage and extreme cystic degeneration. Am J Ophthalmol 1981; 92:691–5.

[31] McLoed AR. Acute blindness in childhood optic glioma caused by hematoma. J Pediatr Ophthalmol Strabismus 1983;20:31–3.

[32] Sanders GS, Allen RA, Straatsma BR. Arachnoidal proliferation of optic nerve simulating extension of intracranial glioma. Arch Ophthalmol 1965;74: 349–52.

[33] Brodski MC. The "pseudo-CSF" signal of orbital optic glioma on magnetic resonance imaging. Surv Ophthalmol 1993;38(3):213–8.

[34] Seiff SR, Brodsky MC, MacDonald G, et al. Orbital optic glioma in neurofibromatosis. Magnetic resonance diagnosis of perineural arachnoidal gliomatosis. Arch Ophthalmol 1987;105(12):1689–92.

[35] Brown PD, Wald JT, McDermott MW, et al. Optic nerve glioma or optic nerve meningioma. Radiographics 2003;23(6):1591–611.

[36] Cooling RJ, Wright JE. Arachnoid hyperplasia in optic nerve glioma: confusion with orbital meningioma. Br J Ophthalmol 1979;63:596–9.

[37] Dekeiser RJW, deWolff-Rouendaall D, Bots GTA, et al. Optic glioma with intraocular tumor and seeding in a child with neurofibromatosis. Am J Ophthalmol 1989;108:717–25.

[38] Brown GC, Shields JA. Tumors of the optic nerve head. Surv Ophthalmol 1985;29:239–64.

[39] Dossetor FM, Landau K, Hoyt WF. Optic disk glioma in neurofibromatosis type 2. Am J Ophthalmol 1989; 108(5):602–3.

[40] Bruggers CS, Friedman HS, Phillips PC, et al. Leptomeningeal dissemination of optic pathway gliomas in three children. Am J Ophthalmol 1991;111(6): 719–23.

[41] Cogan DG, Poppen JL, Hicks SP. Ganglioneuroma of chiasm and optic nerves. Arch Ophthalmol 1961;65: 481–2.

[42] Debus J, Kocagoncu KO, Hoss A, et al. Fractionated stereotactic radiotherapy (FSRT) for optic glioma. Int J Radiat Oncol Biol Phys 1999;44(2):23–8.

[43] Khafaga Y, Hassounah M, Kandil A, et al. Optic gliomas: a retrospective analysis of 50 cases. Int J Radiat Oncol Biol Phys 2003;56(3):807–12.

[44] Wisoff JH. Management of optic pathway tumors of childhood. Neurosurg Clin N Am 1992;3(4):791–802.

[45] Wright JE, McNab AA, McDonald WI. Optic nerve glioma and the management of optic nerve tumours in the young. Br J Ophthalmol 1989;73(12):967–74.

[46] Farmer JP, Khan S, Khan A, et al. Neurofibromatosis type 1 and the pediatric neurosurgeon: a 20-year institutional review. Pediatr Neurosurg 2002;37(3): 122–36.

[47] Tow SL, Chandela S, Miller NR, et al. Long-term outcome in children with gliomas of the anterior visual pathway. Pediatr Neurol 2003;28(4):262–70.

[48] Hoyt WF, Baghdassarian SA. Optic glioma of childhood. Natural history and rationale for conservative management. Br J Ophthalmol 1969;53(12):793–8.

[49] Brodsky MC, Hoyt WF, Newton DR. The "phantom" optic nerve. Demonstration in CT and MR scans 19 years after resection of optic. Clin Neuroophthalmol 1988;8(1):67–8.

[50] Jenkin D, Angyalfi S, Becker L, et al. Optic glioma in children: surveillance or irradiation? Int J Radiat Oncol Phys 1993;25:215–25.

[51] Grabenbauer GG, Schuchardt U, Buchfelder M, et al. Radiation therapy of optico-hypothalamic gliomas (OHG)—radiographic response, vision and late toxicity. Radiother Oncol 2000;54(3):239–45.

[52] Packer RJ, Lange B, Ater J, et al. Carboplatin and vincristine for recurrent and newly diagnosed low-grade glioma of childhood. J Clin Oncol 1993;11(5): 850–6.

[53] Petronio J, Edwards MS, Prados M, et al. Management of chiasmal and hypothalamic gliomas of infancy and childhood with chemotherapy. J Neurosurg 1991;74:701–8.

[54] Lloyd LA. Gliomas of the optic nerve and chiasm

in childhood. Trans Am Ophthalmol Soc 1973;71: 488–535.

[55] Weber AL, Klufas R, Pless M. Imaging evaluation of the optic nerve and visual pathway including cranial nerves affecting the visual pathway. Neuroimaging Clin N Am 1996;6(1):143–77.

[56] Holman RE, Crimson BS, Drayer BP, et al. Magnetic resonance imaging of optic gliomas. Am J Ophthalmol 1985;100:596–601.

[57] Hollander MD, FitzPatrick M, O'Connor SG, et al. Optic gliomas. Radiol Clin North Am 1999;37(1): 59–71.

[58] Imes RK, Hoyt WF. Magnetic resonance imaging signs of optic nerve gliomas in neurofibromatosis type I. Am J Ophthalmol 1991;111:729–34.

[59] Kornreich L, Blaser S, Schwarz M, et al. Optic pathway glioma: correlation of imaging findings with the presence of neurofibromatosis. AJNR Am J Neuroradiol 2001;22(10):1963–9.

[60] Liu GT, Brodsky MC, Phillips PC, et al. Optic radiation involvement in optic pathway gliomas in neurofibromatosis. Am J Ophthalmol 2004;137(3): 407–14.

[61] Lourie GL, Osborne DR, Kirks DR. Involvement of posterior visual pathways by optic nerve gliomas. Pediatr Radiol 1986;16:271–4.

[62] Tekkok IH, Tahta K, Saglam S. Optic nerve glioma presenting as a huge intrasellar mass. Case report. J Neurosurg Sci 1994;38(2):137–40.

[63] Barbaro NM, Rosenblum ML, Maitland CG, et al. Malignant optic glioma presenting radiologically as a "cystic" suprasellar mass: case report and review of the literature. Neurosurgery 1982;11(6):787–9.

[64] Packer RJ, Bilaniuk LT, Cohen BH, et al. Intracranial visual pathway gliomas in children with neurofibromatosis. Neurofibromatosis 1988;1:212–22.

[65] Singhal S, Birch JM, Kerr B, et al. Neurofibromatosis type 1 and sporadic optic gliomas. Arch Dis Child 2002;87(1):65–70.

[66] Arun D, Gutmann DH. Recent advances in neurofibromatosis type 1. Curr Opin Neurol 2004;17(2): 101–5.

[67] Lewis RA, Gerson LP, Axelson KA, et al. Von Recklinghausen neurofibromatosis: II. Incidence of optic gliomata. Ophthalmology 1984;91:929–35.

[68] Brodsky MC. The "pseudo-CSF" signal of orbital optic glioma on magnetic resonance imaging: a signature of neurofibromatosis. Surv Ophthalmol 1993; 38(3):322.

[69] DiMario FJ, Ramsby G, Greenastein R, et al. Neurofibromatosis type I: resonance imaging findings. J Child Neurol 1993;8:32–9.

[70] Liu GT, Brodsky MC, Phillips PC, et al. Optic radiation involvement in optic pathway gliomas in neurofibromatosis. Am J Ophthalmol 2004;137(3): 407–14.

[71] Aoki S, Barkowich AJ, Nishimura K, et al. Neurofibromatosis type 1 and 2: cranial MRI findings. Radiology 1989;172:527–34.

[72] Rosser T, Packer RJ. Intracranial neoplasms in children with neurofibromatosis 1. J Child Neurol 2002; 17(8):630–7.

[73] Erbay SH, Oljeski SA, Bhadelia R. Rapid development of optic glioma in a patient with hybrid phakomatosis: neurofibromatosis type 1 and tuberous sclerosis. AJNR Am J Neuroradiol 2004;25(1):36–8.

[74] Nau JA, Shields CL, Shields JA, et al. Optic nerve glioma in a patient with von Hippel-Lindau syndrome. J Pediatr Ophthalmol Strabismus 2003;40(1): 57–8.

[75] Harper CG, Stewart-Wynn EG. Malignant optic gliomas in adults. Arch Neurol 1978;35:731–5.

[76] Hoyt WF, Meshel LG, Lessell S, et al. Malignant optic glioma of adulthood. Brain 1973;96:121–32.

[77] Manor KS, Israeli J, Sandbank U. Malignant optic glioma in a 70-year-old patient. Arch Ophthalmol 1976;94:1142–4.

[78] Murphy M, Timms C, McKelvie P, et al. Malignant optic nerve glioma: metastases to the spinal neuraxis. Case illustration. J Neurosurg Spine 2003;98(1):110.

[79] Rudd A, Rees JE, Kennedy P, et al. Malignant optic nerve glioma in adults. J Clin Neuroophthalmol 1985; 5:238–43.

[80] Spoor TC, Kennerdell JS, Martinez AJ. Malignant gliomas of the optic nerve pathways. Am J Ophthalmol 1986;89:284–92.

[81] Tapham MJB, deBries-Knoppert WAEJ, Ponssen H, et al. Malignant optic glioma in adults. Neurosurg 1989;70:277–9.

[82] Wabbels B, Demmler A, Seitz J, et al. Unilateral adult malignant optic nerve glioma. Graefes Arch Clin Exp Ophthalmol 2004;242(19):741–8.

[83] Millar WS, Tartaglino LM, Sergott RC, et al. MR of malignant optic glioma of adulthood. AJNR Am J Neuroradiol 1995;16(8):1673–6.

[84] Wright JE, McNab AA, McDonald WI. Primary optic nerve sheath meningioma. Br J Ophthalmol 1989;73(12):960–6.

[85] Dutton JJ. Optic nerve sheath meningiomas. Surv Ophthalmol 1992;37:167–83.

[86] Mehra KS, Khanna S, Dube B. Primary meningiomas of the intraorbital optic nerve. Ann Ophthalmol 1979; 11:758–60.

[87] Saeed P, Rootman J, Nugent RA, et al. Optic nerve sheath meningiomas. Ophthalmology 2003;110(10): 2019–30.

[88] Imes RK, Monteiro ML, Hoyt WF. Optic nerve meningioma with enophthalmos. J Clin Neuroophthalmol 1984;4(3):213–5.

[89] Lloyd GAS. Primary orbital meningioma: a review of 4l patients investigated radiologically. Clin Radiol 1982;33:181–7.

[90] Salazar JL, Bauer J, Frenkel M, et al. Bilateral optic canal meningioma. Surg Neurol 1977;8:11–4.

[91] Rohrbach JM, Wilhelm H, Eichorn M, et al. Optic nerve sheath meningioma with massive intraocular growth. Klin Monatsbl Augenheilkd 1993;203:423–9.

[92] Lindblom B, Norman D, Hoyt WF. Perioptic cyst

distal to optic nerve meningioma: MR demonstration. AJNR Am J Neuroradiol 1992;13(6):1622–4.

[93] Jackson A, Patankar T, Laitt RD. Intracanalicular optic nerve meningioma: a serious diagnostic pitfall. AJNR Am J Neuroradiol 2003;24(6):1167–70.

[94] Sanders MD, Falconer MA. Optic nerve compression by an intracanalicular meningioma. Br J Ophththalmol 1964;48:13–8.

[95] Dervin JE, Beaconsfield M, Wright JE, et al. CT findings in orbital tumours of nerve sheath origin. Clin Radiol 1989;40(5):475–9.

[96] Zimmerman LE, Schatz NJ, Glaser JS. Magnetic resonance imaging of optic nerve meningiomas. Ophthalmology 1990;97:585–91.

[97] Simon J, Szumowski J, Totterman S, et al. Fat suppression MR imaging of the orbit. AJNR Am Neurol Radiol 1988;9:961–8.

[98] Turbin RE, Pokorny K. Diagnosis and treatment of orbital optic nerve sheath meningioma. Cancer Control 2004;11(5):334–41.

[99] Baumert BG, Villa S, Studer G, et al. Early improvements in vision after fractionated stereotactic radiotherapy for primary optic nerve sheath meningioma. Radiother Oncol 2004;72(2):169–74.

[100] Eng TY, Albright NW, Kuwahara G, et al. Precision radiation therapy for optic nerve sheath meningiomas. Int J Radiat Oncol Biol Phys 1992;22(5):1093–8.

[101] Biswas J, Bhushan B, Jayakumar N, et al. Teratoid malignant medulloepithelioma of the optic nerve: report of a case and review of the literature. Orbit 1999;18(3):191–6.

[102] Green WR, Illiff WH, Trotter RE. Malignant teratoid medulloepithelioma of the optic nerve. Arch Ophthalmol 1974;91:451–4.

[103] Bannykh S, Piepmeier J, Baehring J. Melanocytoma. J Neurooncol 2004;70(1):35.

[104] Ahluwalia S, Ashkan K, Casey AT. Meningeal melanocytoma: clinical features and review of the literature. Br J Neurosurg 2003;17(4):347–51.

[105] Painter TJ, Chaljub G, Sethi R, et al. Intracranial and intraspinal meningeal melanocytosis. AJNR Am J Neuroradiol 2000;21(7):1349–53.

[106] Shields JA, Demirci H, Mashayekhi A, et al. Melanocytoma of optic disc in 115 cases: the 2004 Samuel Johnson Memorial Lecture, part 1. Ophthalmology 2004;111(9):1739–46.

[107] Shields JA, Eagle Jr RC, Shields CL, et al. Progressive growth of an iris melanocytoma in a child. Am J Ophthalmol 2002;133(2):287–9.

[108] Meyer D, Ge J, Blinder KJ, et al. Malignant transformation of an optic disk melanocytoma. Am J Ophthalmol 1999;127(6):710–4.

[109] Sharma PM, Sangal K, Malik P, et al. Malignant transformation of optic disc melanocytoma? A clinical dilemma at presentation with a review of the literature. Ophthalmologica 2002;216(4):292–5.

[110] Grasee EA, Wagner JD. Update on diagnostic imaging for melanoma. Facial Plast Surg Clin North Am 2003;11(1):49–60.

[111] Kalkman E, Baxter G. Melanoma. Clin Radiol 2004; 59(4):313–26.

[112] Sugiyama K, Goishi J, Sogabe T, et al. Ganglioglioma of the optic pathway. A case report. Surg Neurol 1992;37(1):22–5.

[113] Bergin DJ, Johnson TE, Spencer WH, et al. Ganglioglioma of the optic nerve. Am J Ophthalmol 1988; 105(2):146–9.

[114] Lu WY, Goldman M, Young B, et al. Optic nerve ganglioglioma. J Neurosurg 1993;78:979–82.

[115] Sadun F, Hinton DR, Sadun AA. Rapid growth of an optic nerve ganglioglioma in a patient with neurofibromatosis. Ophthalmology 1996;103(5):794–9.

[116] Kerr DJ, Scheithauer BW, Miller GM, et al. Hemangioblastoma of the optic nerve: case report. Neurosurgery 1995;36(3):573–80.

[117] Lauten GH, Eatherly JB, Ramirez A. Hemangioblastoma of the optic nerve: radiographic and pathologic features. AJNR Am J Neuroradiol 1981;2:96–9.

[118] Nead J, Kersten R, Anderson R. Hemangioblastoma of the optic nerve: report of a case and review of the literature. Ophthalmology 1988;95:398–401.

[119] Stefani FH, Rothemund E. Intracranial optic nerve angioblastoma. Br J Ophthalmol 1994;58:823–7.

[120] Giannini C, Reynolds C, Leavitt JA, et al. Choristoma of the optic nerve: case report. Neurosurgery 2002; 50(5):1125–8.

[121] Zimmerman LE, Arkfeld DL, Schenken JB, et al. A rare choristoma of the optic nerve and chiasm. Arch Ophthalmol 1983;101:766–70.

[122] Daxer A, Sailer U, Ettl A, et al. Choristoma of the optic nerve: neuroimaging characteristics and association with spinal cord lipoma. Ophthalmologica 1998;212(3):180–3.

[123] Kazim M, Kennerdell JS, Maroon J, et al. Choristoma of the optic nerve and chiasm. Arch Ophthalmol 1992;110(2):236–8.

[124] Christmas NJ, Mead MD, Richardson EP, et al. Secondary optic nerve tumors. Surv Ophthalmol 1991; 36(3):196–206.

[125] Ring HG. Pancreatic carcinoma with metastases to the optic nerve. Arch Ophthalmol 1967;77:798–800.

[126] Garrity JA, Herman DC, Dinapoli RP, et al. Isolated metastasis to optic nerve from medulloblastoma. Ophthalmology 1989;96(2):207–10.

[127] Spagnoli MV, Grossman RI, Packer RJ, et al. Magnetic resonance image determination of gliomatosis cerebri. Neuroradiol 1987;29:15–8.

[128] Arnold AC, Hepler RS, Foos RY. Isolated metastases to the optic nerve. Surv Ophthalmol 1981;26:75–83.

[129] Ginsberg J, Freemond AS, Calhoun JB. Optic nerve involvement in metastatic tumors. Ann Ophthalmol 1970;2:604–17.

[130] Mack HG, Jakobiec FA. Isolated metastases to the retina or optic nerve. Int Ophthalmol Clin 1997;37(4): 251–60.

[131] Mansour AM, Dinowitz K, Chaljub G, et al. Metastatic lesions of the optic nerve. J Clin Neuroophthalmol 1993;13:102–4.

[132] Terry TL, Dunphy EB. Metastatic carcinoma in both optic nerves simulating retrobulbar neuritis. Arch Ophthalmol 1933;10:611.

[133] Ferry AP, Font RL. Carcinoma metastatic to the eye and orbit: a clinicopathologic study of 227 cases. Trans Am Acad Ophthalmol Otolaryngol 1974;72: 877–95.

[134] Lau JJ, Trobe JD, Ruiz RE, et al. Metastatic neuroblastoma presenting with binocular blindness from intracranial compression of the optic nerves. J Neuroophthalmol 2004;24(2):119–224.

[135] Kattah JC, Chrousos GC, Roberts J, et al. Metastatic prostate cancer to the optic canal. Ophthalmology 1993;92:1711–5.

[136] Shields CL, Shields JA, Yarian DL, et al. Intracranial extension of choroidal melanoma via the optic nerve. Br J Ophthalmol 1987;71(3):172–6.

[137] Spencer WH. Optic nerve extension of intraocular neoplasm. Am J Ophthalmol 1975;80:465–71.

[138] Magramm I, Abramson DH, et al. Optic nerve involvement in retinoblastoma. Ophthalmology 1989; 96(2):217–22.

[139] Stannard C, Lipper S, Sealy R, et al. Retinoblastoma: correlation of invasion of optic nerve and choroid with prognosis and metastasis. Br J Ophthalmol 1979;63:560–70.

[140] Shammas HF, Blodi FC. Peripupillary choroidal malignant melanomas: extension along the optic nerve and its sheaths. Arch Ophthalmol 1978;96: 440–5.

[141] Jones DR, Scobie IN, Sarkies NJ. Intracerebral metastases from ocular melanoma. Br J Ophthalmol 1988;72:246–7.

[142] Allen RA, Straatsma BR. Ocular involvement in leukemia and allied disorders. Arch Ophthalmol 1961; 66:490–508.

[143] Kincaid MC, Green WR. Ocular and orbital involvement in leukemia. Surv Ophthalmol 1983;27: 211–32.

[144] Madani A, Christophe C, Ferster A, et al. Perioptic infiltration during leukemic relapse: MRI diagnosis. Pediatr Radiol 2000;30:30–2.

[145] Rosenthal AR, Egbert PR, Wilber JR, et al. Leukemic involvement of the optic nerve. J Pediatr Ophthalmol 1975;12:84–93.

[146] Bullock JD, Yanes B, Kelly M. Non-Hodgkin lymphoma involving the optic nerve. Ann Ophthalmol 1979;11:1477–80.

[147] Lee LC, Howes EL, Bhisitkul RB. Systemic non-Hodgkin's lymphoma with optic nerve infiltration in a patient with AIDS. Retina 2002;22(1):75–9.

[148] Strominger MB, Shatz NH, Glaser JS. Lymphomatous optic neuropathy. Am J Ophthalmol 1993;116: 775–6.

[149] Brazis PW, Menke DM, McLeish WM, et al. Angiocentric T-cell lymphoma presenting with multiple cranial nerve palsies and retrobulbar optic neuropathy. J Neuroophthalmol 1995;15(3):152–7.

[150] Dayan MR, Elston JS, McDonald B. Bilateral lymphomatous optic neuropathy diagnosed on optic nerve biopsy. Arch Ophthalmol 2000;118(10): 1455–7.

[151] Dunker S, Reuter U, Rosler A, et al. Optic nerve involvement in chronic lymphatic leukemia of the B-cell series. [in German]. Ophthalmologe 1996;93(4): 351–3.

[152] Zaman AG, Graham EM, Sanders MD. Anterior visual system involvement in non-Hodgkin's lymphoma. Br J Ophthalmol 1993;77(3):184–7.

[153] Selva D, Rootman J, Crompton J. Orbital lymphoma mimicking optic nerve meningioma. Orbit 2004; 23(2):115–20.

[154] Gudas Jr PP. Optic nerve myeloma. Am J Ophthalmol 1971;71:1085–9.

[155] Little JR, Dale AJD, Okazaki H. Meningeal carcinomatosis: clinical manifestations. Arch Neurol 1984; 30:138–40.

[156] Redman BG, Tapazoglou E, Al-Sarraf M. Meningeal carcinomatosis in head and neck cancer. Cancer 1986; 58:2656–61.

[157] Nakajima T, Kumabe T, Jokura H, et al. Recurrent germinoma in the optic nerve: report of two cases. Neurosurgery 2001;48(1):214–7.

[158] Fujimoto N, Adachi-Usami E, Saito E, et al. Optic nerve blindness due to paranasal sinus disease. Ophthalmologica 1999;213(4):262–4.

[159] Harbison JW, Lessel S, Selhorst JB. Neuro-ophthalmology of sphenoid sinus carcinoma. Brain 1984; 107:855–70.

[160] Maier W, Laubert A, Weinel P. Acute bilateral blindness in childhood caused by rhabdomyosarcoma and malignant lymphoma. J Laryngol Otol 1994; 108(10):873–7.

[161] Postma GN, Chole RA, Nemzek WR. Reversible blindness secondary to acute sphenoid sinusitis. Otolaryngol Head Neck Surg 1995;112(6):742–6.

[162] Balch K, Phillips PH, Newman NJ. Painless orbital apex syndrome from mucormycosis. J Neuroophthalmol 1997;17(3):178–82.

[163] Lee LR, Sullivan TJ. Aspergillus sphenoid sinusitis-induced orbital apex syndrome in HIV infection. Aust N Z J Ophthalmol 1995;23(4):327–31.

[164] Heylbroeck P, Watelet JB, Delbeke P, et al. Vision impairment as presenting symptom of a sphenoidal mucocele. Rhinology 2003;41(3):187–91.

[165] Nerurkar NK, Bradoo R, Muranjan S, et al. Sphenoid sinus mucocele with unilateral blindness. Ann Otol Rhinol Laryngol 2004;113(4):294–6.

[166] Papadopoulos MC, Casey AT, Powell M. Craniofacial fibrous dysplasia complicated by acute, reversible visual loss: report of two cases. Br J Neurosurg 1998; 12(2):159–61.

[167] Carlin L, Biller J, Laster DW, et al. Monocular blindness in nasopharyngeal cancer. Arch Neurol 1981;38(9):600.

[168] Weber AL, al-Arayedh S, Rashid A. Nasopharynx: clinical, pathologic, and radiologic assessment. Neuroimaging Clin N Am 2003;13(3):465–83.

[169] Samii M, Ramina R, Koch G, et al. Malignant teratoma of the optic nerve: case report. Neurosurgery 1985;16(5):696–700.
[170] Backhouse O, Simmons I, Frank A, et al. Optic nerve breast metastasis mimicking meningioma. Aust N Z J Ophthalmol 1998;26(3):247–9.
[171] Brodsky MC, Beck RW. The changing role of MR imaging in the evaluation of acute optic neuritis. Radiology 1994;192(1):22–3.
[172] Levin LA, Lessell S. Optic neuritis and multiple sclerosis. Arch Ophthalmol 2003;121(7):1039–40.
[173] Boomer JA, Siatkowski RM. Optic neuritis in adults and children. Semin Ophthalmol 2003;18(4):174–80.
[174] Howard CW, Archer RH, Tomsak RL. Computed tomographic features in optic neuritis. Am J Ophthalmol 1985;89:699–702.
[175] Miller DH, Newton MK, Vander Poel JC, et al. Magnetic resonance imaging of the optic nerve in optic neuritis. Neurology 1988;38:175–9.
[176] Newbitt GM, Forbes GS, Scheithauer BW, et al. Multiple sclerosis: histopathologic and MR and/or CT correlation in 37 cases at biopsy and three cases at autopsy. Radiology 1991;180:467–74.
[177] Merandi SF, Kudryk BT, Murtagh FR, et al. Contrast enhanced MR imaging of optic nerve lesions in patients with acute optic neuritis. AJNR Am J Neurol Radiol 1999;12:923–6.
[178] Wray SH. Optic neuritis. In: Albert DM, Jakobiec FA, editors. Principles and practice in ophthalmology. Philadelphia: WB Saunders; 1994. p. 2539–68.
[179] Hickman SJ, Miszkiel KA, Plant GT, et al. The optic nerve sheath on MRI in acute optic neuritis. Neuroradiology 2005;47:51–5.
[180] Cornblath WT, Quint DJ. MRI of optic nerve enlargement in optic neuritis. Neurology 1997;48(4):821–5.
[181] Newman LS, Rose CS, Maier LA. Sarcoidosis. N Engl J Med 1997;336:1224–34.
[182] Wachtel AS, Saunders M. Optic nerve sarcoidosis. Mayo Clin Proc 1997;72(8):791.
[183] Westlake, Heath JD, Spalton DJ. Sarcoidosis involving the optic nerve and hypothalamus. Arch Ophthalmol 1995;113(5):669–70.
[184] Frohman LP, Guirgis M, Turbin RE, et al. Sarcoidosis of the anterior visual pathway: 24 new cases. J Neuroophthalmol 2003;23(3):190–7.
[185] Mafee MF, Dorodi S, Pai E. Sarcoidosis of the eye, orbit, and central nervous system. Role of MR imaging. Radiol Clin North Am 1999;37(1):73–87.
[186] Mafee MF, Inoue Y, Mafee RF. Ocular and orbital imaging. Neuroimaging Clin N Am 1996;6(2):291–318.
[187] Simon EM, Zoarski GH, Rothman MI, et al. Systemic sarcoidosis with bilateral orbital involvement: MR findings. AJNR Am J Neuroradiol 1998;19:336–7.
[188] Kosmorsky GS, Prayson R. Primary optic pathway sarcoidosis in a 38-year-old white man. J Neuroophthalmol 1996;16(3):188–90.
[189] Segal EI, Tang RA, Lee AG, et al. Orbital apex lesion as the presenting manifestation of sarcoidosis. J Neuroophthalmol 2000;20(3):156–8.
[190] Yilmazlar S, Kocaeli H, Korfali E. Primary-isolated optic nerve sarcoidosis. Acta Neurochir (Wien) 2004;146(1):65–7.
[191] Bode MK, Tikkakoski T, Tuisku S, et al. Isolated neurosarcoidosis—MR findings and pathologic correlation. Acta Radiol 2001;42(6):563–7.
[192] Engelken JD, Yuh WT, Carter KD, et al. Optic nerve sarcoidosis: MR findings. AJNR Am J Neuroradiol 1992;13(1):228–30.
[193] Beardsley TL, Brown SV, Syndor CF, et al. Eleven cases of sarcoidosis of the optic nerve. Am J Ophthalmol 1994;97:761.
[194] Som PM, Sacher M, Weitzner Jr I, et al. Sarcoidosis of the optic nerve. J Comput Assist Tomogr 1982;6:614–6.
[195] Carmody RF, Mafee MF, Goodwin JA, et al. Orbital and optic pathway sarcoidosis: MR findings. AJNR Am J Neuroradiol 1994;15(4):775–83.
[196] Ing EB, Garrity JA, Cross S, et al. Sarcoid masquerading as optic nerve sheath meningioma. Mayo Clin Proc 1997;72:38.
[197] Jiang GL, Tucker SL, Guttenberger R, et al. Radiation-induced injury to the visual pathway. Radiother Oncol 1994;30(1):17–25.
[198] Kline LB, Kim JY, Ceballos R. Radiation optic neuropathy. Ophthalmology 1985;92:1118–26.
[199] Lessell S. Friendly fire: neurogenic visual loss from radiation therapy. J Neuroophthalmol 2004;24(3):243–50.
[200] Zimmerman CF, Schatz NJ, Glaser JS. Magnetic resonance imaging of radiation optic neuropathy. Am J Ophthalmol 1990;110(4):389–94.
[201] Lessell S. Magnetic resonance imaging signs may antedate visual loss in chiasmal radiation injury. Arch Ophthalmol 2003;121(2):287–8.
[202] Piquemal R, Cottier JP, Arsene S, et al. Radiation-induced optic neuropathy 4 years after radiation: report of a case followed up with MRI. Neuroradiology 1998;40(7):439–41.
[203] Aversa do Souto A, Fonseca AL, Gadelha M, et al. Optic pathways tuberculoma mimicking glioma: case report. Surg Neurol 2003;60(4):349–53.
[204] Iraci C, Giodorano K, Gerosa M, et al. Tuberculoma of the interior optic pathways. J Neurosurg 1980;52:129–33.
[205] Lana-peixoto MA, Bambirra EA, Pitella JE. Optic nerve tuberculoma: a case report. Arch Neurology 1981;37:186–7.
[206] Marco A. Optic nerve tuberculoma. Arch Neurol 1980;37:86.
[207] Schlerrnitzauer DA, Hodges FJ, Bagan M. Tuberculoma of the left optic nerve and chiasm. Arch Ophthalmol 1971;85:75–8.
[208] Celli P, Palma L, Palatisky E. Congenital extradural cyst of the orbital optic nerve: case report. Neurosurgery 1983;13(2):208–10.

[209] Saari M, Mustonen E, Palva A, et al. Arachnoid cyst of the intraorbital portion of the optic nerve with unilateral disc oedema and transient shallowing of the anterior chamber. A case report. Acta Ophthalmol (Copenh) 1977;55(6):959–64.
[210] Akor C, Wojno TH, Newman NJ, et al. Arachnoid cyst of the optic nerve: report of two cases and review of the literature. Ophthal Plast Reconstr Surg 2003; 19(6):466–9.
[211] Harris CJ, Sacks JG, Weinberg PE, et al. Cysts of the intraorbital optic nerve sheath. Am J Ophthalmol 1976;81:656.
[212] Miller NR, Green WR. Arachnoid cysts involving a portion of the intraorbital optic nerve. Arch Ophthalmol 1975;93:1117–21.
[213] Moschos MM, Lymberopoulos C, Moschos M. Arachnoid cyst of the optic nerve: a case report. Klin Monatsbl Augenheilkd 2004;221(5):408–9.
[214] Hayreh SS. Fluids in the anterior part of the optic nerve in health and disease. Surv Ophthalmol 1978; 23:1–25.
[215] Lovblad KO, Remonda L, Ozdoba C, et al. Dural ectasia of the optic nerve sheath in neurofibromatosis type 1: CT and MR features. J Comput Assist Tomogr 1994;18(5):728–30.
[216] Barkovich A, Fram E, Norman D. Septo-optic dysplasia: MR imaging. Radiology 1989;171:189–92.
[217] Ichiyama T, Hayashi T, Nishikawa M, et al. Optic nerve hypoplasia with hypopituitarism and an arachnoid cyst. Brain Dev 1996;18(3):234–5.
[218] Birkebaek NH, Patel L, Wright NB, et al. Optic nerve size evaluated by magnetic resonance imaging in children with optic nerve hypoplasia, multiple pituitary hormone deficiency, isolated growth hormone deficiency, and idiopathic short stature. J Pediatr 2004;145(4):536–41.
[219] Brodsky MC, Glasier CM, Pollock SC, et al. Optic nerve hypoplasia. Identification by magnetic resonance imaging. Arch Ophthalmol 1990;108(11): 1562–7.
[220] Brodsky MC, Glasier CM. Optic nerve hypoplasia. Clinical significance of associated central nervous system abnormalities on magnetic resonance imaging. Arch Ophthalmol 1993;111(1):66–74.

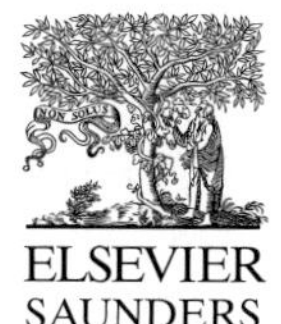
ELSEVIER
SAUNDERS

Neuroimag Clin N Am 15 (2005) 203 – 219

NEUROIMAGING
CLINICS OF
NORTH AMERICA

# Imaging the Sella and Parasellar Region

Mark Pisaneschi, MD[a,b,*], Geetanjali Kapoor, MD[a]

[a]Department of Radiology, John H. Stroger, Jr. Hospital of Cook County, 1901 West Harrison Street, Chicago, IL 60612, USA
[b]Department of Clinical Radiology, University of Illinois Hospital, Chicago, IL, USA

Diagnostic imaging evaluation of a pathologic process suspected to be located within the sellar and parasellar region requires much more than performing a routine CT or MR imaging examination of the brain. An intimate knowledge of the anatomy of the sellar and parasellar region is an essential prerequisite for imaging evaluation of this region. All neural components essential for vision and function of the eye and orbital structures converge in this region and contribute to the anatomic complexity. An understanding of the function of the cranial nerves related to vision and movement of the extraocular muscles aids in developing a more focused imaging examination of this region based on the provided clinical history. Furthermore, familiarity with the type and appearance of the pathologic processes that can be present at this location allows for a more precise and narrow differential diagnosis.

## Anatomy of the sellar and parasellar region

The pituitary fossa lies within the central portion of the sphenoid bone and is bounded anteriorly by the tuberculum sellae and posteriorly by the dorsum sellae. The chiasmatic sulcus lies anterior to the tuberculum sellae and posterior to the planum sphenoidale and medial to the optic nerve canals. The optic strut (inferior root of the lesser wing of the sphenoid), a bridge of bone extending from the anterior clinoid process to the sphenoid body, separates the optic nerve canals from the superior orbital fissure [1]. The optic canal transmits the optic nerve, sympathetic nerves, and ophthalmic artery, a branch arising from the cavernous segment of the internal carotid artery. The superior orbital fissure is a cleft between the greater and lesser sphenoid wings and separates the lateral wall of the orbit from the orbital roof posteriorly [1,2]. The superior orbital fissure is immediately anterior to the cavernous sinus and transmits the superior ophthalmic vein and cranial nerves III, IV, VI, and V.1. The inferior orbital fissure is a cleft between the lateral orbital wall and orbital floor. The inferior orbital fissure lies above the pterygopalatine fossa and is anterior to the cavernous sinus. The inferior orbital fissure transmits the infraorbital nerve (V.2), artery, and vein [2].

The pituitary gland lies within the pituitary fossa and is composed of the anterior lobe (adenohypophysis); intermediate lobe; and posterior lobe (neurohypophysis) (Fig. 1A). The average height of the adult pituitary gland is 5.4 ± 9 mm [3]. This may increase during puberty or pregnancy but in general should not exceed 10 mm [4]. The anterior lobe is relatively isointense to brain parenchyma on T1-weighted MR images and enhances intensely with contrast because of its highly vascular nature and lack of a blood-brain barrier. The intermediate lobe sometimes can be identified on postcontrast T1-weighted MR images and is hypointense to the anterior and posterior lobes related to its relatively avascular nature. The posterior lobe can frequently be identified by an area of increased signal on precontrast T1-weighted MR images in 90% of healthy patients and almost 100% of normal infants, the so-called "bright spot." The high signal is likely related

* Corresponding author. Department of Radiology, John H. Stroger, Jr. Hospital of Cook County, 1901 West Harrison Street, Chicago, IL 60612.

*E-mail address:* mjpisa@aol.com (M. Pisaneschi).

1052-5149/05/$ – see front matter 
doi:10.1016/j.nic.2005.02.007

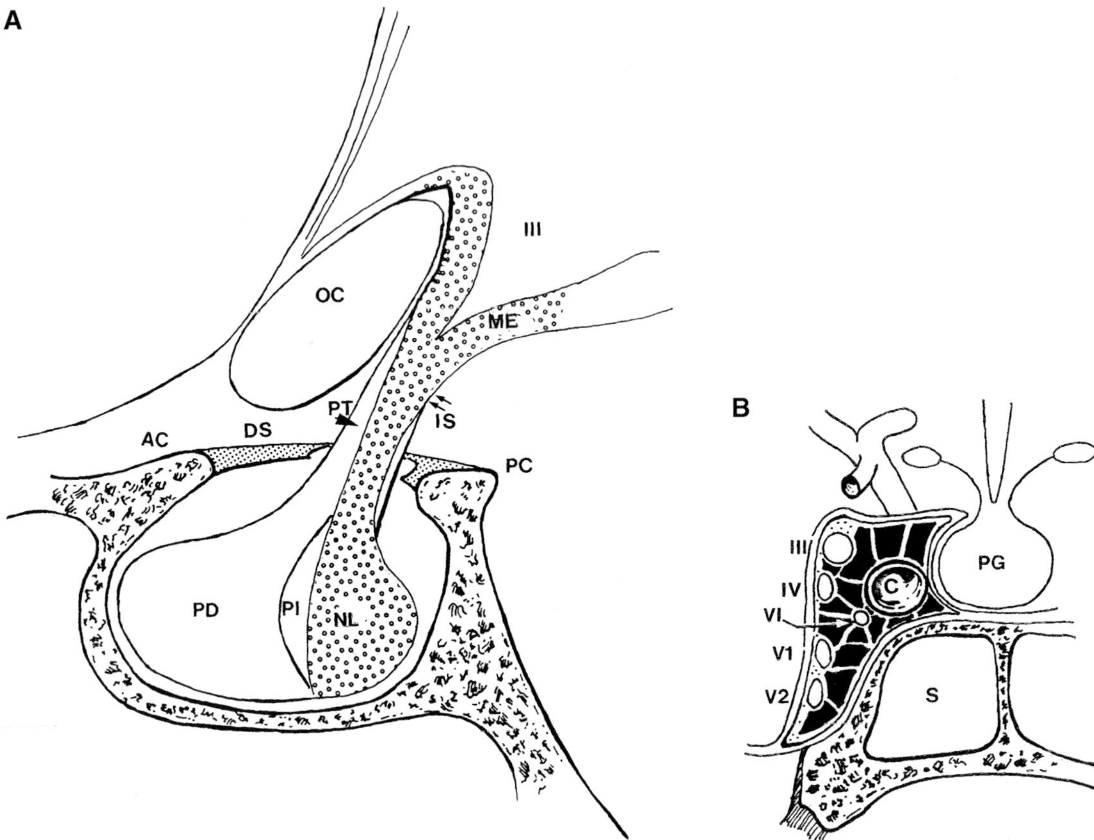


Fig. 1. (*A*) Sagittal schematic view of the pituitary. AS, anterior clinoid; DS, diaphragma sella; III, third ventricle; IS, infundibular stem; ME, median eminence; NL, neural lobe; OC, optic chiasm; PC, posterior clinoid; PD, pars distalis; PI, pars intermedia; PT, pars tuberalis. (*B*) Coronal cavernous sinus diagram. Roman numerals correspond to cranial nerves. Note the position of CN VI with respect to the cavernous carotid artery (C). PG, pituitary gland; S, sphenoid sinus. (*From* FitzPatrick M, Tartaglino LM, Hollander MD, et al. Imaging of sellar and parasellar pathology. Radiol Clin North Am 1999;37:102.)

to antidiuretic hormone neurosecretory granules and its presence implies a normal transport of antidiuretic hormone from the hypothalamus to the posterior gland by the pituitary infundibulum [4–6]. At times, the posterior lobe may be ectopic.

The pituitary stalk or infundibulum extends from the hypothalamus, posterior to the optic chiasm, through the diaphragm sellae, and to the pituitary gland (see Fig. 1A). The pituitary stalk is composed of the supraoptic hypophyseal tract, tuberohypophyseal tract, and hypophyseal portal system. The supraoptic hypophyseal tract contains fibers from the supraoptic and paraventricular nuclei that project to the neurohypophysis. The tuberohypophyseal tract (tuberoinfundibular tract) extends mainly from the arcuate nucleus of the tuberal region to the median eminence and infundibular stem. It ends near the capillary loops adjacent to the sinusoids of the hypophyseal portal system. The fibers of the tuberohypophyseal tract convey releasing hormones that are transported by the hypophyseal portal system to the adenohypophysis. The adenohypophysis secretes growth hormone, thyroid-stimulating hormone, adrenocorticotropic hormone, follicle-stimulating hormone, luteinizing hormone, and prolactin. The neurohypophysis secretes vasopressin and oxytocin. The median lobe produces melanocyte-stimulating hormone [7].

The optic chiasm is located approximately 10 mm above the pituitary gland (see Fig. 1A). The pituitary infundibulum is located immediately posterior to the chiasm. In 80% of individuals, the chiasm is directly above the gland. In 5% to 15% of individuals, the chiasm is prefixed and located anteriorly over the tuberculum sellae. The remainder has a postfixed chiasm located over the dorsum sellae. The variable location of the chiasm with respect to the pituitary gland partly determines the type of neurophthalmalogic symptoms experienced by patients with pituitary tumors.

Within the chiasm, the nasal retinal fibers (including the macular fibers), which provide sight to the temporal fields, cross and continue in the contralateral optic tract. The temporal fibers, which provide sight to the nasal field, continue directly without crossing into the optic tracts. The central portion of the chiasm contains crossing fibers and the lateral portion of the chiasm contains uncrossed fibers. The superior retinal fibers are superior within the chiasm; the inferior retinal fibers are inferior within the chiasm. Wilbrand's knee is a small anterior bend of the inferior nasal retinal fibers into the posterior aspect of the contralateral optic nerve at its junction with the optic chiasm. Wilbrand's knee occurs before the fibers continue posteriorly into the optic tracts. Macular fibers compose almost 90% of the optic nerves and cross in the posterior and central portions of the chiasm [8,9].

The size of tumor, the rate and direction of growth, the chiasm anatomy with respect to the pituitary gland, and the presence of hemorrhage influence the type of visual loss in patients with a pituitary tumor. Classically, pituitary macroadenomas growing through the diaphragm sellae into the suprasellar cistern compressing the chiasm produce bitemporal hemianopsia secondary to compression of the inferonasal fibers from below, which are usually affected first. The superotemporal fields are affected first, progressing inferiorly and medially in both eyes. Lastly, the superonasal field is affected. When the chiasm is postfixed or the mass grows anteriorly, one or both optic nerves may be affected. This may produce a central scotoma in the involved optic nerve. If a single optic nerve and its junction with the chiasm are affected, potentially a junctional syndrome or scotoma can occur because of compression of a prechiasmatic optic nerve and Wilbrand's knee. This results in an ipsilateral central scotoma because of the affected ipsilateral optic nerve and a contralateral superior temporal field defect caused by the involvement of the inferior nasal fibers from the contralateral globe within Wilbrand's knee. When the chiasm is prefixed or the sellar mass grows posteriorly, one or both of the optic tracts may be affected. If a single tract is affected, a homonymous hemianopsia can occur involving the contralateral visual field. Bitemporal hemianoptic scotomas with or without inferior field defects indicate involvement of the posterior chiasmal notch where there is a higher concentration of macular crossing fibers [8,9].

Posteriorly, the dorsum sellae is continuous with the clivus, which forms the anterior aspect of the posterior cranial fossa. The posterior clinoid processes are two bony tubercles along the superior margin of the dorsum sellae, which give attachment to the fixed margin of the tentorium cerebelli [10]. Bridged by the spheno-occipital synchondrosis, the upper portion of the clivus is formed by the sphenoid bone (basiphenoid), whereas the lower portion is formed by the occipital bone (basiocciput) [1]. Dorello's canal is a dural reflection along the posterior clivus, which transmits the abducens nerve to the cavernous sinus.

The centrally located sphenoid sinus is a potential site for the spread of inflammation or neoplasm, which can affect vision or the nerves that are integral in vision function (Fig. 2). The sphenoid sinus lies below the pituitary gland and separates it from the nasal cavity. The cavernous sinuses are lateral to the sphenoid sinus (Fig. 1B). The carotid sulcus is along the lateral surface of the sphenoid body (see Fig. 1B). The optic nerve canals protrude into the superolateral portion of the sinus. The maxillary nerve canal (foramen rotundum and canal) protrudes into the inferolateral aspect of the sphenoid sinus. The vidian nerve canal contains the vidian nerve, which provides parasympathetic fibers to the lacrimal gland and nasal mucosa. The vidian nerve is a combination of parasympathetic fibers from the greater petrosal branch of CN VII and sympathetic fibers from the deep petrosal nerve. The vidian canal protrudes superiorly from the floor of the sphenoid sinus. During developmental

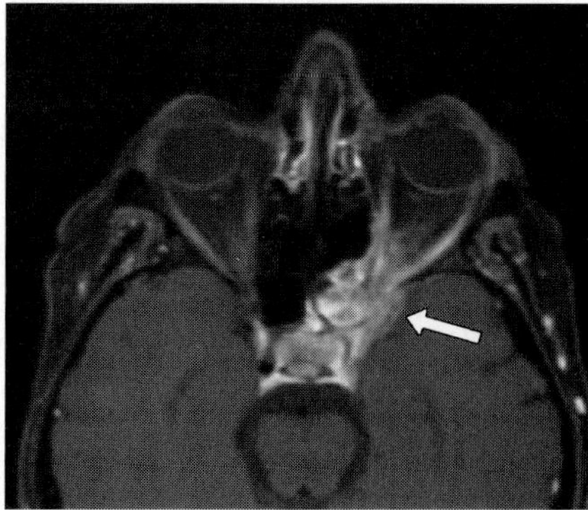

Fig. 2. Aspergillus sinusitis with cavernous sinus and orbital involvement. Immunocompetent patient presented with left vision loss, left periorbital pain, and ptosis. Axial enhanced T1-weighted MR image demonstrates soft tissue enhancement in left posterior ethmoid cells (sphenoid sinus was also involved), abnormal enhancement of the left cavernous sinus (*arrow*), and left orbital apex. Note the loss of signal void of the left internal carotid artery.

expansion of the sphenoid sinus, the bone covering these structures may become very thin or frankly dehiscent predisposing them to inflammatory or neoplastic spread or damage during surgery [1].

The diaphragm sellae is a rectangular dural structure forming the roof of the sella turcica, which has a central opening that transmits the pituitary infundibulum (see Fig. 1A). The size of the opening is large when compared with the size of the infundibulum. A deficiency of the diaphragm is believed to predispose patients to developing an empty sella [1]. The dura of the diaphragm sella is continuous with the dura covering of the cavernous sinus.

The cavernous sinus is a dural-covered venous sinus located along the lateral aspect of the sella turcica and sphenoid sinus (see Fig. 1B). Below, the sphenoid bone, which forms the floor of the cavernous sinus, is superior to the nasopharynx. The cavernous sinus extends posteriorly from the superior orbital fissure to the petrous apex. The location of the cavernous sinuses and their potential connections makes them a potential conduit of spread of inflammation and neoplasm.

Variable intercavernous venous connections can exist along the margins of the diaphragm sellae and around the pituitary gland. The anterior intercavernous sinus passes anterior to the pituitary gland and the posterior intercavernous sinus passes posterior to the gland within the sella. If both are present, the whole structure constitutes a circular sinus. A large intercavernous connection called the basilar sinus, the most constant of the formed sinuses, is located posterior to the dorsum sellae. The intercavernous connections can allow inflammatory or thrombophlebotic processes to cross the midline to involve the contralateral sinus. They can be damaged and account for hemorrhage during transphenoidal surgery [1].

The ophthalmic vein and sphenoparietal dural venous sinus drain into the cavernous sinus. The cavernous sinus drains posteriorly into the greater and lesser petrosal sinuses, which then drain into the transverse sinus and jugular bulb, respectively. Venous connections with the pterygoid (usually through the foramen ovale) and pharyngeal venous plexuses are also present [7]. Because the ophthalmic vein drains into the cavernous sinus, any pathologic process resulting in venous congestion of the cavernous sinus can potentially produce proptosis and chemosis [1].

The cavernous segments of the internal carotid arteries, cranial nerves III, IV, V.1, V.2, and VI, are located within the cavernous sinus (see Fig. 1B). Meckel's cave, a dural reflection located at the posterior aspect of the cavernous sinus, contains the trigeminal sensory ganglion and trigeminal (gasserian) cistern. Meckel's cave is located at the Meckel's impression (cavity) of the petrous apex [10,11].

## Pathologic processes in the sellar and parasellar region

### *Pituitary macroadenoma*

Pituitary adenomas account for approximately 10% of all intracranial neoplasms and between one third to one half of sellar and parasellar masses [11]. Pituitary macroadenomas are twice as common as microadenomas and are the most common suprasellar masses, and the most common mass resulting in visual symptoms in this region [9,11]. Among the secretory adenomas, visual loss is rarely the initial complaint. Nonsecretory adenomas account for 60% of patients with visual complaints having an adenoma [9].

Because pituitary microadenomas do not produce visual symptoms typically, they are not discussed. A pituitary macroadenoma is defined as an adenoma greater than 10 mm. A slow-growing macroadenoma expands the bony sella and extends into the suprasellar cistern. Often, these lesions have a "figure eight" or "snowmanlike" appearance because the rigid dura of the diaphragm sellae results in a waist to the mass (Fig. 3). On precontrast CT scanning, macroadenomas are isointense to brain and demon-

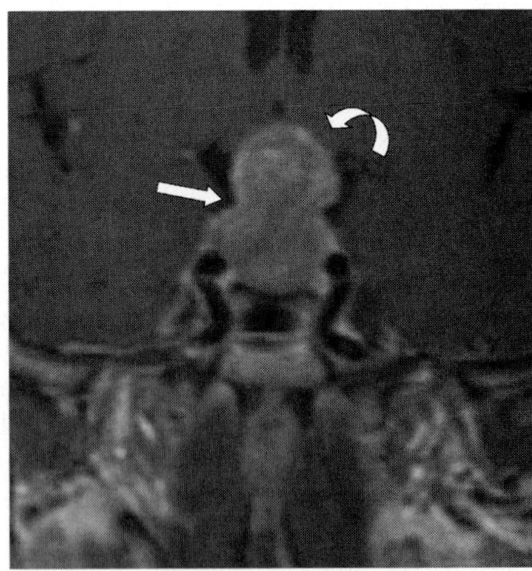

Fig. 3. Macroadenoma with suprasellar extension. Coronal enhanced T1-weighted MR image demonstrates an enhancing sellar mass with suprasellar extension compressing the optic chiasm (*curved arrow*). The indentation of the diaphragm sellae (*straight arrow*) produces the snowmanlike appearance.

strate moderate contrast enhancement. On MR imaging, a macroadenoma appears isointense to gray matter on T1- and T2-weighted MR images, and usually demonstrates intense contrast enhancement unless there are areas of necrotic degeneration or small amounts of hemorrhage [11].

Macroadenomas are usually well defined and slow growing. Typically, they extend through the diaphragm sellae and affect the optic chiasm or nerves; however, sometimes if the adenoma is significantly large or invasive, it may extend into the sphenoid bone and sinus or may extend into the cavernous sinuses affecting the carotid arteries or cranial nerves. Invasive adenomas are usually prolactin-excreting tumors. If prolactin levels are greater than 1000 ng/dL, cavernous sinus invasion is likely [4,12]. Cavernous sinus invasion by an adenoma is almost certain if the vessel is more than 67% encased [12]. Invasion is highly likely if the carotid sulcus venous compartment (the space between the cavernous carotid artery and the carotid sulcus of the sphenoid bone) is obliterated or a line drawn along the lateral margins of the intracavernous and supracavernous segments of the internal carotid artery is crossed (Fig. 4). Invasion is nearly excluded if the vessel is less than 25% encased or a line drawn along the medial margins of the intracavernous and supracavernous segments of the internal carotid artery is not crossed [12]. Invasive adenomas cannot be distinguished from rare pituitary carcinomas by imaging studies

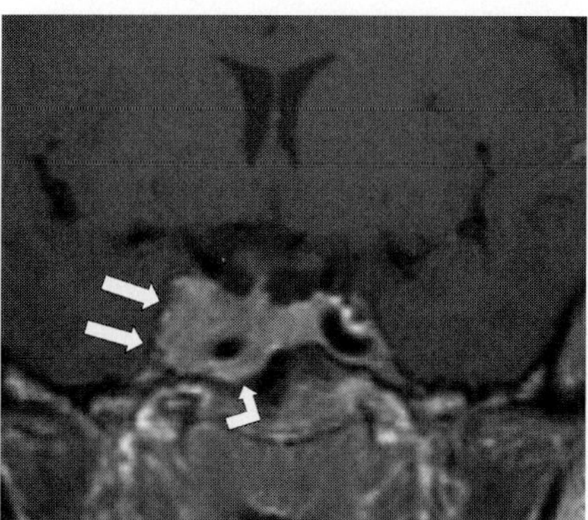

Fig. 4. Invasive macroadenoma extending into the right cavernous sinus. The patient presented with headache, right ptosis, galactorrhea, and blurry vision. Coronal enhanced T1-weighted MR image demonstrates an enhancing mass in the right aspect of the sella extending into the right cavernous sinus (*arrows*) encasing and extending lateral to the right cavernous internal carotid artery. Note the widened carotid sulcus venous compartment (*angled arrow*) compared with the left. The pituitary stalk is deviated to the right.

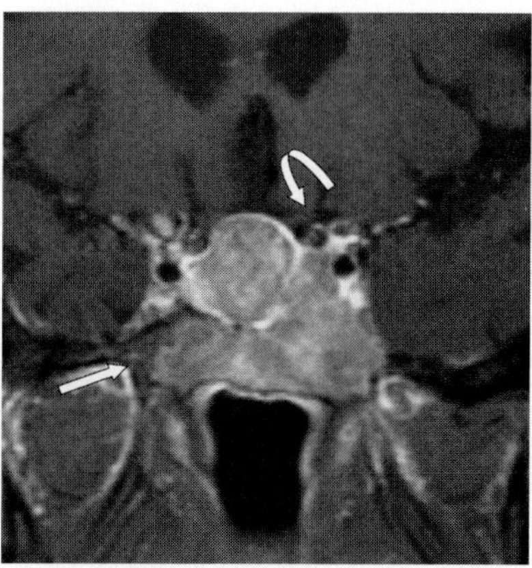

Fig. 5. Invasive macroadenoma. The patient presented with right eye blindness, poor peripheral vision, and left-sided partial visual field defect. Coronal enhanced T1-weighted MR image demonstrates a large, infiltrating, enhancing mass extending into the suprasellar cistern between the prechiasmatic optic nerves (*curved arrow*), extending into the left cavernous sinus, sphenoid sinus, and also extending into the bone of the sphenoid body. A small amount of normal marrow signal remains in the right sphenoid body at the junction of the pterygoid plates (*straight arrow*).

alone (Fig. 5) [11]. Pituitary carcinomas that metastasize within the neural axis tend to be nonfunctioning and exhibit suprasellar extension. Pituitary carcinomas that tend to metastasize to extraneural sites, usually corticotropin-secreting tumors, tend not to enlarge the sella but exhibit early extension through the floor gaining access to extracranial vessels and lymphatics [4].

Involvement of the ocular motor nerves occurs in 1% to 14% of patients with a pituitary tumor. This may occur late in the disease with a very large adenoma or may be less commonly an earlier symptom before visual loss. CN III is the most commonly involved followed by CN VI. The proposed mechanism for CN III palsy is mass effect from the growing tumor compressing the third nerve against the interclinoid ligament. Fourth cranial nerve palsies are usually associated with other cranial nerve palsies; however, isolated fourth nerve palsies have been described [9,13].

### *Pituitary apoplexy*

The anterior pituitary gland receives its blood supply mainly by the hypophyseal portal system; the lack of direct arterial supply makes it susceptible to ischemia and subsequent hemorrhage. Because pituitary adenomas have a tenuous blood supply, they are more prone to hemorrhage and necrosis, which can

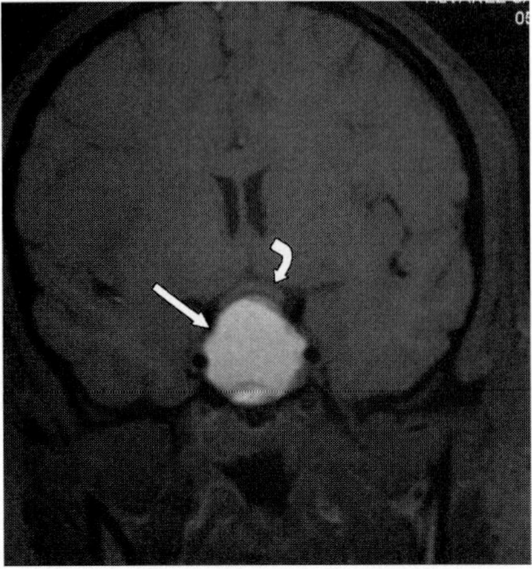

Fig. 6. Pituitary apoplexy. The patient presented with headache, photophobia, amenorrhea, and chemosis. No visual field defects were reported. Coronal enhanced T1-weighted fat-suppressed MR image demonstrates a rounded high signal mass consistent with blood product within the sella, extending into the suprasellar cistern (*straight arrow*). The optic chiasm (*curved arrow*) is deformed by the mass. Note the smooth remodeled sella and splayed internal carotid arteries indicating that this represents hemorrhage into a chronic macroadenoma.

be life threatening, a condition known as pituitary apoplexy. Pituitary apoplexy is characterized by headache, vomiting, ophthalmoplegia, or visual loss [4]. The classic visual field defect is a bitemporal superior quadrantic defect. Ocular paresis can occur in 78% of patients, usually affecting CN III. Rapid enlargement of the hemorrhagic adenoma tends to compress the optic chiasm. Surgical decompression performed within 1 week of onset has been shown to improve recovery of visual acuity [14]. Sheehan's syndrome, postpartum or peripartum pituitary necrosis and hemorrhage, results from hypovolemia and shock [15]. Hemorrhage associated with apoplexy from an existing adenoma exhibiting an enlarged sella can be distinguished from Sheehan's syndrome exhibiting a normally sized sella. MR imaging findings can vary depending on hemoglobin state of oxygenation with apoplexy; however, a large high-signal mass on T1- and T2-weighted MR images is typical (Fig. 6) [11,16]. High signal within an adenoma on diffusion-weighted MR imaging scan may indicate early apoplexy [17].

### *Rathke's cleft cyst*

Rathke's pouch is an evagination of stomodeum (primitive mouth) ectoderm, which loses connection with the oral cavity at about the second month of development. Rathke's pouch extends dorsally and is induced by a downward extension of the diencephalon, the infundibulum, to develop into the adenohypophysis [18]. Both Rathke's cleft cysts and craniopharyngiomas are derived from Rathke's pouch.

Rathke's cleft cysts are rare and frequently asymptomatic. Visual disturbances may be present, usually bitemporal hemianopsia. Pituitary dysfunction may be present in up to 69% of symptomatic cases. In contrast to craniopharyngiomas, Rathke's cleft cysts are usually smaller, intrasellar, and noninvasive. They rarely calcify. They are lined by a single layer of columnar or cuboidal epithelium. Treatment is usually by transphenoidal drainage and partial resection of the wall. There is a low incidence of recurrence and good visual prognosis [4,19,20].

Rathke's cleft cysts may contain serous or mucoid material, which influences imaging studies. Serous-containing cysts are low density on CT scan and appear hypointense on T1-weighted and hyperintense on T2-weighted MR images (Fig. 7). Mucoid-containing cysts are higher attenuating on CT scan and can be hyperintense on T1-weighted MR images. There is only mild enhancement to the wall of the cyst after contrast administration [4,21,22].

### *Craniopharyngioma*

Craniopharyngiomas are benign neoplasms believed to arise within squamous epithelial remnants of Rathke's pouch. Although benign, craniopharyngiomas tend to recur and invade adjacent structures. Tumor adhesion to surrounding vascular structures

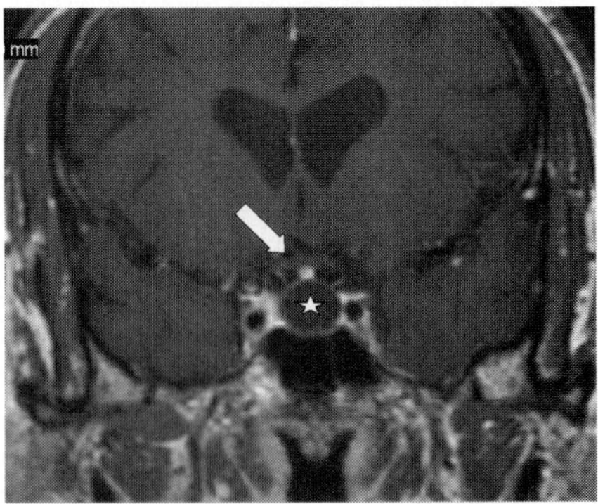

Fig. 7. Rathke's cleft cyst. Coronal enhanced T1-weighted MR image demonstrates a mass (*star*) isointense to cerebrospinal fluid with a thin enhancing wall protruding into the suprasellar cistern. The optic chiasm is indicated by the arrow.

represents the most common cause of incomplete resection. Presenting symptoms include headaches, endocrine dysfunction, and visual disturbances. The age of presentation is bimodal: 5 to 14 years in children and 65 to 74 years in adults. Survival rate is excellent for patients younger than 20 years (99% at 5 years) and poor for patients older than 65 years (38% at 5 years) [4,23]. There are two main histologic subtypes: adamantinomatous, mainly in children, and squamous, mainly in adults. The squamous subtype has a better prognosis [24].

Craniopharyngiomas are typically suprasellar in location and can extend into the sella. Prechiasmatic craniopharyngiomas usually result in optic atrophy. Retrochiasmatic craniopharyngiomas are commonly associated with signs of increased intracranial pressure (papilledema) caused by compression of the hypothalamus and protrusion into the third ventricle (Fig. 8) [25].

Classical visual presentation is bitemporal hemianopsia or inferior quadrantanopia caused by chiasmal compression. Pleomorphism, defined as change of one type of visual field defect to another, can also be a feature. Possibly this is related to intermittent enlargement or decompression of the cystic components [24,25]. Craniopharyngiomas vary in size and composition having cystic and solid components identified on CT and MR imaging examination. Rim or nodular calcifications are present in about 80% of cases. Cystic components are present in about 85%. Focal areas of high signal can sometimes be identified on T1-weighted MR images, which correspond to machine oil–like cysts, which contain proteinaceous debris, cholesterol, and hemoglobin (Fig. 9) [4].

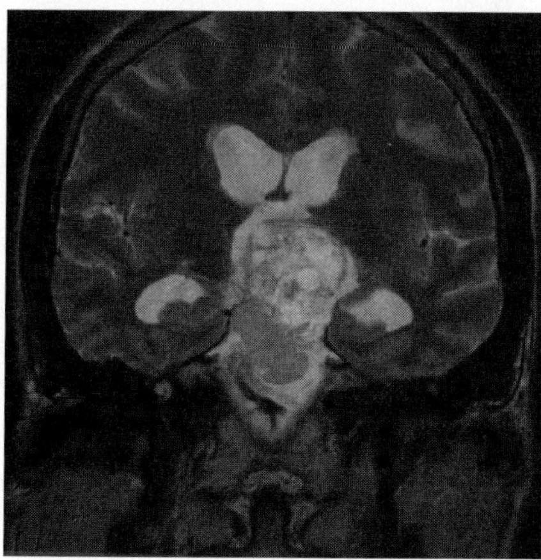

Fig. 8. Craniopharyngioma extending into the third ventricle. Coronal T2-weighted MR image demonstrates a cystic and solid mass in the suprasellar region extending superiorly and displacing the third ventricle. Note the hydrocephalus apparent in the lateral ventricles.

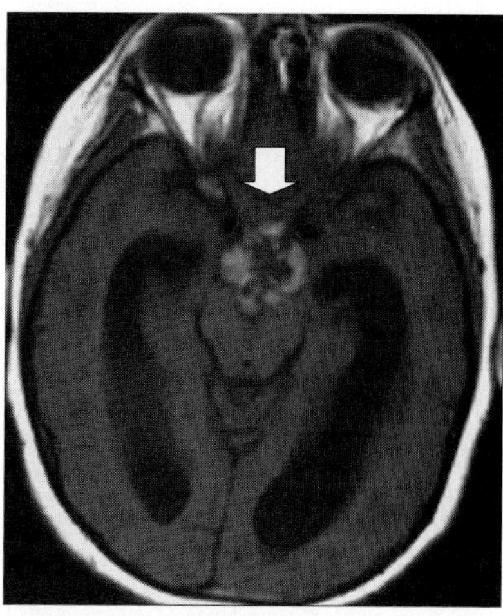

Fig. 9. Craniopharyngioma. Axial nonenhanced T1-weighted MR image demonstrates a heterogenous mass with hyperattenuating areas within the mass corresponding to increased protein within the machine oil-like cysts. The mass is retrochiasmatic (*arrow* represents chiasm) and protrudes into the interpeduncular cistern posteriorly. Note the dilated lateral ventricles more frequently identified with retrochiasmatic lesions.

### *Meningioma*

Meningioma is the most common nonglial primary brain tumor and accounts for 15% of all intracranial neoplasms [26]. Five percent to 10% of all meningiomas occur in the sellar region, where they are the second most common lesion in adults exceeded only by the pituitary adenoma. Based on clinical presentation, a sellar meningioma can be distinguished from a pituitary adenoma. The presence of visual symptoms without evidence of endocrine abnormalities or bitemporal hemianopsia with the presence of a normal-sized sella favors the diagnosis of a meningioma [27]. Meningiomas may arise from the suprasellar (tuberculum sella, anterior clinoid processes, planum sphenoidale, upper clivus, diaphragm sellae); parasellar (cavernous sinus); or intrasellar regions (diaphragm sellae).

Suprasellar meningioma arises close to the optic chiasm displacing it posteriorly and superiorly (Fig. 10). This usually results in vision loss, the most common and earliest complaint. The clinical presentation of this slow-growing tumor usually involves monocular vision loss progressing to binocular vision loss. Because of the typically asymmetric growth of

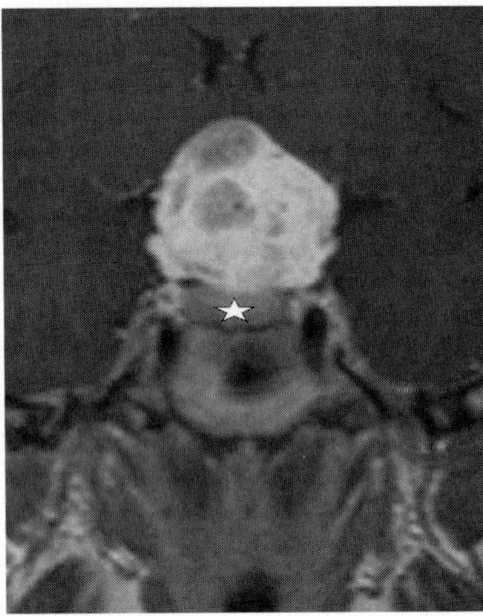

Fig. 10. Meningioma arising from the diaphragm sellae. The patient presented with a history of gradual vision loss and photophobia. There was no light perception in the left eye, with a large temporal field defect in the right eye on examination. Coronal enhanced T1-weighted MR image demonstrates a large contrast enhancing mass centered on the diaphragm sellae, extending into the suprasellar cistern obscuring the optic chiasm. Note the normal-appearing pituitary gland (*star*) within the sella.

the tumor, initially only a portion of the chiasm or only one optic nerve may be affected causing a distinct asymmetric variant of a bitemporal hemianopsia, specifically amaurosis of one eye with temporal hemianopia of the other eye (caused by unilateral involvement of the optic nerve and the anterior angle of the chiasm, Wilbrand's knee). A variety of other visual field deficits and optic atrophy can occur [8,27]. Other common symptoms include headaches, seizures, and mental changes. Visual loss associated with meningioma, which can be confused with retrobulbar neuritis, does not involve pain on eye movement and is gradual in nature [27].

Meningiomas can arise laterally from the medial sphenoid ridge or cavernous sinus. Parasellar meningioma of the lesser sphenoid wing can expand medially and affect the ipsilateral optic nerve and the superior orbital fissure (Fig. 11). Involvement of the optic nerve can result in unilateral loss of vision. Depending on the extent of optic nerve involvement, a variety of visual field deficits can occur. Diplopia may be present because of paresis of the extrinsic ocular muscles (ie, the oculomotor, abducens, and trochlear nerves). Extension of the tumor into the superior orbital fissure can also affect the branches of these nerves and the ophthalmic division of the trigeminal nerve resulting in the superior orbital fissure syndrome. The superior orbital fissure syndrome is characterized by the combination of a variety of cranial nerve palsies with no one particular nerve predominating. Pupillary dysfunction is not uncommon. In contrast to ischemic cranial neuropathies, nerve palsies associated with superior orbital fissure syndrome are chronic in nature [28]. Exophthalmos can result either from direct invasion of the orbit through the superior orbital fissure or obstruction of the draining venous system of the orbit and the cavernous sinus [8].

Cavernous sinus meningioma [8] can involve the cavernous sinus, Meckel's cave, or the sella turcica resulting in the cavernous sinus syndrome. This is clinically similar to the superior orbital fissure syndrome because almost the same neural structures are involved. Unlike the superior orbital fissure syndrome, which only affects the first branch of the trigeminal nerve, the cavernous sinus syndrome may involve all branches of the trigeminal nerve.

Foster Kennedy syndrome is a rare condition characterized by ipsilateral optic atrophy and contralateral papilledema. Classically, it was described with frontobasal intracranial lesions, usually meningiomas of the tuberculum sellae; however, craniopharyngiomas and pituitary adenoma have been reported [29]. The exact mechanism is unclear. It may be caused by unilateral optic nerve compression with increased intracranial pressure, bilateral

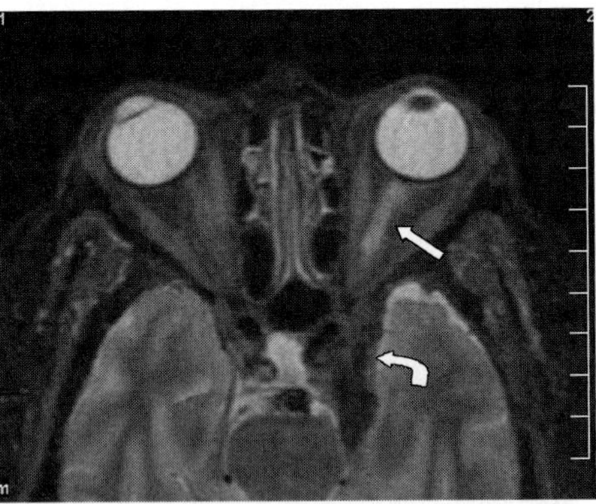

Fig. 11. Meningioma involving left cavernous sinus. The patient had no light perception in the left eye. Axial short tau inversion recovery (STIR) MR image demonstrates a low signal extra-axial mass (*curved arrow*) involving the left cavernous sinus extending to the orbital apex. High signal is present along the left intraorbital optic nerve (*straight arrow*) consistent with increased cerebrospinal fluid within the optic nerve sheath secondary to long-standing optic atrophy. Note the absent low signal lens in the right globe from prior cataract surgery.

optic nerve compression, or increased intracranial pressure alone.

Intrasellar meningiomas are rare and probably originate from the diaphragm sellae causing the diaphragm to be depressed if arising from above and elevated if arising from below [30].

The characteristic features of meningiomas can help distinguish them from other sellar lesions. Imaging features of their extra-axial origin include obtuse dural margins, hyperostosis, and cerebrospinal fluid (CSF) clefts (Fig. 12). A linear dural tail enhancement may be seen. They are homogeneously solid tumors but may occasionally contain areas of necrosis, scarring, cystic degeneration, and calcifications. Meningiomas are slightly hyperdense to brain parenchyma on nonenhanced CT and isointense to gray matter on T1-weighted and variable on T2-weighted MR images. Postcontrast CT and MR imaging reveal intense homogeneous enhancement [26]. Angiography shows a tumoral blush.

*Schwannoma*

Schwannomas can occur in the parasellar region and involve any of the cranial nerves. Trigeminal schwannomas represent one third of primary trigeminal and Meckel's cave tumors. These tumors originate from the Schwann cells of nerve sheaths [31]. Involvement and expansion of the foramen rotundum or ovale is common if they are of trigeminal origin [32]. Patients usually present with progressive facial numbness, pain, and paresthesia.

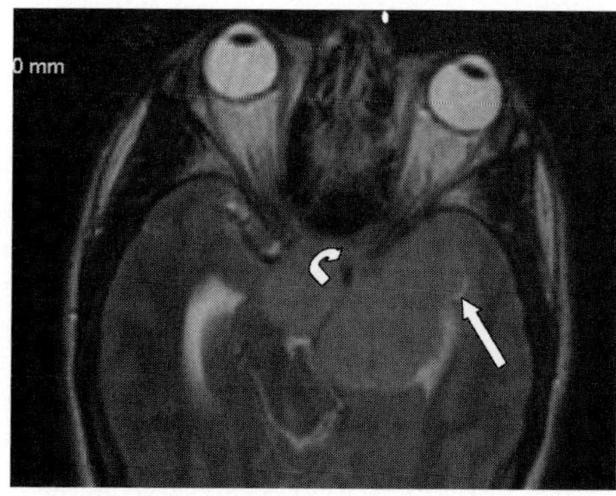

Fig. 12. Meningioma arising adjacent to the lesser wing of sphenoid. The patient presented with progressive blindness with a nonfocal ophthalmologic examination and inaccurate finger counting. Axial T2-weighted MR image demonstrates a large, lobulated, extra-axial, suprasellar and parasellar mass isointense to gray matter encasing the left supraclinoid internal carotid artery (*curved arrow*). Note the cerebrospinal fluid high signal cleft (*straight arrow*) between the meningioma and left temporal lobe.

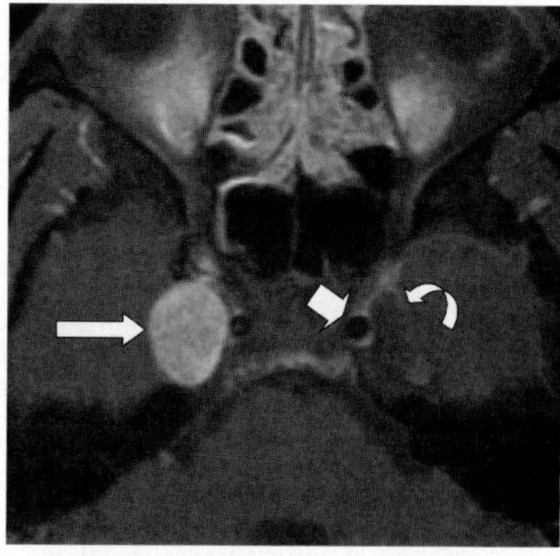

Fig. 13. Schwannoma of the cavernous sinus. The patient presented with gradual onset of diplopia with isolated right CN VI palsy and right facial numbness on examination. Axial enhanced T1-weighted fat-suppressed MR image demonstrates a well-defined, ovoid contrast enhancing mass (*long arrow*) in the right cavernous sinus contacting the right cavernous internal carotid artery and obliterating the cerebrospinal fluid in Meckel's cave. The short arrow indicates the left cavernous carotid artery and the curved arrow indicates the left gasserian cistern with the Meckel's cave.

CT demonstrates a mass that is isodense to the brain parenchyma and enhances homogeneously with contrast. On MR imaging, schwannomas are well-marginated and fusiform in appearance (Fig. 13). They are isointense or slightly hypointense to gray matter on T1-weighted MR images and hypointense to CSF on T2-weighted MR images and enhance homogeneously after contrast administration. Occasionally, they may appear heterogeneous with variable contrast enhancement patterns depending on cystic, necrotic, and hemorrhagic components [33].

*Aneurysm*

Aneurysms of the cavernous or supraclinoid portions of the internal carotid artery, posterior communicating artery, and ophthalmic artery can present as parasellar and suprasellar masses. Although intracavernous aneurysms account for only 2% to 3% of all intracranial aneurysms, they represent almost one fourth of all cavernous sinus syndrome–producing lesions [28]. An aneurysm can cause a posterior cavernous sinus syndrome with involvement of the first and second branches of the trigeminal nerve and frequently the sixth nerve. An anterior cavernous sinus syndrome can result when

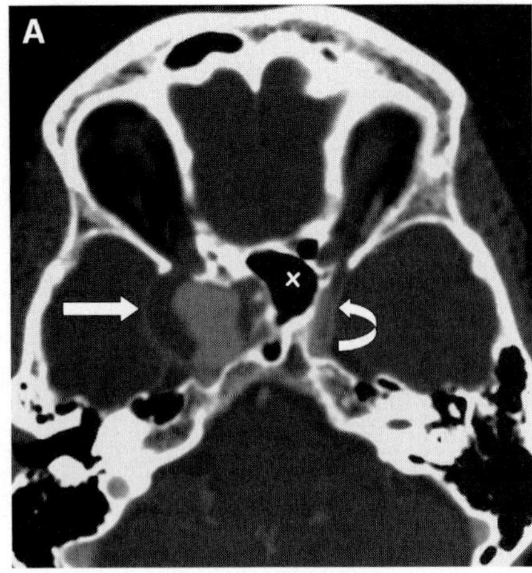


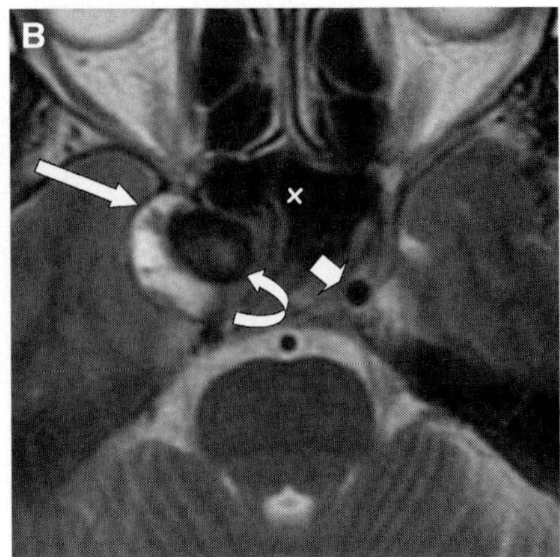


Fig. 14. Cavernous carotid aneurysm. The patient presented with severe right retro-orbital pain, right optic nerve atrophy, diplopia, right chemosis, right lid lag, right V.1 and V.2 paresthesias, and right lateral gaze palsy. (*A*) Axial enhanced CT examination demonstrates a rounded parasellar mass (*straight arrow*), remodeling the sphenoid bone and protruding into the sphenoid sinus (X). The central portion of the lesion enhances similar to other vascular structures. The nonenhancing areas represent mural thrombus; conventional and MR angiography can underestimate the size of the aneurysm because these modalities only demonstrate flowing blood. Normal left cavernous sinus (*curved arrow*). (*B*) Axial T2-weighted MR image demonstrates the dark flow void (*curved arrow*) of the flowing portion of the aneurysm, which is difficult to distinguish from the signal void of the sphenoid sinus (X), a potential pitfall. Note the semilunar-shaped high signal region (*long arrow*) corresponding to the mural thrombus. Normal left cavernous carotid flow void (*short arrow*).

only the first branch of the trigeminal nerve and third cranial nerve are affected with or without associated fourth or sixth nerve paresis [8,34]. Clinical manifestations include hypesthesia or hypalgesia of the face, diplopia, and ptosis caused by trigeminal nerve involvement and ocular motor nerve palsies. Unlike trigeminal neuralgia, however, the pain is constant. In some cases, the only sign of trigeminal nerve involvement may be the absence of a corneal reflex. Large aneurysms may affect the ipsilateral optic nerve causing atrophy and subsequent vision loss [8]. Contrary to ischemic causes of third nerve palsies, compression of the third nerve by an aneurysm does not present with pupil sparing. Because the pupillomotor fibers are located peripherally in the third nerve, an aneurysm impinging on the third nerve affects the pupil first [35].

Imaging features vary greatly depending on the amount of calcification and thrombosis present within the aneurysm. CT may reveal a hyperdense mass with curvilinear calcifications and enhancement of a patent lumen. There may be evidence of bone remodeling of the sella turcica. On MR imaging, a nonthrombosed aneurysm may appear as a rounded flow void that is contiguous with an adjacent arterial signal void. A thrombosed aneurysm may be heterogeneous in signal intensity on T1- and T2-weighted MR images because of the various stages of hemoglobin and amount of calcification. Flow-related artifacts, such as signal misregistration artifact in the phase-encoding axis, may also be present (Fig. 14) [26,36]. The exclusion of an aneurysm is essential in evaluating a sellar mass because of its high morbidity. In indeterminate cases where MR angiography is not diagnostic, conventional angiography may be necessary.

### *Carotid-cavernous fistula*

Carotid-cavernous fistulas can be classified into two types: traumatic and spontaneous. Traumatic carotid-cavernous fistulas are caused by a ruptured internal carotid artery or one of its branches as a result of a head injury. The spontaneous type most commonly results from a ruptured carotid aneurysm but can be caused by a congenital arteriovenous malformation that opens from atherosclerotic disease, hypertension, collagen vascular disease, or childbirth [37].

Because the cavernous sinus communicates with the ophthalmic veins, the veins become arterialized and develop increased pressure. At the same time, arterial blood flow to the cranial nerves in the cavernous sinus is diminished. Consequently, patients may develop ophthalmic signs including palsies of cranial nerves III, IV, V, and VI and decreased visual acuity. They may present with pulsatile exophthalmos, ocular bruit, and chemosis, and be misdiagnosed as conjunctivitis [38]. Secondary glaucoma is noted frequently. In addition, diplopia and ophthalmoplegia can occur because of venous congestion of orbital muscles or compression of cranial nerves in the cavernous sinus from mass effect [37].

CT reveals enlargement of the ipsilateral cavernous sinus, ophthalmic veins, and extraocular muscles. MR imaging and MR angiography demonstrate abnormal flow voids in the cavernous sinus, dilated cavernous sinus vessels and ophthalmic veins, a convex lateral wall of the cavernous sinus, and orbital edema. On angiography, shunting of blood from the carotid artery into the cavernous sinus may be seen [39].

*Arachnoid cyst*

Most arachnoid cysts occur in the middle cranial fossa. Approximately 15%, however, are located in the suprasellar region. Intrasellar arachnoid cysts are rare but have been reported [40]. The exact mechanism of pathogenesis is unknown. One theory is that they result secondary to an inflammatory process, such as postinfectious arachnoiditis. Another theory is that they develop from the splitting of arachnoid membranes and progressively enlarge. Because of lack of communication with the subarachnoid space, the cyst is under pressure thereby causing mass effect on the parasellar structures. If the optic nerves, chiasm, or tracts are compressed, visual disturbances can occur. If the pituitary stalk or hypothalamus is compressed, endocrine dysfunction can occur. Lastly, hydrocephalus can result from obstruction of the foramen of Monroe because of mass effect on the third ventricle [41]. Occasionally, an intrasellar arachnoid cyst may be confused with an empty sella. An empty sella, however, does not demonstrate mass effect because of its free communication with the subarachnoid space [40].

Arachnoid cysts are smooth, well-defined lesions. The density and signal characteristics are identical to CSF on CT and all MR imaging sequences. Because of their slow growth, CT may demonstrate bone remodeling. Unlike craniopharyngioma and Rathke's cleft cyst, there is lack of calcification or enhancement (Fig. 15) [27].

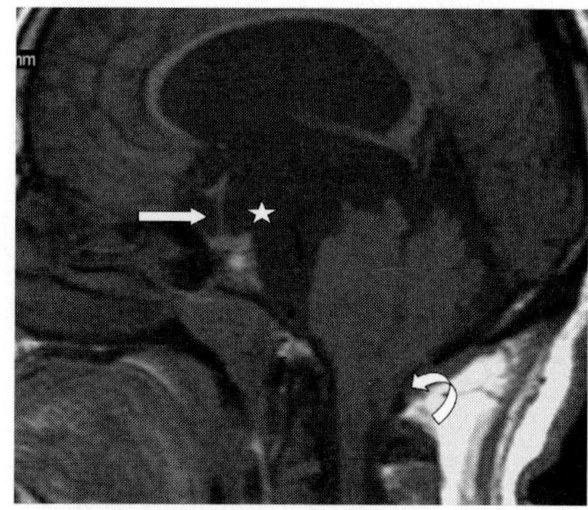

Fig. 15. Arachnoid cyst. The patient presented with horizontal nystagmus, inability of lateral gaze, and left facial droop. Sagittal T1-weighted MR image demonstrates a cerebrospinal fluid signal intensity, transtentorial mass (*star*) extending from the retrochiasmatic, suprasellar cistern inferiorly to the prepontine cistern displacing the brain stem and basilar artery. Note the ectopic cerebellar tonsils (*curved arrow*) consistent with a Chiari I malformation. The straight arrow indicates the pituitary stalk.

*Epidermoid*

Epidermoids are congenital epithelial inclusion cysts that contain desquamated epithelial lining consisting of cellular debris, keratin, and cholesterol crystals. They represent 2% of all intracranial masses and occur usually in the fourth to fifth decades [26]. They can be found in the sellar and parasellar regions where their mass effect can lead to visual disturbances, hypopituitarism, diabetes insipidus, and cranial nerve palsies [27].

Epidermoids are usually isointense to CSF on T1- and T2-weighted MR images and do not enhance. They may contain a calcified rim. Unlike arachnoid cysts, which displace surrounding structures and are identical to CSF on all sequences, epidermoid cysts insinuate between structures and are hyperintense to CSF on fluid-attenuated inversion recovery and diffusion-weighted imaging [11].

*Dermoid*

Dermoids are similar to epidermoids in their appearance and developmental origin. They are benign congenital inclusion cysts lined with stratified squamous epithelium. The tumors are composed of ectodermal elements. Unlike epidermoids, however, dermoids may contain hair follicles, sebaceous glands, and sweat glands [42]. They predominantly occur in young men under the age of 20 and are midline typically. The most common locations include the posterior fossa and suprasellar region [11]. Because of mass effect in the sella and suprasellar regions, dermoids can result in optic neuropathy, visual disturbances, diabetes insipidus, and hypopituitarism.

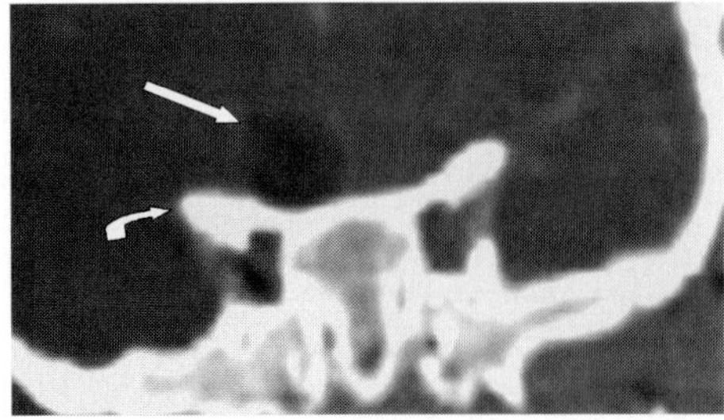

Fig. 16. Dermoid. Coronal reformatted postcontrast CT image demonstrates a well-defined, fat-attenuating, round mass (*straight arrow*) superior to the right anterior clinoid process (*curved arrow*) consistent with a dermoid.

Dermoids are well-circumscribed cystic lesions. On CT, they appear heterogeneous with decreased attenuation because of their fat content (Fig. 16). Calcification is occasionally seen and contrast enhancement is uncommon. Similarly, dermoids have signal intensities characteristic of fat and are high on T1-weighted and low on T2-weighted MR images [43]. In addition, fat-fluid levels may be seen. Dermoids may also appear heterogenous because of the presence of additional ectodermal elements [44].

### *Germinoma*

Germinomas are the most common intracranial germ cell tumors. They affect primarily children and young adults. Germinomas are midline tumors and most frequently arise in the pineal and suprasellar regions. Unlike pineal germinomas, which have a male predilection, primary suprasellar germinomas have no sex prevalence [45]. Suprasellar germinoma may be primary or secondary to metastasis from pineal lesions. They commonly invade the hypothalamus and extend into the third ventricle. They may also involve the optic chiasm and optic nerves or extend into the sella to involve the pituitary gland. Classically, patients present with diabetes insipidus, hypopituitarism, and visual symptoms. The visual disturbances include visual field deficits, optic atrophy, diplopia, and decreased visual acuity.

Noncontrast CT demonstrates a hyperdense suprasellar mass that enhances strongly with contrast administration. On MR imaging, a germinoma usually appears as a well-defined, homogeneous, and infiltrative mass. It is isointense to gray matter on T1- and T2-weighted MR images and enhances intensely with contrast [45]. Cystic change and hemorrhage are rare. Contrast-enhanced studies may reveal enhancement of the subarachnoid spaces indicating tumor spread.

### *Infiltrating lesions*

Infiltrating lesions of the sellar and parasellar region include metastatic disease, sarcoidosis, lymphoma and leukemia, pseudotumor, lymphocytic hypophysitis, and other granulomatous disease including tuberculosis. These entities can have a very similar appearance and are best detected on postcontrast MR imaging examinations. Frequently, clinical history helps narrow the differential diagnosis.

### *Metastatic disease*

Metastatic disease to the sella and parasellar region can be from distant sites; CSF dissemination of a primary central nervous system malignancy; leptomeningeal spread (carcinomatosis, melanomatosis); or from local extension of lesions of the central skull base, sinuses, and head and neck (Fig. 17).

Metastatic disease to the pituitary gland is a relatively common finding in cancer patients at autopsy with a reported incidence up to 26% [46]. Breast cancer is the most common malignancy to metastasize to the pituitary followed by lung cancer

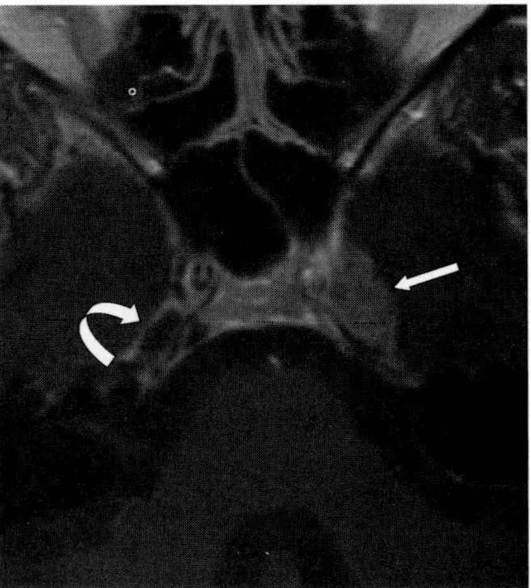

Fig. 17. Metastatic disease to left cavernous sinus. The patient had a history of breast cancer, left ophthalmoplegia, and left trigeminal neuralgia. Axial enhanced T1-weighted MR image demonstrates asymmetric enlargement of the left cavernous sinus with obliteration of the gasserian cistern within Meckel's cave (*straight arrow*). The curved arrow indicates the normal right Meckel's cave.

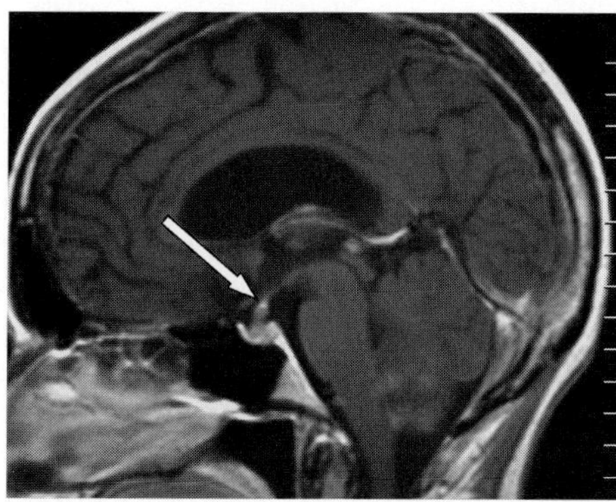

Fig. 18. Metastatic disease to pituitary stalk. The patient had a history of metastatic breast cancer. Sagittal enhanced T1-weighted MR image demonstrates diffuse thickening of the pituitary stalk (*arrow*) and additional areas of nodular enhancement along the surface of the brain stem and cerebellum consistent with metastatic disease.

(Fig. 18) [46–48]. Pituitary metastases are more commonly identified in patients with bone or widespread metastases. Pituitary metastases are more common to the posterior pituitary, likely because of its direct systemic blood supply from the meningohypophyseal trunk as opposed to the anterior pituitary, which receives its blood supply indirectly by the hypophyseal portal system. It has been hypothesized that the hormonal-rich environment of the anterior pituitary is the preferred environment for breast cancer cells and enhances their proliferation [46].

Frequently, the patient's history helps to distinguish metastatic disease from other similar-appearing pituitary lesions, usually macroadenomas. Cranial nerve palsies and diabetes insipidus are more common with metastatic lesions. Rapid onset and progression of symptoms, failed bromocriptine therapy, history of cancer, and advanced age favor metastatic lesions. Pathologic examination of metastatic lesions can be difficult and misdiagnosed as pituitary adenomas. Cases considered to be possibly metastatic should be given special pathologic review and consideration for special staining techniques [49].

The diagnostic imaging appearance of pituitary metastases can be similar to pituitary adenomas. If there is an intrasellar and suprasellar lesion and the sella turcica is not enlarged or eroded, metastatic disease is favored. Dumbbell-shaped lesions with only a small connection between the suprasellar and intrasellar component favor metastatic disease. This is likely related to the slowly growing expanding adenoma widening and destroying the diaphragm sella. The suprasellar portion of a pituitary adenoma is usually located anterior to the infundibular recess of the third ventricle, which becomes displaced posteriorly. Metastatic disease tends to invade the infundibular recess [48].

Nasopharyngeal carcinomas are the most common tumors to invade the skull base. The tumor may directly involve the sphenoid sinus, sella turcica, or middle cranial fossa. Perineural extension along CN V.3 through foramen ovale or direct extension through foramen lacerum can result in cavernous sinus involvement and subsequent ophthalmoplegia (Fig. 19) [50]. Sinonasal neoplasms may extend through the sphenopalatine foramen into the pterygopalatine fossa with subsequent involvement of the orbit by the inferior orbital fissure or the cavernous sinus.

*Lymphocytic infiltration*

Tolosa-Hunt syndrome is an idiopathic inflammatory granulomatous process involving the cavernous sinus with possible extension into the superior orbital fissure and orbital apex. The inflammation causes extrinsic compression of the cranial nerves that transit the cavernous sinus (III, IV, V1, VI, and infrequently V2); the cavernous carotid artery; and the oculosympathetic fibers. The patient presents with

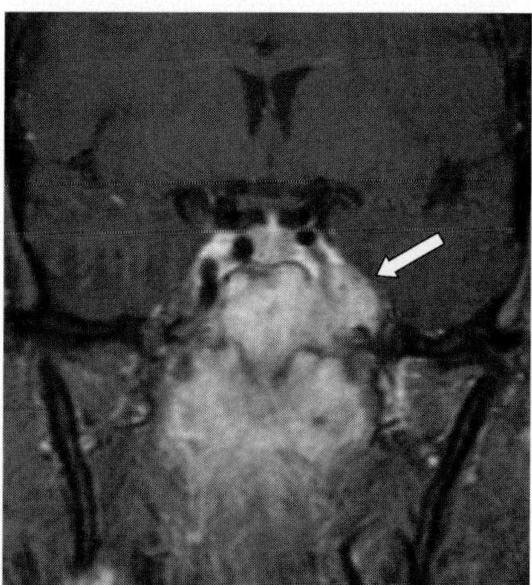

Fig. 19. Nasopharyngeal carcinoma. The patient had a history of known poorly differentiated nasopharyngeal carcinoma with headache, diplopia, and bilateral conductive hearing loss secondary to obstruction of the eustachian tubes. Coronal T1-weighted fat-suppressed postcontrast MR image demonstrates an ill-defined enhancing mass in the nasopharynx extending superiorly to involve the sphenoid body, sphenoid sinus, and left cavernous sinus (*arrow*). The left cavernous internal carotid artery is elevated.

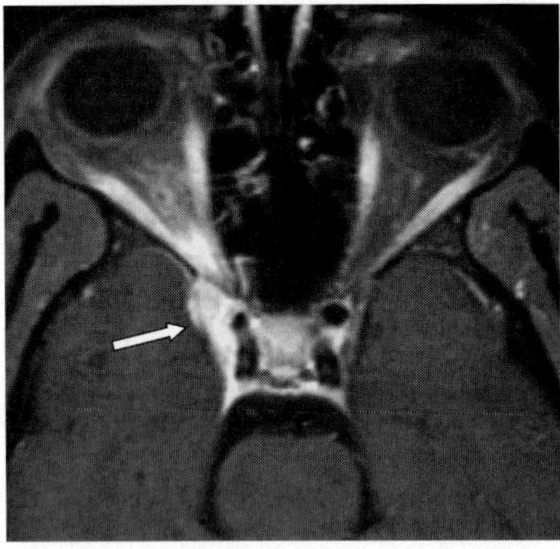

Fig. 20. Tolosa-Hunt syndrome. The patient had a history of right orbital pain, decreased vision of the right eye, and diplopia. Axial enhanced T1-weighted fat-suppressed MR image demonstrates abnormal enhancement in the right orbital apex, mildly thickened extraocular muscles, and asymmetric enlargement of the anterior right cavernous sinus (*arrow*). The patient's symptoms responded to steroid therapy.

severe retro-orbital pain and cranial nerve ophthalmoplegia, which is responsive to steroid therapy. The symptoms usually last for days or weeks and may recur or spontaneous remit [51,52].

Tolosa-Hunt syndrome can be diagnosed when all other infectious, inflammatory, neoplastic, and vascular entities are excluded. CT and MR imaging may demonstrate abnormal enlargement and enhancement of the cavernous sinus (Fig. 20). On MR imaging, the granulation tissue is isointense to muscle on T1-weighted and isointense to gray matter on T2-weighted MR images [53]. Angiography demonstrates narrowing of the cavernous portion of the internal carotid artery that reverses after steroid administration. Erosive changes of the sella turcica have also been described [54].

Lymphocytic hypophysitis is chronic idiopathic inflammation in the sella turcica. It is pathologically similar to orbital pseudotumor; inflammation in the orbit; and Tolosa-Hunt syndrome, inflammation in the cavernous sinus. It may involve an autoimmune pathogenesis and is most common in pregnant and postpartum women [55].

Lymphocytic hypophysitis is an infiltrative process of lymphocytes and plasma cells [56]. Usually, it involves the adenohypophysis and can mimic a pituitary adenoma. Because of compression of nearby neural structures, the inflammation may cause cranial neuropathy and visual disturbance. Endocrine abnormalities, such as loss of anterior pituitary function and hyperprolactinemia, may ensue [55,56]. When the infundibulum and posterior lobe are involved, a rare condition called infundibular neurohypophysitis occurs. Diabetes insipidus may result. Hormone replacement and steroids have proved to be effective in the management of lymphocytic hypophysitis [27].

MR imaging may demonstrate an enhancing mass in the pituitary gland with extension into the suprasellar region or cavernous sinus. There may be loss of the posterior pituitary bright spot, enlargement and thickening of the pituitary stalk, or dural enhancement [26].

### *Lymphoma*

Lymphoma arising from the sellar and parasellar region is considered a rare entity. Primary pituitary lymphomas are more common in males and have a peak incidence around the sixth decade [57]. Clinically, they can present like any other sellar mass and cause cranial neuropathy. On MR imaging, they are typically hypointense on both T1- and T2-weighted MR images [26]. More commonly, lymphoma can involve the skull base, cavernous sinus, and leptomeninges with a similar appearance to metastatic disease or other granulomatous diseases (Figs. 21 and 22).

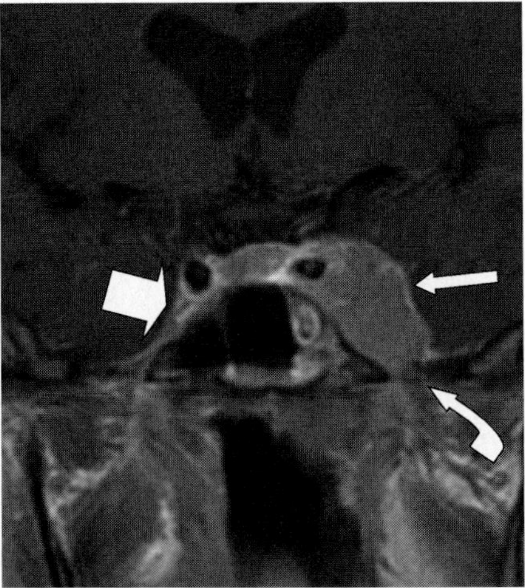

Fig. 21. Lymphoma of the cavernous sinus. The patient had a history of known lymphoma with ptosis and left CN III (oculomotor) nerve palsy. Coronal enhanced T1-weighted MR image demonstrates asymmetric enlargement of the left cavernous sinus by an enhancing mass (*thin straight arrow*) partially encasing the left carotid artery. Normal right cavernous sinus (*fat straight arrow*), mandibular nerve extending through foramen ovale (*curved arrow*). The patient's symptoms resolved with radiation therapy.

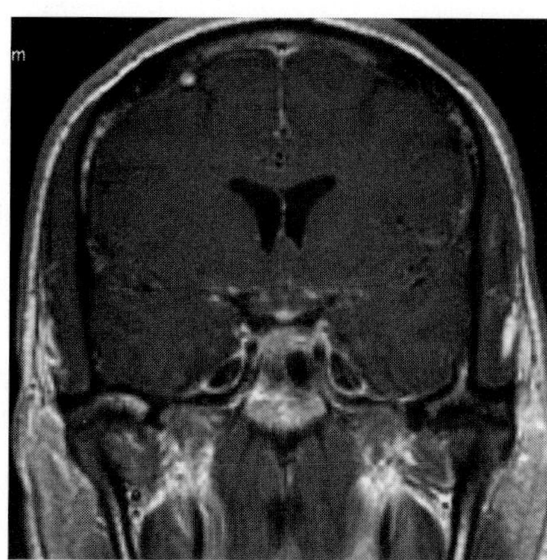

Fig. 22. Leptomeningeal lymphomatosis. Coronal enhanced T1-weighted MR image demonstrates diffuse nodular contrast enhancement of the leptomeninges of the basal cistern, surface of the optic chiasm, and upper pituitary stalk.

*Sarcoid*

Sarcoid is a multisystem disease that affects the central nervous system in 5% to 15% of cases [58]. It is an infiltrative disease characterized by noncaseating granulomas. Neurosarcoidosis affects predominately the leptomeninges but may involve the hypothalamus, pituitary stalk, and optic chiasm. Patients may present with hypopituitarism, diabetes insipidus, and visual symptoms [27].

On MR imaging, sarcoidosis can appear as a pituitary mass simulating a pituitary adenoma or cause diffuse thickening of the pituitary stalk (Fig. 23). Lesions are isointense on T1-weighted and variable on T2-weighted MR images and demonstrate uniform enhancement. There is usually associated leptomeningeal enhancement [59].

*Tuberculosis*

Tuberculosis can spread to the central nervous system, most commonly causing basilar meningitis. Tuberculomas may result presenting as masslike lesions in the sellar, parasellar, and suprasellar regions producing endocrine dysfunction, cranial neuropathies, or diabetes insipidus. MR imaging reveals lesions that are isointense on T1-weighted and variable on T2-weighted with strong enhancement. There may be thickening of the stalk and leptomeningeal enhancement [27].

*Chordoma*

Clival chordomas develop from the primitive notochord and are usually located in the clivus near the spheno-occipital synchondrosis. Other sites of origin include the basion, sella, and parasellar regions. Diplopia is the most frequent initial complaint usually secondary to involvement of CN VI because of the proximity of the posterior clivus to

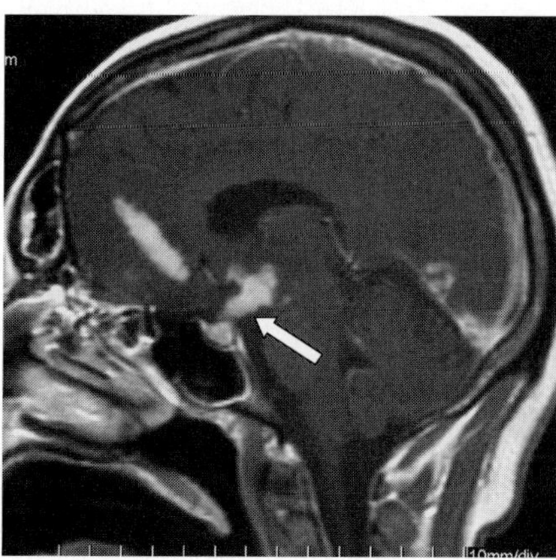

Fig. 23. Sarcoid. The patient presented with photophobia, uveitis, and blurry vision with left superior quadrantopia on physical examination. Sagittal enhanced T1-weighted MR image demonstrates marked enhancing nodular thickening of the optic chiasm, pituitary stalk, and optic tracts (*arrow*) with additional enhancement involving the falx and tentorium.

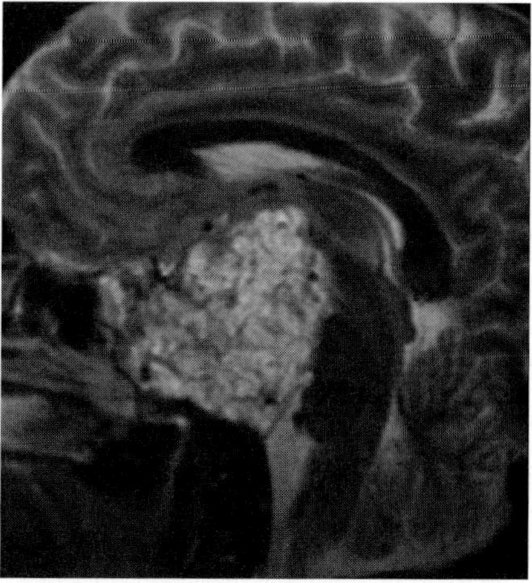

Fig. 24. Clival chordoma. The patient presented with blurry vision, right greater than left, and diplopia. Sagittal STIR image demonstrates a large multilobulated high signal mass destroying the clivus and obscuring the definition of the pituitary gland and optic chiasm.

Dorello's canal. The chondroid subtype has a slight female predominance, usually manifests earlier, more typically calcifies, and has a better prognosis.

CT and MR imaging are complementary. CT, providing superior bony anatomic detail, demonstrates the bony extent of this destructive lesion of the clivus and tumoral calcification. MR imaging scanning provides superior detail regarding localized effect on the adjacent brain parenchyma and involvement of the cavernous sinus, cranial nerves, and optic chiasm. Typically, chordomas are of moderate signal intensity on T1-weighted and high signal intensity on T2-weighted MR images with variable contrast enhancement (Fig. 24) [60].

## References


[1] Rhoton A. The sellar region. Neurosurgery 2002;51: 335–74.

[2] Ettl A, Zwrtek K, Daxer A, et al. Anatomy of the orbital apex and cavernous sinus on high-resolution magnetic resonance images. Surv Ophthalmol 2000; 44:303–23.

[3] Wiener SN, Rzeszotarski MS, Droege RT, et al. Measurement of pituitary gland height with MR imaging. AJNR Am J Neuroradiol 1985;6:717–22.

[4] Elster AD. Modern imaging of the pituitary. Radiology 1993;187:1–14.

[5] Kucharczyk W, Lenkinski RE, Kucharczyk J, et al. The effect of phospholipids vesicles on the NMR relaxation of water: an explanation for the MR appearance of the neurohypophysis. AJNR Am J Neuroradiol 1990;11:693–700.

[6] Colombo N, Berry I, Kucharczyk J, et al. Posterior pituitary gland: appearance on MR images in normal and pathologic states. Radiology 1987;165:481–5.

[7] Carpenter MB. Core text of neuroanatomy. 3rd edition. Baltimore (MD): Williams and Wilkins; 1985.

[8] Huber A. Eye signs and symptoms in brain tumors. 3rd edition. St. Louis (MO): Mosby; 1976.

[9] Chung SM. Neuro-ophthalmic manifestations of pituitary tumors. Neurosurg Clin N Am 1999;10:717–29.

[10] Snell RS. Clinical anatomy for medical students. 3rd edition. Boston/Toronto: Little, Brown and Co.; 1986.

[11] Osborn AG. Diagnostic neuroradiology. St. Louis (MO): Mosby-YearBook; 1994.

[12] Cottier JP, Destrieux C, Brunereau L, et al. Cavernous sinus invasion by pituitary adenoma: MR imaging. Radiology 2000;215:463–9.

[13] Petermann S, Newman N. Pituitary macroadenoma manifesting as an isolated fourth nerve palsy. Am J Ophthalmol 1999;127:235–6.

[14] Bills D, Meyer F, Laws E, et al. A retrospective analysis of pituitary apoplexy. Neurosurgery 1993;33: 602–8.

[15] Berkow R. The Merck manual of diagnosis and therapy. 15th edition. Rahway (NJ): Merck Sharp & Dome; 1987.

[16] Lacomis D, Johnson LN, Mamourian AC. Magnetic resonance imaging in pituitary apoplexy. Arch Ophthalmol 1988;106:207–9.

[17] Rogg J, Tung G, Anderson G, et al. Pituitary apoplexy: early detection with diffusion-weighted MR imaging. AJNR Am J Neuroradiol 2002;23:1240–5.

[18] Sadler TW. Langman's medical embryology. 5th edition. Baltimore: Williams & Wilkins; 1985.

[19] Rao G, Blyth C, Jeffreys R. Ophthalmic manifestations of Rathke's cleft cyst. Am J Ophthalmol 1995; 119:86–91.

[20] Ross DA, Norman D, Wilson CB. Radiologic characteristics and results of surgical management of Rathke's cysts in 43 patients. Neurosurgery 1992;30: 173–8.

[21] Nakasu Y, Isozumi T, Nakasu S, et al. Rathke's cleft cyst: computed tomographic scan and magnetic resonance imaging. Acta Neurochir (Wien) 1990;103: 99–104.

[22] Sumida M, Uozumi T, Mukada K, et al. Rathke cleft cysts: correlation of enhanced MR and surgical findings. AJNR Am J Neuroradiol 1994;15:525–32.

[23] Bunin GR, Surawicz TS, Witman PA. The descriptive epidemiology of craniopharyngioma. J Neurosurg 1998;89:547–51.

[24] Chen C, Okera S, Davies P, et al. Craniopharyngioma: a review of long-term visual outcome. Clin Experiment Ophthalmol 2003;31:220–8.

[25] Kennedy H, Smith R. Eye signs in craniopharyngioma. Br J Ophthalmol 1975;59:689–95.

[26] Zee C, Go J, Kim P, et al. Imaging of the pituitary and parasellar region. Neurosurg Clin N Am 2003;14: 55–80.

[27] Freda PU, Post KD. Differential diagnosis of sellar masses. Endocrinol Metab Clin North Am 1999;28: 81–117.

[28] Trobe JD, Glaser JS, Post JD. Meningiomas and aneurysms of the cavernous sinus. Arch Ophthalmol 1978;96:457–67.

[29] Ruben S, Elston J, Hayward R. Pituitary adenoma presenting as the Foster-Kennedy syndrome. Br J Ophthalmol 1992;76:117–9.

[30] Kinjo T, Al-Mefty O, Ciric I. Diaphragma sellae meningiomas. Neurosurgery 1995;36:1082–92.

[31] Majoie CB, Verbeeten B, Dol JA, et al. Trigeminal neuropathy: evaluation with MR imaging. Radiographics 1995;15:795–811.

[32] Caldemeyer KS, Mathews VP, Righi PD, et al. Imaging features and clinical significance of perineural spread or extension of head and neck tumors. Radiographics 1998;18:97–110.

[33] Yuh WT, Wright DC, Barloon TJ, et al. MR imaging of primary tumors of trigeminal nerve and Meckel's cave. AJR Am J Roentgenol 1988;151:577–82.

[34] Jefferson G. Concerning injuries, aneurysms and tumors involving the cavernous sinus. Trans Ophthalmol Soc U K 1952;73:117–52.

[35] Lee A, Beaver H, Brazis P. Painful ophthalmologic disorders and eye pain for the neurologist. Neurol Clin 2004;22:75–97.
[36] Donovan J, Nesbit G. Distinction of masses involving the sella and suprasellar space: specificity of imaging features. AJR Am J Roentgenol 1996;167:597–603.
[37] Phillips PH. Carotid-cavernous fistulas. Neurosurg Clin N Am 1999;10:653–65.
[38] Biousse V, Newman NJ. Intracranial vascular abnormalities. Ophthalmol Clin North Am 2001;14:243–64.
[39] Uchino A, Hasuo K, Matsumoto S, et al. MRI of dural carotid-cavernous fistulas: comparisons with postcontrast CT. Clin Imaging 1992;16:263–8.
[40] Hasegawa M, Yamashima T, Yamashita J, et al. Symptomatic intrasellar arachnoid cyst: case report. Surg Neurol 1991;35:355–9.
[41] Post KD, McCormick PC, Bello JA. Differential diagnosis of pituitary tumors. Endocrinol Metab Clin North Am 1987;16:609–45.
[42] Smirniotopoulos JG, Chiechi MV. Teratomas, dermoids, and epidermoids of the head and neck. Radiographics 1995;15:1437–55.
[43] Lee SH, Rao K, Zimmerman RA. Cranial MRI and CT. 4th edition. New York: McGraw–Hill; 1999.
[44] Smith AS, Benson JE, Blaser SI, et al. Diagnosis of ruptured intracranial dermoid cyst: value of MR over CT. AJNR Am J Neuroradiol 1991;12:175–80.
[45] Chong BW, Newton H. Hypothalamic and pituitary pathology. Radiol Clin North Am 1993;31:1147.
[46] Morita A, Meyer F, Laws E. Symptomatic pituitary metastases. J Neurosurg 1998;89:69–73.
[47] Sioutos P, Yen V, Arbit E. Pituitary gland metastases. Ann Surg Oncol 1996;3:94–9.
[48] Schubiger O, Haller D. Metastases to the pituitary-hypothalamic axis. Neuroradiology 1992;34:131–4.
[49] Aaberg T, Kay M, Sternau L. Metastatic tumors to the pituitary. Am J Ophthalmol 1995;119:779–85.
[50] Valvassori GE, Mafee MF. Imaging of the head and neck. New York: Thieme Medical; 1995.
[51] Tolosa E. Periarteritic lesions of the carotid siphon with clinical features of carotid intraclinoid aneurysms. J Neurol Neurosurg Psychiatry 1954;17:300–2.
[52] Hunt WE, Meager JN, LeFever H. Painful ophthalmoplegia: its relation to indolent inflammation of the cavernous sinus. Neurology 1961;11:56–62.
[53] Yousem DM, Atlas SW, Grossman RI, et al. MR imaging of Tolosa-Hunt syndrome. AJR Am J Roentgenol 1990;154:167–70.
[54] Drevelengas A, Kalaitzoglou I, Tsolaki M. Tolosa-Hunt syndrome with sellar erosion: case report. Neuroradiology 1993;35:451–3.
[55] Cheung C, Ezzat S, Smyth H, et al. The spectrum and significance of primary hypophysitis. J Clin Endocrinol Metab 2001;86:1048–53.
[56] Thodou E, Asa SL, Kontogeorgos G, et al. Lymphocytic hypophysitis: clinicopathological findings. J Clin Endocrinol Metab 1995;80:2302–11.
[57] Giustina A, Gola M, Doga M, et al. Clinical review 136: primary lymphoma of the pituitary: an emerging clinical entity. J Clin Endocrinol Metab 2001;86: 4567–75.
[58] Freda PU, Silverberg SJ, Post KD, et al. Hypothalamic-pituitary sarcoidosis. Trends Endocrinol Metab 1992; 3:321–5.
[59] Sherman JL, Stern BJ. Sarcoidosis of the CNS: comparison of unenhanced and enhanced MR images. AJNR Am J Neuroradiol 1990;11:915–23.
[60] Larson T, Houser O, Laws E. Imaging of cranial chordomas. Mayo Clin Proc 1987;62:886–93.

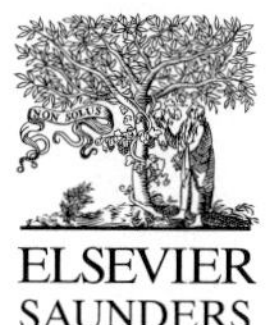

ELSEVIER
SAUNDERS

Neuroimag Clin N Am 15 (2005) 221 – 237

NEUROIMAGING CLINICS OF NORTH AMERICA

# Pathology and Imaging of the Lacrimal Drainage System

Sameer A. Ansari, MD, PhD[a], John Pak, MD, PhD[b], Marc Shields, MD[c,*]

[a]*Department of Radiology, University of Illinois Hospital at Chicago, University of Illinois College of Medicine, 1801 West Taylor Street, MC 711, Chicago, IL 60612, USA*
[b]*Division of Oculoplastic and Reconstructive Surgery, Department of Ophthalmology, University of Illinois Eye and Ear Infirmary, 1855 West Taylor Street, Chicago, IL 60610, USA*
[c]*Department of Ophthalmology, University of Virginia, Charlottesville, VA, USA*

The lacrimal drainage apparatus is a complex system that pumps and drains tears and debris away from the globe. The complexity of the system is compounded by the complicated structures with which it is contiguous. The globe, lids, orbit, sinuses, and nasal passages are all intimately related to the lacrimal drainage system and contribute to the wide variety of pathologic conditions that can affect it. Symptoms associated with lacrimal drainage pathology are relatively limited but can signify a simple obstructive, infectious, inflammatory, or neoplastic disease process. A thorough clinical history, physical examination, laboratory testing, and appropriate radiologic imaging can assist in differentiating these processes.

## Anatomy of the lacrimal drainage system

The lacrimal drainage system consists of three major structures: the canaliculi, the lacrimal sac, and the nasolacrimal duct (Fig. 1). One canaliculus is present in superior and inferior each lid. The most proximal ends of the canalicular system are the punctum, and it is the punctum through which tears are first pumped away from the eye into the lacrimal drainage apparatus. The punctum are approximately 0.2 mm in diameter and are directed posteriorly such that there is in contact with the tear meniscus. Just distal to the punctum are the vertical canaliculi, approximately 2 mm in length, which is directed perpendicular to the lid margin. The superior and inferior canaliculi then turn medially, travel horizontally for 8 mm, and join to form a common canaliculus in more than 90% of individuals [1]. Less commonly, each canaliculus empties directly into the lacrimal sac. The valve of Rosenmüller is located at the junction between the canaliculi and the lacrimal sac. It is this valve that prevents the retrograde flow of tears from the lacrimal sac back toward the globe.

The lacrimal sac is a 13- to 15-mm vertically oriented structure that sits in the bony lacrimal fossa. This fossa is formed by the frontal processes of the maxillary bone and the lacrimal bone. The body of the lacrimal sac extends from the medial canthal tendon inferiorly to the nasolacrimal duct. It is the nasolacrimal duct that enters the osseous nasolacrimal canal of the maxillary bone and empties into the inferior meatus. The valve of Hasner is present at the distal end of the nasolacrimal duct. In approximately 6% of newborns, the valve of Hasner is imperforate [2].

## Physiology of the lacrimal drainage system: the lacrimal pump

Tears do not passively drain from the eyes, but are actively pumped out of the lacrimal drainage system.

* Corresponding author. 70 Medical Center Circle, Suite 114, Fishersville, VA 22939.
*E-mail address:* marcdshields@yahoo.com (M. Shields).

1052-5149/05/$ – see front matter 
doi:10.1016/j.nic.2005.02.001

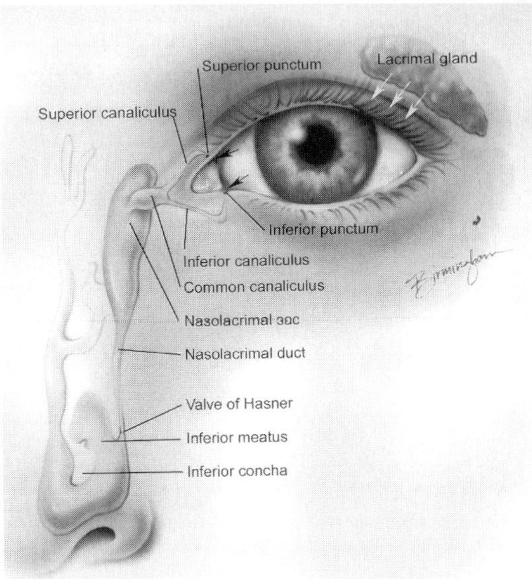


Fig. 1. Normal anatomy of the nasolacrimal drainage system. Frontal view of the eye highlights the lacrimal gland and nasolacrimal drainage system. (Illustrations by Adrienne J. Boutwell and Lisa J. Birmingham, copyright University of Illinois at Chicago Board of Trustees 2002; with permission.)

Positive pressure in the lacrimal sac is created with the contraction of the orbicularis oculi muscle during eyelid closure. The valve of Rosenmüller closes, and tears are forced down the nasolacrimal duct. As the eyelids open, negative pressure develops in the lacrimal sac. The valve of Rosenmüller opens, and tears are drawn through the puncta and down the canaliculi to the lacrimal sac, where the cycle starts again [3]. In addition to the active pumping mechanism, capillary action and gravity may play a role in the drainage of tears. This is reflected in the fact that the lower lid puncta and canalicular systems are usually larger and drain more than their upper lid counterparts.

Lacrimal pump disorders are functional disorders of tear drainage with a deficiency of the pump system as opposed to obstructive disorders with an anatomic blockage of the drainage system. Lacrimal pump disorders include seventh nerve palsy and stiff lids from burn injuries, scar tissue, ocular cicatricial pemphigoid, and scleroderma. This type of pathologic finding is poorly demonstrated by dacryocystography (DCG), CT–DCG, and MR–DCG in which contrast material is injected into the lacrimal system, because there is no anatomic obstruction and the injection obviates the need for a lacrimal pump.

## Diagnostic imaging

### *Dacryocystography*

DCG is the irrigation of contrast material through the lacrimal drainage system with subsequent serial radiography [4]. It was the first radiologic method for evaluating the lacrimal outflow system [5]. DCG provides details about nasolacrimal duct stenosis, fistulae, mucoceles, neoplasms, and lacrimal system stones or dacryoliths. The information is qualitative in nature, but not quantitative.

DCG is performed on patients with epiphora, medial canthal masses, and purulent or bloody discharge from the lacrimal puncta. There are multiple methods for performing DCG [6]. At our institution, baseline anterior-posterior and lateral films of the orbits are taken. If necessary, the lower lid punctum is dilated. A lacrimal cannula is then inserted into the lower lid canalicular system, and water-soluble contrast material is injected into the lacrimal drainage system. If the lower lid punctum or canalicular system is not patent, the upper lid system may be used. Serial anterior-posterior and lateral films are taken with the patient in a sitting position immediately after injection and then 15 minutes later [7]. In a normal dacryocystogram, contrast material is seen immediately flowing through the lacrimal drainage system and onto the floor of the nasal cavity. The delayed films show no retention of contrast material in the lacrimal sac or nasolacrimal duct. Although abnormal DCG confirms lacrimal outflow obstruction, a normal examination can be seen with partial obstruction or functional abnormalities [8].

### *CT and CT–dacryocystography*

CT and CT–DCG provide additional cross-sectional information in comparison to conventional DCG (Fig. 2). In CT–DCG, preliminary images are still obtained and water-soluble contrast material is injected into the canalicular system as described or may be administered as an eye drop [9] prior to axial and/or coronal CT scanning. CT–DCG delineates not only the patency of the lacrimal drainage system, but also the adjacent soft tissue and osseous abnormalities seen with pathologic conditions like sinusitis, mucoceles, nasal polyposis, and dacryoliths

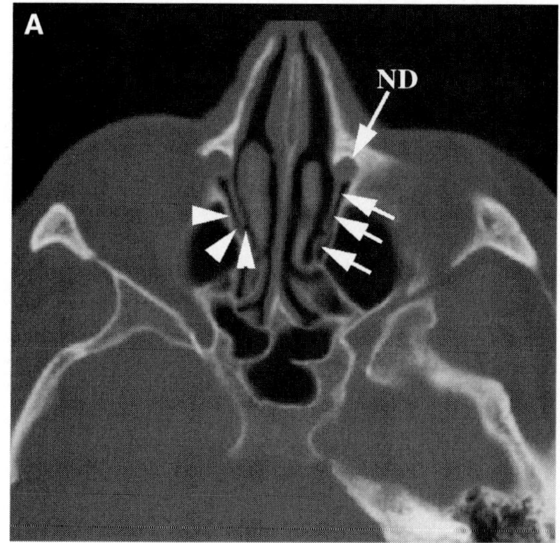


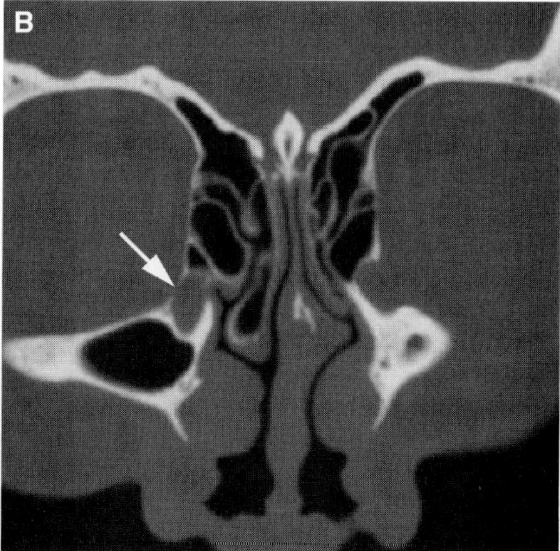


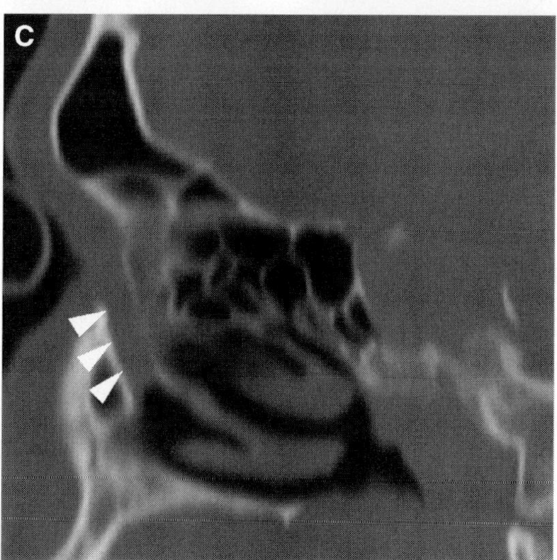


Fig. 2. Normal CT anatomy of the nasolacrimal drainage system. (*A*) Axial CT scan shows the normal nasolacrimal duct (ND, *arrow*). Note uncinate process (*arrows*) and its attachment to the lacrimal bone. The infundibulum (*arrowheads*) is visualized lateral to the uncinate process. (*B*) Coronal CT scan shows the normal lacrimal sac fossa (*arrow*). (*C*) Reformatted sagittal CT reconstructions show the osseous nasolacrimal canal (*arrowheads*) entering into the inferior meatus.

[10]. This is the radiologic study of choice for evaluating the patency of the ostomy in a patient after a dacryocystorhinostomy [11]. One study indicates that CT–DCG is superior for imaging the small lacrimal draining structures compared with MR–DCG [12].

### *MR imaging and MR–dacryocystography*

MR imaging and MR–DCG provide further imaging modalities to evaluate the lacrimal drainage system [13]. MR imaging alone can be helpful in identifying the subtle lacrimal drainage anatomy (Fig. 3) and determining the extent and specific type of pathology when soft tissue lesions such as neoplasms, papillomas, and mucoceles are suspected. Diluted gadolinium–diethylenetriamine penta-acetic acid (Gd–DTPA) can be instilled into the inferior cul-de-sac as an eye drop prior to performing MR–DCG. Imaging with head or surface coils allows for increased soft tissue resolution of the lacrimal outflow apparatus, improving MR imaging or MR–DCG.

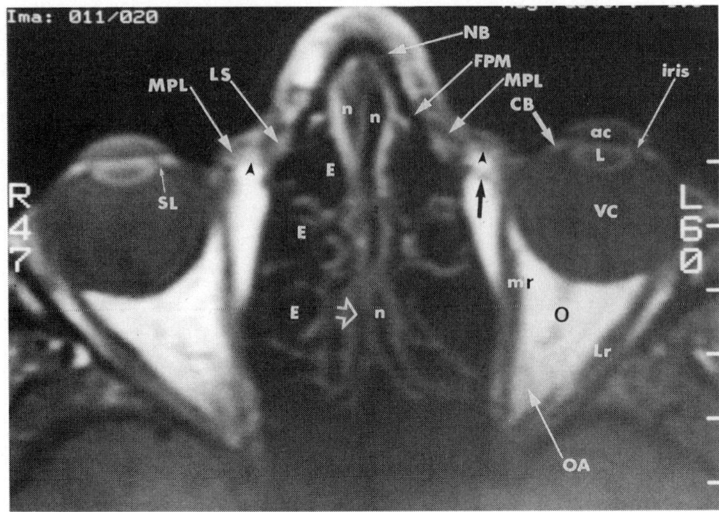


Fig. 3. Normal MR imaging anatomy of the lacrimal sac. Note the expansion of the fascial sleeve of the medial rectus as it forms the medial check ligament (*black arrow*). The medial check ligaments are attached to the lacrimal bone. The orbital septum (*arrowheads*) is anterior to the medial check ligament. The orbital septum at the level of the lacrimal groove splits to enclose the lacrimal sac (LS) and continues inferiorly to the periosteum of the nasolacrimal canal. The medial palpebral ligament (MPL) is anterior to the lacrimal sac, and the ligament attaches to the medial ends of the tarsi to the lacrimal crest and the frontal process of the maxilla (FPM). The MPL is approximately 4 mm long and 2 mm wide. It is separated from the lacrimal sac by the lacrimal fascia. Anterior chamber (ac), ciliary body (CB), ethmoid air cells (E), lateral rectus (Lr), lens (L), medial rectus (mr), nasal bone (NB), nasal cavity (n), nasal septum (*open white arrow*), ophthalmic artery (OA), optic nerve (O), suspensory ligament of lens (SL), vitreous chamber (VC). (*From* Mafee MF, Valvassori GE, Becker M. Imaging of the head and neck. Stuttgart (Germany): Thieme; 2004. p. 207; with permission.)

Multiple studies have demonstrated the adequacy of MR–DCG to identify obstruction of the lacrimal drainage system [14,15]. Because of its high cost, however, it should not be considered a first-line diagnostic test at this time [16].

### *Dacryoscintigraphy*

Dacryoscintigraphy was developed in the early 1970s [17]. Technetium-99m pertechnetate solution is instilled into each eye, and sequential analog images are then taken. This test exposes patients to less radiation than DCG and has been shown to be as sensitive as DCG in determining nasolacrimal duct obstruction [18,19]. Dacryoscintigraphy is useful in children because of the ease with which it can be performed and because there is no need to inject the lacrimal apparatus [20,21].

### *Ultrasonography*

Although ultrasonography is not ideal for the evaluation of canaliculi or the nasolacrimal duct, it can be used to examine the lacrimal sac and surrounding tissues as a diagnostic adjunct or in postoperative situations. Lacrimal disease, including a dacryocele, may be encountered during routine ultrasonography in utero [22], and recent literature documents the prenatal detection of an orbital rhabdomyosarcoma by ultrasonography.

## Pathologic findings

### *Congenital abnormalities of the lacrimal drainage system*

Multiple congenital abnormalities may result in the disruption of tear flow [23–25]. The most common congenital abnormality is partial or complete obstruction at the distal end of the nasolacrimal duct as the result of an impatent valve of Hasner or osseous obstruction [26,27]. The diagnosis is usually made on clinical grounds without need for radiologic assessment. However, congenital craniofacial deformities, for which imaging studies may be ordered, can involve the distal end of the nasolacrimal duct.

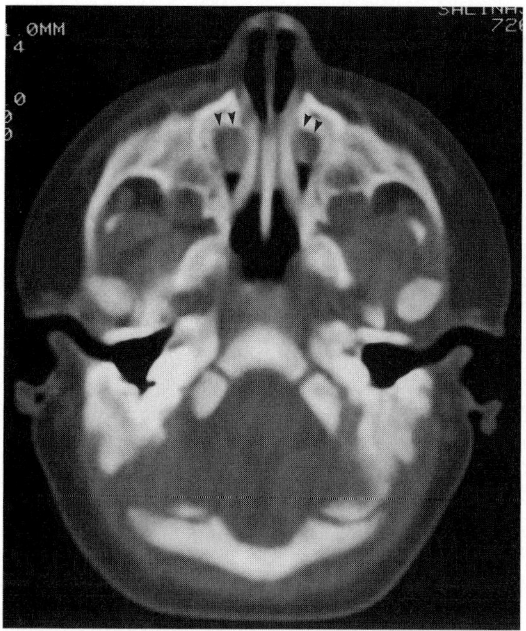

Fig. 4. Bilateral congenital dacryoceles (mucoceles). Axial CT scan shows marked dilation of both nasolacrimal ducts (*arrowheads*).

With complete obstruction of the valve of Hasner, a sterile accumulation of mucus or amniotic fluid may become trapped in the lacrimal sac and nasolacrimal duct. This entity has been named a congenital dacryocele, mucocele, dacrocystocele, or amniotocele [28], even occurring bilaterally (Fig. 4). Grossly, it appears as a blue mass inferior to the medial canthal tendon. On CT, dacryoceles are described as hypodense lesions or cystlike structures originating from the lacrimal sac fossa and associated with a dilated nasolacrimal duct. Rand et al [29] described the triad for diagnosis of a dacryocele by CT as the following: a cystic medial canthus mass, dilation of the nasolacrimal canal, and a submucosal nasal cavity mass. Furthermore, Freitag et al [30] used CT–DCG to demonstrate that the lacrimal sacs of patients with complete nasolacrimal duct obstructions are statistically larger than those with no obstruction or partial obstruction. On MR imaging, a dacryocele is described as a well-encapsulated, multilobulated, and septated mass in the lacrimal sac fossa exhibiting hypointensity on T1-weighted images and hyperintensity on T2-weighted images (Fig. 5) [31].

Congenital atresia of the lacrimal puncta in which the puncta are absent but the remaining lacrimal drainage system is patent, duplication of a canaliculus, and diverticulae of the lacrimal drainage system may all be seen in young patients as well as in older individuals. CT and MR imaging findings may be nonspecific for characterizing diverticulae, which can be mistaken for cysts. All the above may be diagnosed using conventional DCG with improved sensitivity when B-mode ultrasonography [32].

### *Infectious disease of the lacrimal drainage system*

The most common infectious process of the lacrimal drainage system is dacryocystitis. In nearly all cases, it is a result of obstruction at some level of the lacrimal drainage system that causes decreased

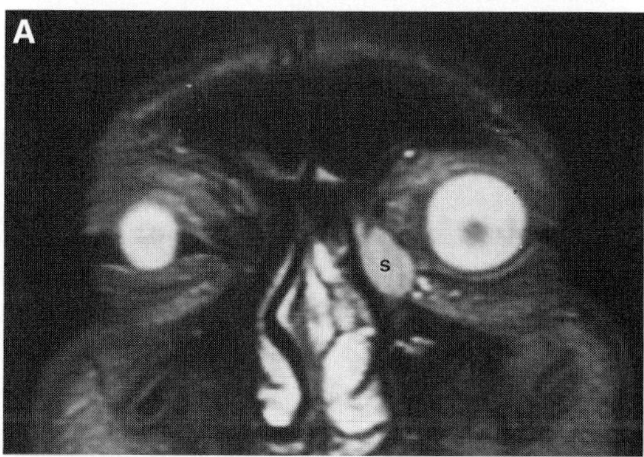



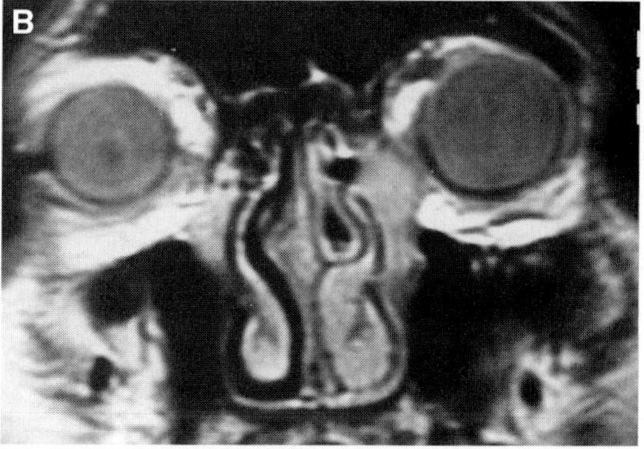



Fig. 5. Dacryocele (mucocele) with nasolacrimal duct obstruction. (*A*) Coronal T2-weighted (repetition time [TR]/echo time [TE]: 2000/70 ms) MR image demonstrates a dilated left lacrimal sac (S) consistent with a dacryocele (mucocele). (*B*) Coronal proton density-weighted (TR/TE: 2000/20 ms) MR image shows a dilated left lacrimal sac and nasolacrimal duct consistent with obstruction in the same patient.

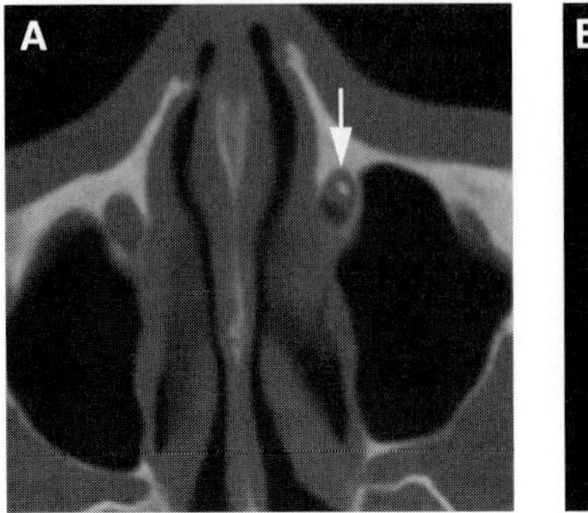


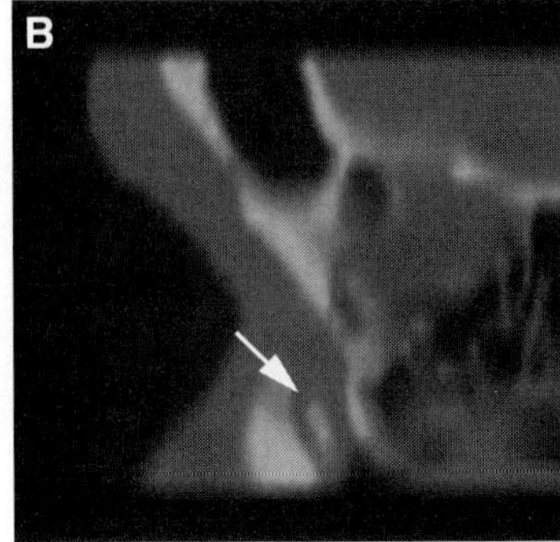


Fig. 6. Partial nasolacrimal duct obstruction. Following DCG, an axial CT scan (*A*) and a reformatted sagittal CT reconstruction (*B*) demonstrate delayed and/or residual contrast in the left nasolacrimal duct (*arrows*) related to primary acquired stenosis and partial obstruction at the distal end of the nasolacrimal duct. The patient's symptoms resolved status post left dacryocystorhinostomy.

tear outflow, bacteria proliferation, and infection. Acquired nasolacrimal duct obstruction has been divided into primary (idiopathic) and secondary causes [33]. Primary acquired nasolacrimal duct obstruction is most often seen in women (Fig. 6). Several causes have been postulated, including inflammatory changes, hormonal changes, and inherent anatomic differences between men and women. CT studies have shown that women have a narrower inferior bony nasolacrimal canal in comparison with men [34]. Secondary acquired nasolacrimal duct obstruction may be caused by dacryoliths (Fig. 7) seen in

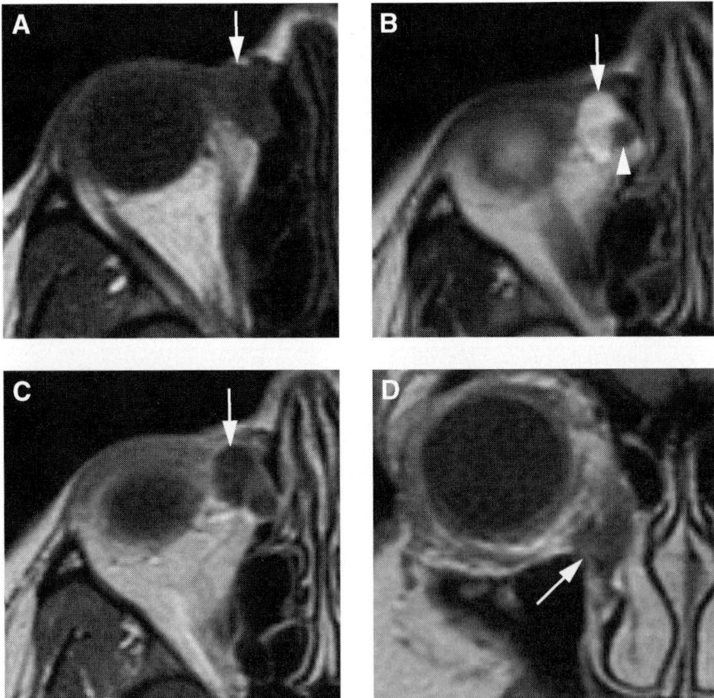


Fig. 7. Dacryolith-induced dacryocele (mucocele). Axial T1-weighted (TR/TE: 400/14 ms) (*A*), axial T2-weighted (TR/TE: 4000/88 ms) (*B*), axial T1-weighted (TR/TE: 400/14 ms) post–Gd-DTPA contrast (*C*), and coronal T1-weighted (TR/TE: 550/20 ms) post–Gd-DTPA contrast (*D*) MR images demonstrate a dilated right lacrimal sac (*arrows*) secondary to a surgically proven dacryolith (*arrowhead*).

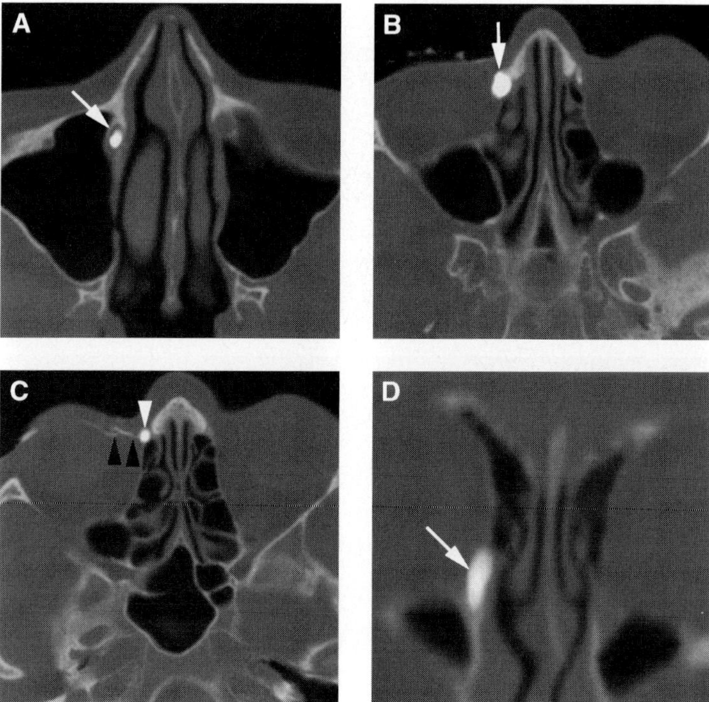


Fig. 8. Nasolacrimal duct obstruction. Following DCG, contiguous axial (*A–C*) and coronal (*D*) CT scans demonstrate retained contrast in the dilated right nasolacrimal duct (*arrows*), right lacrimal sac (*white arrowhead*), and inferior lacrimal canaliculus (*black arrowheads*) consistent with right nasolacrimal duct obstruction in a patient who subsequently required a right dacryocystorhinostomy.

conjunction with fungal and actinomyces infections or without dacryoliths in conjunction with Epstein-Barr viral infections. Other foreign bodies, such as lashes and deposits from certain eye drops containing epinephrine, may precipitate secondary obstruction of the lacrimal drainage apparatus. Many other eye drops have been associated with lacrimal system obstruction as a result of cicatricial changes [35]. Chemotherapy with fluorouracil, docetaxel, radioactive iodine therapy, and topical mitomycin-C can cause secondary punctal, canalicular, or nasolacrimal duct stenosis and/or obstruction [36,37]. Furthermore, secondary causes of lacrimal system obstruction include previous trauma, entrapped migrated punctal plugs used to treat dry eye syndromes, intranasal use of cocaine, mechanical obstruction, and neoplastic disease [38–40].

The most common infectious agents responsible for dacryocystitis are *Streptococcus pneumoniae*, *Staphylococcus*, and *Pseudomonas* bacterial strains [41,42]. Chronic infections are characterized by tearing, discharge, and unilateral conjunctivitis. Acute infections are characterized by similar symptoms with additional redness, swelling, and tenderness over the medial canthal area. Left untreated, acute dacryocystitis may progress into a preseptal cellulitis, necrotizing fasciitis [43], or even orbital cellulitis [44].

In acute and chronic dacryocystitis, DCG demonstrates distention of the lacrimal sac with at least partial obstruction of the nasolacrimal duct (Figs. 8 and 9) [45]. The expansion of the lacrimal drainage system can extend into the canaliculi, and filling defects may be noted secondary to pus or dacryoliths. Dacryocystitis may lead to lacrimal sac fistulas, which can be demonstrated by DCG. On CT, chronic dacryocystitis appears as an inferior medial orbital mass with cystic dilation of the lacrimal sac (Fig. 10) [46]. With acute dacryocystitis, additional postseptal inflammation is often present and a peripheral enhancing mass may be seen in the lacrimal sac fossa compatible with an abscess. Using MR imaging, acute dacryocystitis exhibits the imaging characteristics of an abscess in the region of the lacrimal sac with hypointensity on T1-weighted images,

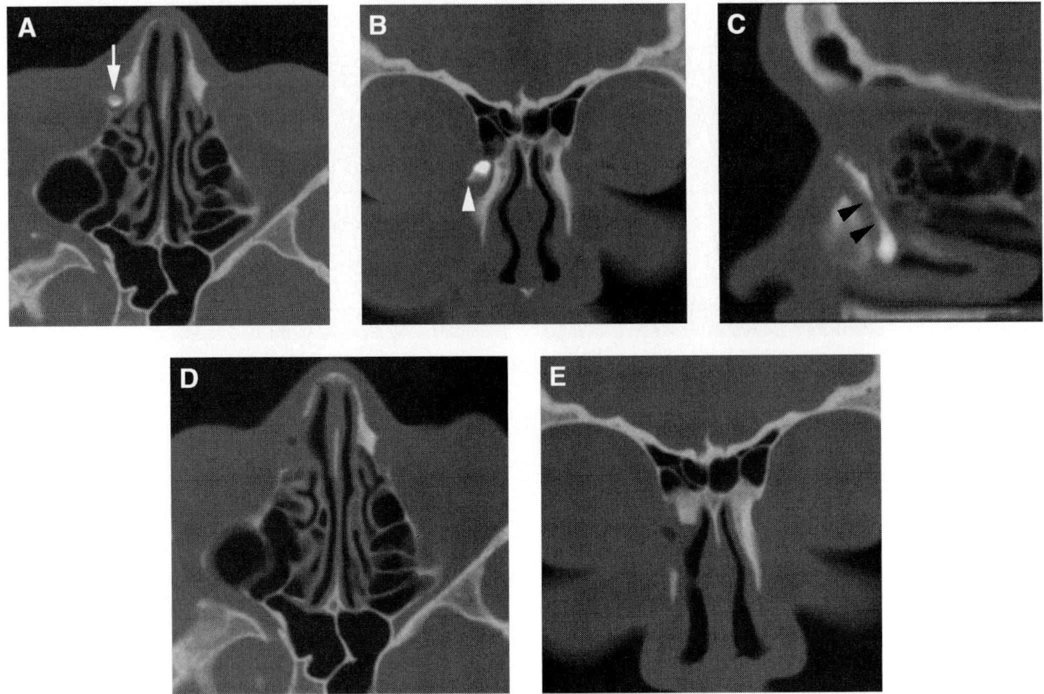

Fig. 9. Nasolacrimal duct obstruction. After DCG, axial (*A*) and coronal (*B*) CT scans with a reformatted sagittal CT reconstruction (*C*) show retained contrast in the right inferior canaliculus (*white arrowhead*), lacrimal sac (*arrow*), and nasolacrimal duct (*black arrowheads*) consistent with distal nasolacrimal duct obstruction causing biopsy-proven dacryocystitis of the right lacrimal sac. Axial (*D*) and coronal (*E*) follow-up CT scans demonstrate postsurgical osteotomy changes 8 months status post right dacryocystorhinostomy in the same patient.

hyperintensity on T2-weighted images, and peripheral gadolinium-DTPA contrast enhancement.

Congenital dacryoceles caused by distal nasolacrimal duct obstruction and congenital dacryocystoceles caused by obstruction at both valves of Rosenmüller and Hasner [47] are prone to superimposed infection. The CT and/or MR imaging characteristics of congenital infected dacryoceles or dacryocystoceles parallel the findings for acute dacryocystitis (Fig. 11).

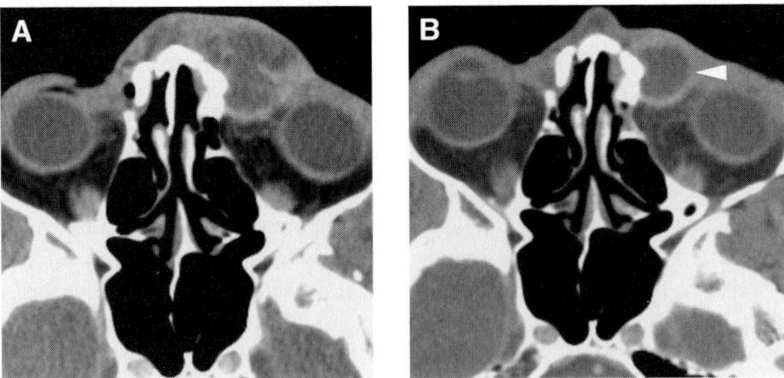

Fig. 10. Dacryoadenitis/chronic dacryocele. (*A*) Axial postcontrast CT scan demonstrates an enlarged left lacrimal sac and edema of the left eyelid in a patient with *Proteus*-positive eye cultures consistent with suppurative dacryoadenitis. (*B*) Following treatment, an axial postcontrast CT scan shows a persistent abscess (*arrowhead*) or chronic dacryocele 10 months later in the same patient.

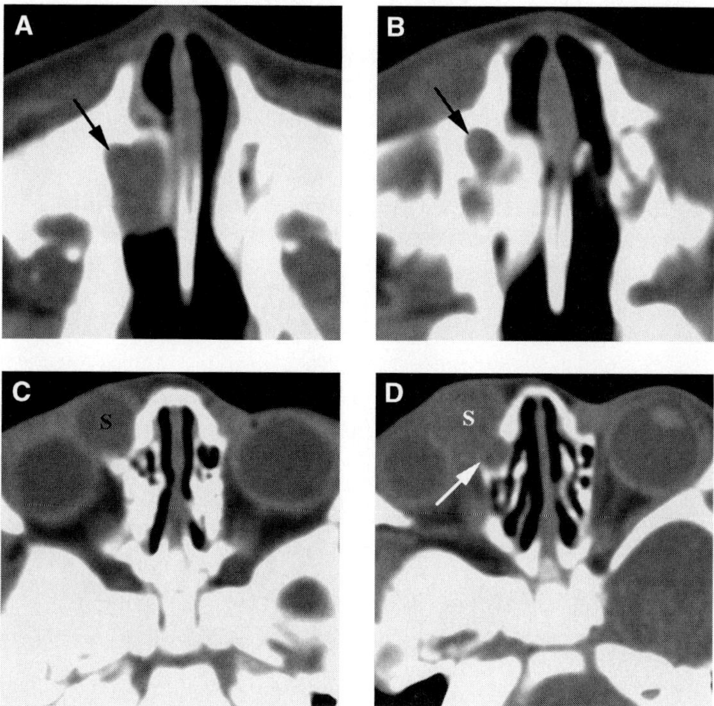


Fig. 11. Congenital infected dacryocele and/or dacryocystocele. Contiguous axial (*A–C*) and single axial (*D*) CT scans demonstrate markedly dilated right lacrimal sacs (S) and nasolacrimal ducts (*arrows*) in a 5-day-old infant with *Staphylococcus*-positive eye cultures (*A–C*) and in a 3-week-old infant with *Staphylococcus aureus* (MRSA)-positive eye cultures (*D*) consistent with congenital infected dacryoceles and/or dacryocystoceles. The second patient underwent immediate abscess drainage but still required a right dacryocystorhinostomy 8 months later for chronic dacryocystitis.

Canaliculitis is another less common infection of the lacrimal drainage apparatus presenting with acute or chronic conjunctivitis, a "pouting" inflamed punctum, tearing, and purulent discharge. Associated with *Actinomyces israelii* infection and canalicular stones [48], the diagnosis of canaliculitis is usually made on clinical grounds, but can be aided with high-resolution ultrasonography [49].

## *Inflammatory disease of the lacrimal drainage system*

The lacrimal drainage system is susceptible to several systemic inflammatory conditions. Many have characteristic clinical and pathologic findings that aid in their diagnosis and treatment. In contrast, most display nonspecific radiologic findings in the region of the lacrimal drainage system, however.

Sarcoidosis may involve almost every organ system, including multiple ocular and orbital sites as well as the lacrimal drainage system [50–52]. Orbital and lacrimal symptoms associated with sarcoidosis include pain, tearing, exophthalmos, restricted motility, palpable masses, conjunctival masses [53], diminished visual acuity, and visual field deficits. DCG findings are nonspecific and may show partial or complete obstruction of the lacrimal drainage system. CT and/or MR imaging of the orbit and CT and/or MR–DCG studies may identify additional findings more suggestive of sarcoidosis [54]. These include sinus opacification and osseous destruction [55], bilateral lacrimal gland enlargement [56], optic nerve tumors [57], and orbital masses [58]. Treatment of sarcoidosis involving the lacrimal drainage system is predicated first on treatment of the underlying disease. If nasolacrimal duct obstruction or lacrimal sac irregularities are present and a dacryocystorhinostomy is planned, biopsy of the lacrimal sac wall should be undertaken.

Another inflammatory disease associated with significant lacrimal drainage pathology is Wegener granulomatosis (Fig. 12). Wegener granulomatosis is

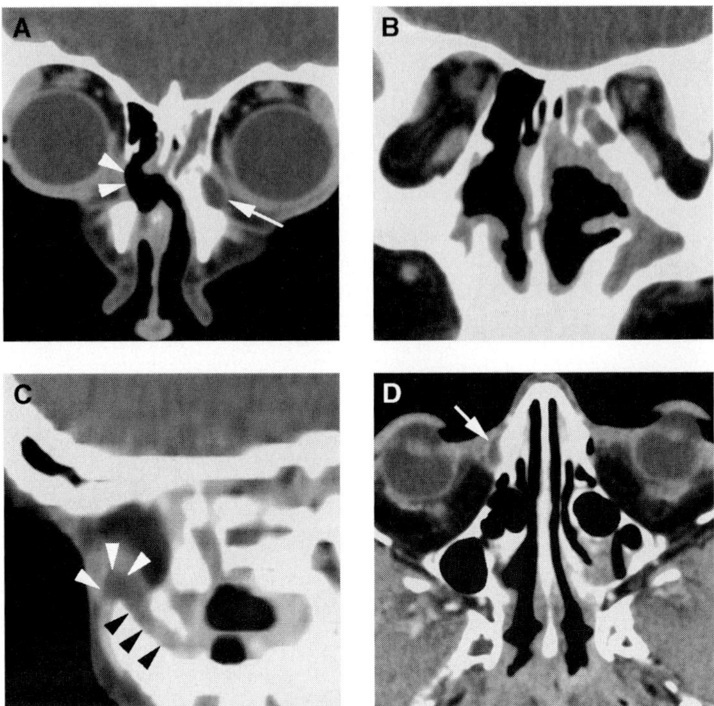


Fig. 12. Wegener granulomatosis. (*A*) Coronal CT scan demonstrates postsurgical changes after a right dacryocystorhinostomy (*arrowheads*) and a dilated left lacrimal sac (*arrow*). (*B*) Coronal CT scan demonstrates posteriorly the postsurgical changes of the nasal cavities, soft tissue thickening of the left nasal cavity, and opacification of the left ethmoid air cells in this patient with Wegener granulomatosis. (*C*) Reformatted sagittal CT reconstruction in same patient demonstrates the dilated lacrimal sac (*white arrowheads*) and fluid within the nasolacrimal duct (*black arrowheads*). (*D*) Axial CT scan in another patient with Wegener granulomatosis shows a dilated and fluid-filled right lacrimal sac (*arrow*).

a multisystem disease, but typically presents with severe upper respiratory tract findings including paranasal sinus disease, purulent or bloody drainage, and mucosal ulceration. Pulmonary involvement manifests as cough, hemoptysis, dyspnea, and chest discomfort. Renal involvement is present in 77% of individuals with symptoms related to glomerulonephritis. Eye manifestations occur in 50% of patients presenting with dacryocystitis, lacrimal sac masses, and tearing [59]. Wegener granulomatosis is often

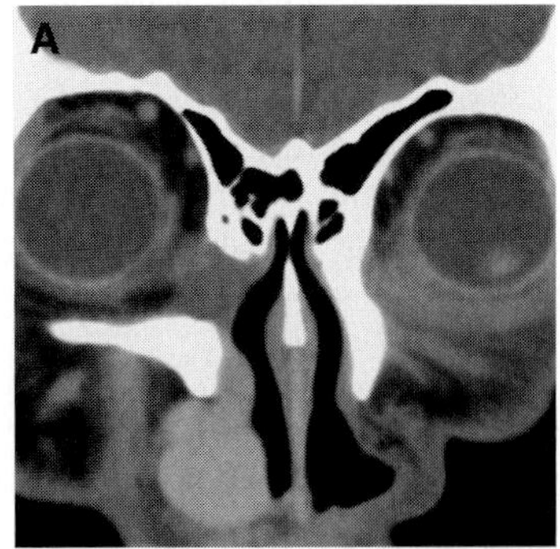


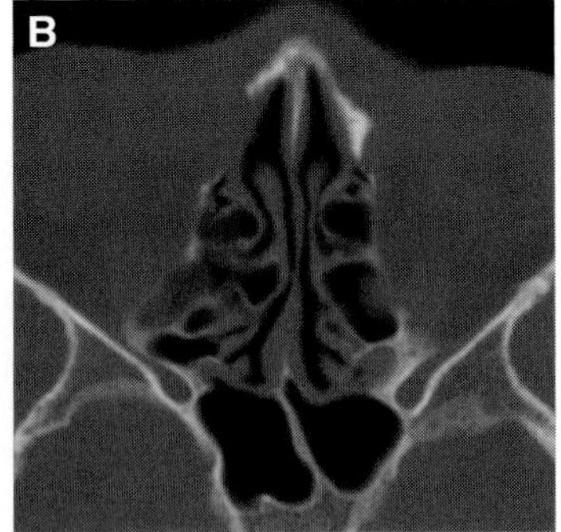


Fig. 13. Status post dacryocystorhinostomy. Coronal (*A*) and axial (*B*) CT scans demonstrate recent postsurgical changes after a right dacryocystorhinostomy with notable osteotomy and soft tissue edema.

difficult to diagnose using radiologic means alone, unless sinus involvement and bone destruction are extensive [60,61]. Various medical and surgical approaches are used to treat Wegener granulomatosis. The systemic disease is often amenable to cyclophosphamide in conjunction with glucocorticoids. More aggressively, lacrimal drainage pathology may be treated with dacryocystorhinostomy or dacryocystectomy depending on the activity of the disease and the patient's symptoms (see Figs. 9D and E, 12, and 13) [62,63].

*Neoplastic disease of the lacrimal drainage system*

Lacrimal drainage system tumors are extremely rare [64] (Box 1). A recent series by Shields et al [65] evaluated 1264 orbital tumors, of which only 2 originated from the lacrimal sac. A French study that included all eye and adnexal tumors corroborated this low prevalence with characterization of only 2 lacrimal sac tumors out of 1705 malignant tumors [66]. Given their rare occurrence, few large series studies of lacrimal drainage system tumors have been published. The largest and most recent report by Stefanyszyn et al [67] characterized 115 lacrimal sac neoplasms in adults; the tumors were divided into epithelial and nonepithelial neoplasms. Epithelial tumors comprised 71% of all tumors and were further divided into benign and malignant neoplasms. The most common benign epithelial lesions were squamous and transitional cell papillomas, which constituted 28% of all lesions. Other benign epithelial lesions included oncocytomas and benign mixed tumors. The most common malignant epithelial neoplasm was squamous cell carcinoma, which comprised 19% of all tumors. Stefanyszyn et al [67] identified 370 lacrimal sac tumors reported throughout the literature, of which 202 (55%) were malignant.

**Box 1. Neoplasms of the lacrimal sac**

*Epithelial*

- *Benign*
  - Squamous/transitional cell papilloma
  - Oncocytoma
  - Benign mixed tumors
- *Malignant*
  - Squamous/transitional cell carcinoma
  - Adenocarcinoma
  - Oncocytic adenocarcinoma
  - Mucoepidermoid carcinoma
  - Undifferentiated carcinoma
  - Adenoid cystic carcinoma
  - Eccrine adenocarcinoma

*Nonepithelial*

- Lymphoma
- Melanoma
- Granulocytic sarcoma
- Neurofibroma
- Pyogenic granuloma
- Fibrous histiocytoma
- Hemangiopericytoma
- Lipoma
- Solitary fibrous tumor
- Angiofibroma

Patients with lacrimal drainage system tumors present with symptoms of epiphora, bloody epiphora, nasal obstruction, and purulent or bloody discharge. With larger or more aggressive tumors, the presentation includes a medial canthal or lacrimal sac mass; inflammation; and orbital signs of proptosis, dysmotility, and globe displacement [68].

Benign epithelial tumors of the lacrimal drainage system (Box 1) expand into the lumen of the lacrimal sac and lacrimal drainage apparatus [69,70]. On clinical examination, they are generally well circumscribed, mobile beneath the skin, and firm on palpation. The most common benign epithelial tumor is a papilloma, which has been associated with human papillomavirus (HPV) type 11 and type 18 [71]. On DCG, a papilloma appears as an irregular filling defect within the lumen of the lacrimal sac. Other benign lesions, such as oncocytoma and benign mixed tumors, appear as sharply defined filling defects within the lacrimal sac. Although the lacrimal drainage system may be patent, residual contrast material can be seen on delayed films along with lacrimal sac distention, indicating partial obstruction by the tumor. Using CT, benign lesions typically do not demonstrate bone erosion, which indicates a primary osseous lesion or a more malignant process. Epithelial cysts may mimic neoplasms of the lacrimal drainage system [72] and appear as fluid-filled hypodense masses on CT.

Malignant epithelial tumors of the lacrimal drainage system (Box 1) are most commonly squamous

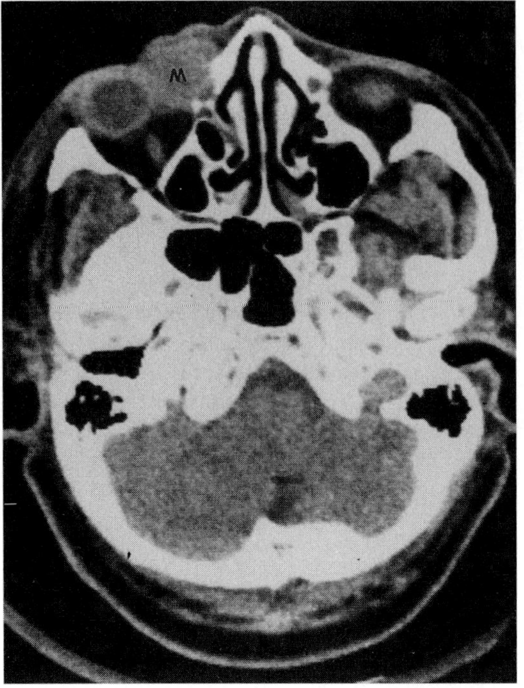


Fig. 14. Squamous cell carcinoma. Axial CT scan demonstrates a mass (M) involving the right lacrimal sac consistent with pathologically proven squamous cell carcinoma.

cell carcinomas [73]. On clinical examination, malignant tumors usually exhibit rapid growth, skin fixation, and a firm texture with irregular borders. On DCG, malignant lesions tend to appear as sharply or irregularly defined filling defects within the lumen of the lacrimal drainage apparatus. Using CT, a mass involving the lacrimal drainage system that is large, irregular, and associated with bone destruction is highly suggestive of malignancy (Figs. 14 and 15). MR imaging of epithelial tumors usually demonstrates hypointensity on T1-weighted images and isointensity on T2-weighted sequences (Fig. 16), but, in general, these findings are nonspecific in differentiating benign from malignant lesions. Interestingly, squamous cell carcinomas may characteristically appear hypointense on T2-weighted images [74]. Nevertheless, the irregular margins and infiltration of adjacent soft tissues by malignant tumors may be better appreciated using MR imaging because of superior contrast resolution (Figs. 16 and 17).

Nonepithelial tumors of the lacrimal drainage system (Box 1) may present as well-defined masses with nonspecific CT characteristics, which causes difficulty in diagnosis and differentiation from epithelial tumors before lacrimal surgery and pathologic evaluation [75]. In contrast, a subset of melanomas exhibit unique imaging characteristics with hyper-

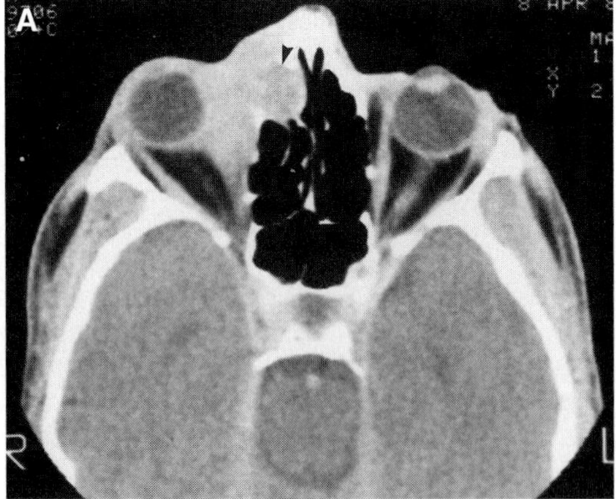


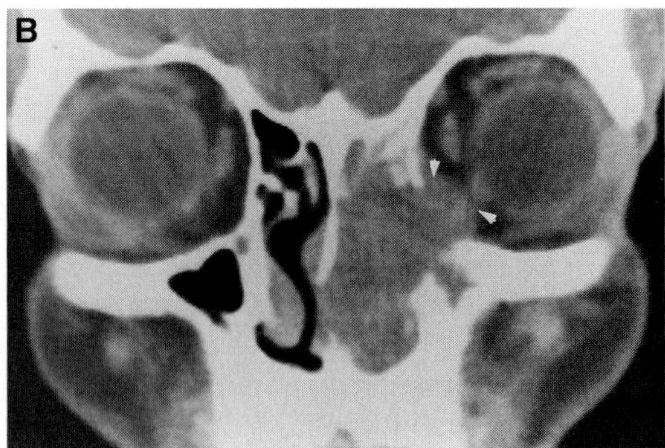


Fig. 15. Squamous cell carcinoma. (*A*) Axial postcontrast CT scan demonstrates an enhancing right lacrimal sac tumor (*black arrowhead*) invading the adjacent orbit, including the right medial rectus muscle, consistent with pathologically proven squamous cell carcinoma. (*B*) Coronal postcontrast CT scan shows a large enhancing tumor in the left nasal cavity extending into and involving the left lacrimal sac (*white arrowheads*) with osteolysis of the medial orbital rim, consistent with pathologically proven squamous cell carcinoma.

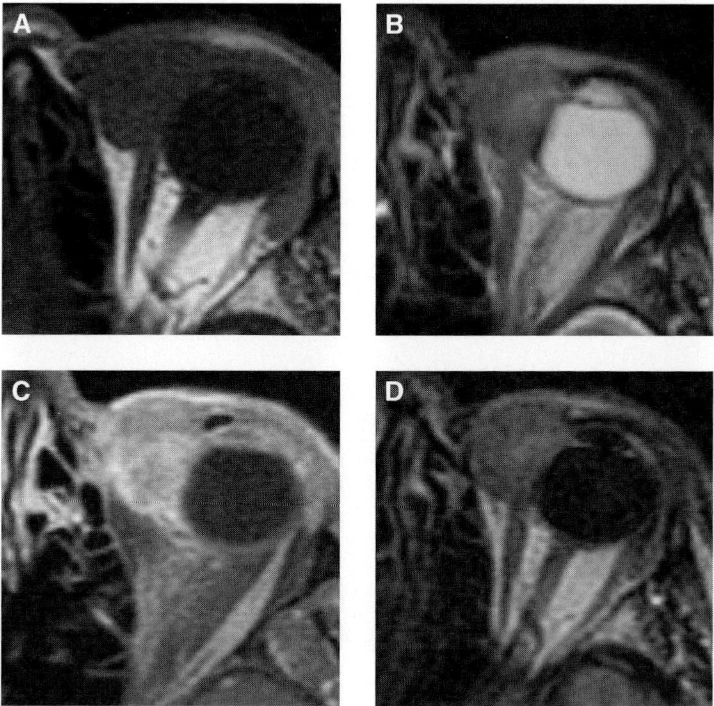


Fig. 16. Mucoepidermoid carcinoma. Axial T1-weighted (TR/TE: 366/9 ms) (*A*), axial T2-weighted (TR/TE: 4200/99 ms) (*B*), axial T1-weighted (TR/TE: 600/9 ms) post–Gd-DTPA contrast (*C*), and axial fluid-attenuated inversion recovery (FLAIR)–weighted (TR/TE: 10,000/157 ms) (*D*) MR images demonstrate a contrast-enhancing mass involving the left eyelid and soft tissue in proximity to the left lacrimal sac consistent with pathologically proven high-grade mucoepidermoid carcinoma of the left eyelid with chronic inflammation, fibrosis, and granulation tissue of the left nasolacrimal duct.

intensity on T1-weighted images, hypointensity on T2-weighted images, and prominent Gd–DTPA contrast enhancement (Fig. 17) [76,77].

Secondary tumors involving or extending into the lacrimal drainage system include osteomas, mucoceles, dermoids, fibro-osseous lesions, sinus tumors, eyelid tumors, and lymphomas (Fig. 18). Benign tumors in this group usually cause mass effect with displacement of the lacrimal drainage apparatus and secondary obstruction. The most common benign secondary tumor is a mucocele. Mucoceles, possibly arising from the sinuses, may be confused with lacrimal sac neoplasms (Fig. 19). Using MR imaging, the signal intensity of mucoceles can be highly variable depending on the water and protein content of the mucus. Mucoceles are depleted of water and increase in protein content over time, becoming more hyperintense on T1-weighted images and less hyperintense on T2-weighted images [78]. Second-

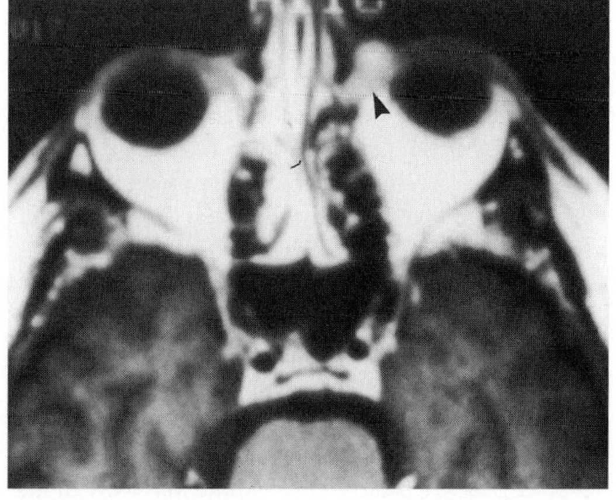

Fig. 17. Malignant melanoma. Axial T1-weighted post–Gd-DTPA contrast MR image demonstrates recurrence of pathologically proven conjunctival malignant melanoma involving the left lacrimal sac (*arrowhead*). (*From* Mafee MF, Valvassori GE, Becker M. Imaging of the head and neck. Stuttgart (Germany): Thieme; 2004. p. 290; with permission.)

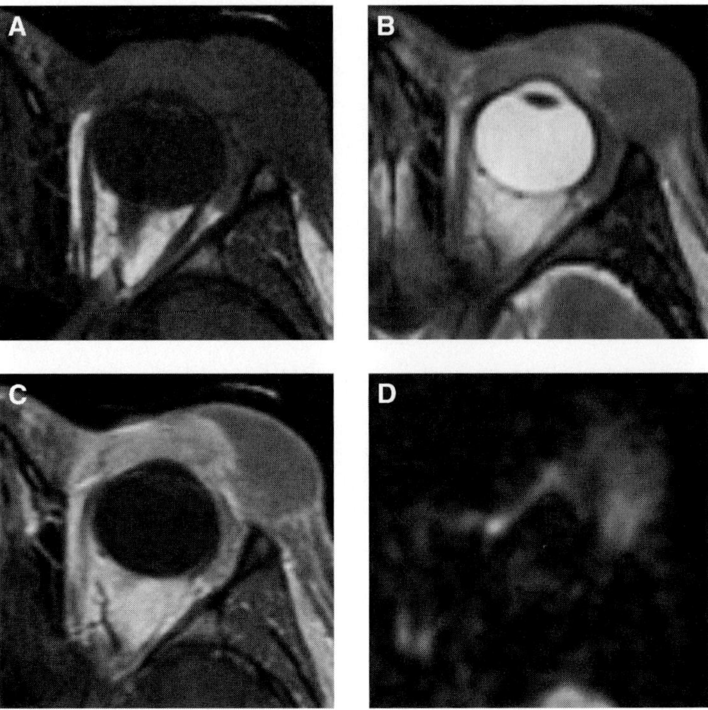


Fig. 18. Burkitt lymphoma. Axial T1-weighted (TR/TE: 400/14 ms) (*A*), axial T2-weighted (TR/TE: 4000/88 ms) (*B*), axial T1-weighted (TR/TE: 400/14 ms) post–Gd-DTPA contrast (*C*), and axial diffusion-weighted (TR/TE: 10,000/93 ms) (*D*) MR images demonstrate a bulky contrast-enhancing mass involving the left eyelid and lacrimal sac consistent with pathologically proven high-grade Burkitt type B-cell lymphoma in a 16-year-old patient. Note area of restricted diffusion (D) compatible with lymphoma.

ary malignant tumors often invade the lacrimal drainage system, causing lacrimal symptoms in addition to the symptoms from their primary site. Secondary infiltrative processes, such as amyloid or venous-lymphatic malformations (Fig. 20), can be mistaken for secondary tumors involving the lacrimal drainage system. If radiologic assessment is necessary to define the extent of these diseases, contrast CT or MR imaging provides superior cross-sectional resolution.

Management of lacrimal system tumors is as varied as the histopathology that the tumors represent. Some benign lesions can be treated with dacryocystorhinostomy and excision of the lesions. More aggressive lesions necessitate removal of the entire lacrimal drainage apparatus, including the canaliculi, lacrimal sac, and entire nasolacrimal duct to the inferior meatus. Ni et al [68] have shown that patients with premalignant and malignant lesions have decreased recurrence rates with a lateral rhinostomy and wide excision as compared with those without (12.5% versus 43.7%). Secondary tumors invading the lacrimal system require more complicated surgery, including paranasal sinus resection, orbital exenteration, and cervical lymph node dissection, depending on the primary site and extent of metastasis. Depending on the histopa-

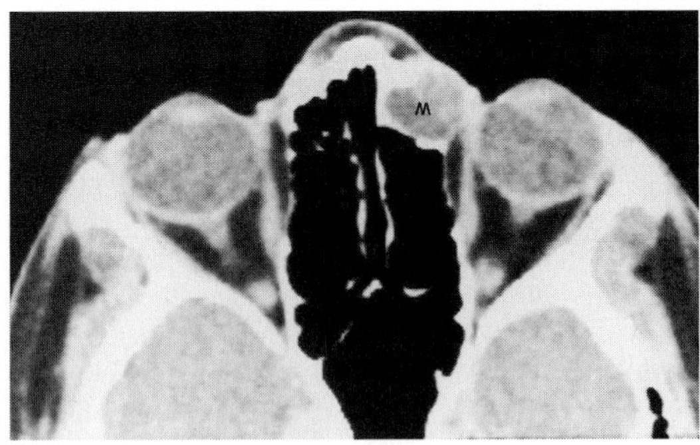


Fig. 19. Anterior ethmoid mucocele involving the lacrimal sac. Axial CT scan shows a left anterior ethmoid sinus mucocele (M) secondarily invading the adjacent left lacrimal sac.

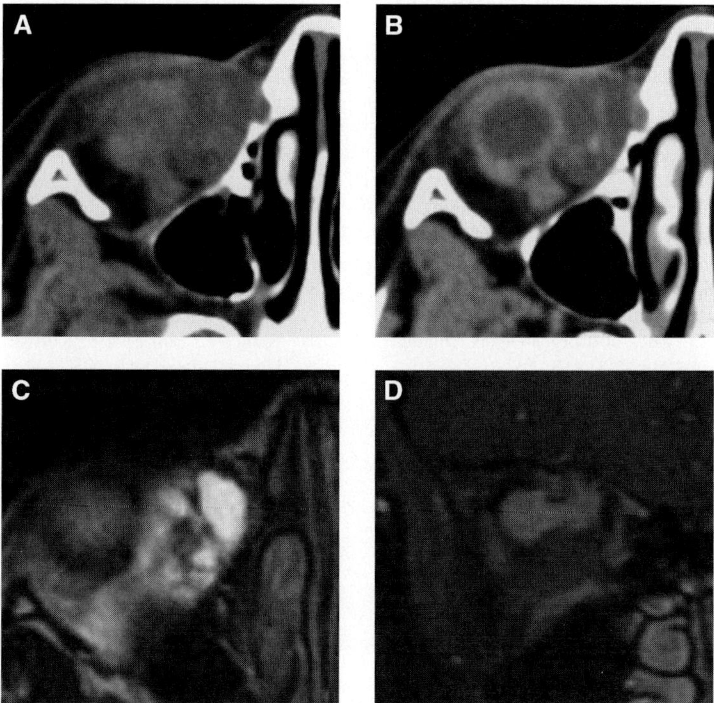


Fig. 20. Venous-lymphatic malformation (lymphangioma). Contiguous axial CT scans (*A, B*) as well as axial T2-weighted (TR/TE: 4200/99 ms) (*C*) and coronal T1-weighted (TR/TE: 300/20 ms) post–Gd-DTPA (*D*) contrast fat-suppressed MR images demonstrate a multiloculated orbital lesion with minimal contrast enhancement involving the right lacrimal sac compatible with a venous-lymphatic malformation in an 8-year-old girl.

thology, local radiation and chemotherapy may be warranted [79].

## Summary

Lacrimal drainage pathology encompasses obstructive, infectious, inflammatory, and neoplastic disease, which can present clinically with overlapping and nonspecific symptoms. In such cases, a thorough history, physical examination, laboratory workup, and radiologic assessment are essential for accurate diagnosis, evaluation of disease extension, and treatment planning.

## Acknowledgments

The authors wish to thank the Departments of Radiology and Ophthalmology at the University of Illinois at Chicago Hospital for great assistance in preparing this manuscript, specifically Dr. Nikhil Balakrishnan, Yassir Aich, and Aura Smith. This work was approved by the Institutional Review Board of the University of Illinois at Chicago.

## References

[1] Yazici B, Yazici Z. Frequency of the common canaliculus: a radiological study. Arch Ophthalmol 2000; 118(10):1381–5.

[2] Jordan DR, Anderson RL. The lacrimal drainage system. In: Surgical anatomy of the ocular adnexa: a clinical approach. San Francisco: American Academy of Ophthalmology, Palace Press; 1996.

[3] Doane MG. Blinking and the mechanics of the lacrimal drainage system. Ophthalmology 1981;88:850.

[4] Milder B, Demorest BH. Dacryocystography: the normal lacrimal apparatus. Arch Ophthalmol 1954;51: 180–95.

[5] Ewing AE. Roentgen ray demonstration of the lacrimal abscess cavity. Am J Ophthalmol 1909;24:1.

[6] Weber AL, Rodriquez-DeVelasquez A, Lucarelli MJ, et al. Normal anatomy and lesions of the lacrimal sac and duct: evaluated by dacryocystography, computed tomography, and MR imaging. Neuroimaging Clin N Am 1996;6(1):199–216.

[7] Millman AL, Liebeskind A, Putterman AM. Dacryocystography: the technique and its role in the practice of ophthalmology. Radiol Clin N Am 1987;25(4):781–6.

[8] Guzek JP, Ching AS, Hoang TA, et al. Clinical and radiologic lacrimal testing in patients with epiphora. Ophthalmology 1997;104(11):1875–81.

[9] Sarac K, Hepsen IF, Bayramlar H, et al. Computed tomography dacryocystography. Eur J Radiol 1995;19(2):128–31.

[10] Francis IC, Kappagoda MB, Cole IE, et al. Computed tomography of the lacrimal drainage system: retrospective study of 107 cases of dacryostenosis. Ophthal Plast Reconstr Surg 1999;15(3):217–26.

[11] Glatt HJ, Chan AC, Barrett L. Evaluation of dacryocystorhinostomy failure with computed tomography and computed tomographic dacryocystography. Am J Ophthalmol 1991;112(4):431–6.

[12] Caldemeyer KS, Stockberger Jr SM, Broderick LS. Topical contrast-enhanced CT and MR dacryocystography: imaging the lacrimal drainage apparatus of healthy volunteers. AJR Am J Roentgenol 1998;171(6):1501–4.

[13] Rubin PA, Bilyk JR, Shore JW, et al. Magnetic resonance imaging of the lacrimal drainage system. Ophthalmology 1994;101(2):235–43.

[14] Hoffmann KT, Hosten N, Anders N, et al. High-resolution conjunctival contrast-enhanced MRI dacryocystography. Neuroradiology 1999;41(3):208–13.

[15] Karagulle T, Erden A, Erden I, et al. Nasolacrimal system: evaluation with gadolinium-enhanced MR dacryocystography with a three-dimensional fast spoiled gradient-recalled technique. Eur Radiol 2002;12(9):2343–8.

[16] Goldberg RA, Heinz GW, Chiu L. Gadolinium magnetic resonance imaging dacryocystography. Am J Ophthalmol 1993;115(6):738–41.

[17] Rossomondo R, Carlton W, Trueblood J. A new method of evaluating lacrimal drainage. Arch Ophthalmol 1972;88:523.

[18] Wearne MJ, Pitts J, Frank J, et al. Comparison of dacryocystography and lacrimal scintigraphy in the diagnosis of functional nasolacrimal duct obstruction. Br J Ophthalmol 1999;83(9):1032–5.

[19] Rose JD, Clayton CB. Scintigraphy and contrast radiography for epiphora. Br J Radiol 1985;58(696):1183–6.

[20] Heyman S, Katowitz JA, Smoger B. Dacryoscintigraphy in children. Ophthalmic Surg 1985;16(11):703–9.

[21] Foster JA, Katowitz JA, Heyman S. Results of dacryoscintigraphy in passage of congenitally blocked nasolacrimal duct. Ophthalmol Plast Reconstr Surg 1996;12:27–32.

[22] Kivikoski AI, Amin N, Cornell C. Antenatal sonographic diagnosis of dacryocystocele. J Matern Fetal Med 1997;6(5):273–5.

[23] Busse H, Miller KM, Kroll P. Radiologic and histological findings of the lacrimal passages of newborns. Arch Ophthalmol 1980;98:528.

[24] Veirs ER. Disorders of the nasolacrimal apparatus in infants and children. J Pediatr Ophthalmol 1966;3.

[25] Ahn Yuen SJ, Oley C, Sullivan T. Lacrimal outflow dysgenesis. Ophthalmology 2004;111(9):1782–90.

[26] Kushner BJ. Congenital nasolacrimal system obstruction. Arch Ophthalmol 1982;100:597.

[27] Raul TO, Shepherd R. Congenital nasolacrimal duct obstruction: natural history and the timing of optimal intervention. J Pediatr Ophthalmol Strabismus 1994;31:362–7.

[28] Winstein GS, Biglan AW. Congenital lacrimal sac mucoceles. Am J Ophthalmol 1982;94(1):106–10.

[29] Rand PK, Ball Jr WS, Kulwin DR. Congenital nasolacrimal mucoceles: CT evaluation. Radiology 1989;173:691–4.

[30] Freitag SK, Woog JJ, Kousoubris PD, et al. Helical computed tomographic dacryocystography with three-dimensional reconstruction: a new view of the lacrimal drainage system. Ophthal Plast Reconstr Surg 2002;18(2):121–32.

[31] Farrer RS, Mohammed TL, Hahn FJ. MRI of childhood dacryocystocele. Neuroradiology 2003;45(4):259–61.

[32] Polito E, Leccisotti A, Menicacci F, et al. Imaging techniques in the diagnosis of lacrimal sac diverticulum. Ophthalmologica 1995;209(4):228–32.

[33] Bartley GB. Acquired lacrimal drainage obstruction: an etiologic classification system, case reports and a review of the literature, I. Ophthal Plast Reconstr Surg 1992;4:237–42.

[34] Groessl SA, Sires BS, Lemke BN. An anatomical basis for primary acquired nasolacrimal duct obstruction. Arch Ophthalmol 1997;115(1):71–4.

[35] McNab AA. Lacrimal canalicular obstruction associated with topical ocular medication. Aust NZ J Ophthalmol 1998;26(3):219–23.

[36] Shepler TR, Sherman SI, Faustina MM, et al. Nasolacrimal duct obstruction associated with radioactive iodine therapy for thyroid carcinoma. Ophthal Plast Reconstr Surg 2003;19(6):479–81.

[37] Esmaeli B, Hidaji L, Adinin RB, et al. Blockage of the lacrimal drainage apparatus as a side effect of docetaxel therapy. Cancer 2003;98(3):504–7.

[38] Becelli R, Renzi G, Mannino G, et al. Posttraumatic obstruction of lacrimal pathways: a retrospective analysis of 58 consecutive naso-orbitoethmoid fractures. J Craniofac Surg 2004;15(1):29–33.

[39] White WL, Bartley GB, Hawes MJ, et al. Iatrogenic complications related to the use of Herrick Lacrimal Plugs. Ophthalmology 2001;108(10):1835–7.

[40] Alexandrakis G, Tse DT, Rosa Jr RH, et al. Nasolacrimal duct obstruction and orbital cellulitis associated with chronic intranasal cocaine abuse. Arch Ophthalmol 1999;117(12):1617–22.

[41] DeAngelis D, Hurwitz J, Mazzulli T. The role of bacteriologic infection in the etiology of nasolacrimal duct obstruction. Can J Ophthalmol 2001;36(3):134–9.

[42] Brook I, Frazier EH. Aerobic and anaerobic micro-

biology of dacryocystitis. Am J Ophthalmol 1998; 125(4):552–4.
[43] Lin PW, Lin HC. Facial necrotizing fasciitis following acute dacryocystitis. Am J Ophthalmol 2003;136(1): 203–4.
[44] Kikkawa DO, Heinz GW, Martin RT, et al. Orbital cellulitis and abscess secondary to dacryocystitis. Arch Ophthalmol 2002;120(8):1096–9.
[45] Agarwal ML. Dacryocystography in chronic dacryocystitis. Am J Ophthalmol 1961;52:245–9.
[46] Russell EJ, Czervionke L, Huckman M, et al. CT of the inferomedial orbit and the lacrimal drainage apparatus: normal and pathologic anatomy. AJR Am J Roentgenol 1985;145(6):1147–54.
[47] Mafee MF, Valvassori GE, Becker M. Imaging of the head and neck. Stuttgart: Thieme; 2004.
[48] McKellar MJ, Aburn NS. Cast-forming Actinomyces israelii canaliculitis. Aust NZ J Ophthalmol 1997;25(4): 301–3.
[49] Tost F, Bruder R, Clemens S. Clinical diagnosis of chronic canaliculitis by 20-MHz ultrasound. Ophthalmologica 2000;214(6):433–6.
[50] Garcia GH, Harris GJ. Sarcoid inflammation and obstruction of the nasolacrimal system. Arch Ophthalmol 2000;118(5):719–20.
[51] Vasquez RJ, Linberg JV, McCormick SA. Histopathology of nasolacrimal duct obstruction compatible with localized sarcoidosis. Ophthal Plast Reconstr Surg 1988;4(3):147–51.
[52] Chapman KL, Bartley GB, Garrity JA, et al. Lacrimal bypass surgery in patients with sarcoidosis. Am J Ophthalmol 1999;127(4):443–6.
[53] Nichols CW, Mishkin M, Yanoff M. Presumed orbital sarcoidosis: report of a case followed by computerized axial tomography and conjunctival biopsy. Trans Am Ophthalmol Soc 1978;76:67–75.
[54] Freitag SK, Woog JJ, Kousoubris PD, et al. Helical computed tomographic dacryocystography with three-dimensional reconstruction: a new view of the lacrimal drainage system. Ophthal Plast Reconstr Surg 2002; 18(2):121–32.
[55] Wolk RB. Sarcoidosis of the orbit with bone destruction. AJNR Am J Neuroradiol 1984;5(2):204–5.
[56] Sacher M, Lanzieri CF, Sobel LI, et al. Computed tomography of bilateral lacrimal gland sarcoidosis. J Comput Assist Tomogr 1984;8(2):213–5.
[57] Azar-Kia B, Naheedy MH, Elias DA, et al. Optic nerve tumors: role of magnetic resonance imaging and computed tomography. Radiol Clin N Am 1987;25(3): 561–81.
[58] Nichols CW, Mishkin M, Yanoff M. Presumed orbital sarcoidosis: report of a case followed by computerized axial tomography and conjunctival biopsy. Trans Am Ophthalmol Soc 1978;76:67–75.
[59] Kuchar A, Novak P, Steinkogler FJ. Manifestation of Wegener's granulomatosis as lacrimal sac tumor. Klin Monatsbl Augenheilkd 1998;212(1):59–60.
[60] O'Sullivan RM, Nugent RA, Satorre J, et al. Granulomatous orbital lesions: computed tomographic features. Can Assoc Radiol J 1992;43(5):349–58.
[61] Yang C, Talbot JM, Hwang PH. Bony abnormalities of the paranasal sinuses in patients with Wegener's granulomatosis. Am J Rhinol 2001;15(2):121–5.
[62] Glatt HJ, Putterman AM. Dacryocystorhinostomy in Wegener's granulomatosis. Ophthal Plast Reconstr Surg 1990;6(3):207–10.
[63] Holds JB, Anderson RL, Wolin MJ. Dacryocystectomy for the treatment of dacryocystitis patients with Wegener's granulomatosis. Ophthalmic Surg 1989;20(6): 443–4.
[64] Flanagan JC, Stokes DP. Lacrimal sac tumors. Ophthalmology 1978;85(12):1282–7.
[65] Shields JA, Shields CL, Scartozzi R. Survey of 1264 patients with orbital tumors and simulating lesions: the 2002 Montgomery Lecture, part 1. Ophthalmology 2004;111(5):997–1008.
[66] Scat Y, Liotet S, Carre F. Epidemiological study of 1705 malignant tumors of the eye and adnexa. J Fr Ophtalmol 1996;19(2):83–8.
[67] Stefanyszyn MA, Hidayat AA, Pe'er JJ, et al. Lacrimal sac tumors. Ophthal Plast Reconstr Surg 1994; 10(3):169–84.
[68] Ni C, D'Amico D, Fan CQ, et al. Tumors of the lacrimal sac: a clinicopathological analysis of 82 cases. Int Ophthalmol Clin 1982;22(1):121–40.
[69] Pe'er J, Hidayat AA, Ilsar M, et al. Glandular tumors of the lacrimal sac. Their histopathologic patterns and possible origins. Ophthalmology 1996;103(10):1601–5.
[70] Ryan SJ, Font RL. Primary epithelial neoplasms of the lacrimal sac. Am J Ophthalmol 1973;76(1):73–88.
[71] Madreperla SA, Green WR, Daniel R, et al. Human papillomavirus in primary epithelial tumors of the lacrimal sac. Ophthalmology 1993;100(4):569–73.
[72] Hsu HC, Lin SA. Orbital epithelial cyst derived from the lacrimal sac. Ophthalmologica 2001;215(4):318–20.
[73] Katircioglu YA, Altiparmak UE, Akmansu H, et al. Squamous cell carcinoma of the lacrimal sac. Orbit 2003;22(3):151–3.
[74] Rahangdale SR, Castillo M, Shockley W. MR in squamous cell carcinoma of the lacrimal sac. AJNR Am J Neuroradiol 1995;16(6):1262–4.
[75] Pe'er JJ, Stefanyszyn M, Hidayat AA. Nonepithelial tumors of the lacrimal sac. Am J Ophthalmol 1994; 118(5):650–8.
[76] Billing K, Malhotra R, Selva D, et al. Magnetic resonance imaging findings in malignant melanoma of the lacrimal sac. Br J Ophthalmol 2003;87(9):1187–8.
[77] McNab AA, McKelvie P. Malignant melanoma of the lacrimal sac complicating primary acquired melanosis of the conjunctiva. Ophthalmic Surg Lasers 1997; 28(6):501–4.
[78] Som PM, Dillon WP, Fullerton GD. Chronically obstructed sinonasal secretions: observation on T1 and T2 shortening. Radiology 1989;172:515–20.
[79] Parmar DN, Rose GE. Management of lacrimal sac tumours. Eye 2003;17(5):599–606.

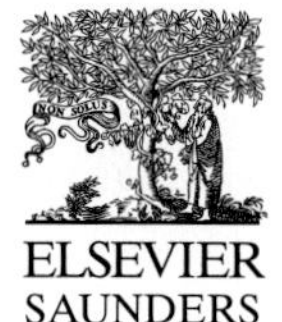

ELSEVIER
SAUNDERS

Neuroimag Clin N Am 15 (2005) 239–244

NEUROIMAGING
CLINICS OF
NORTH AMERICA

# Index

*Note:* Page numbers of article titles are in **boldface** type.



1052-5149/05/$ – see front matter 
doi:10.1016/S1052-5149(05)00024-9

*neuroimaging.theclinics.com*

## D



## E



## F



## G



## H

## I



## L



## M

## N



## O



## P

## T



## U



## V



## W



## X

## *Changing Your Address?*

Make sure your subscription changes too! When you notify us of your new address, you can help make our job easier by including an exact copy of your Clinics label number with your old address (see illustration below.) This number identifies you to our computer system and will speed the processing of your address change. Please be sure this label number accompanies your old address and your corrected address—you can send an old Clinics label with your number on it or just copy it exactly and send it to the address listed below.

We appreciate your help in our attempt to give you continuous coverage. Thank you.

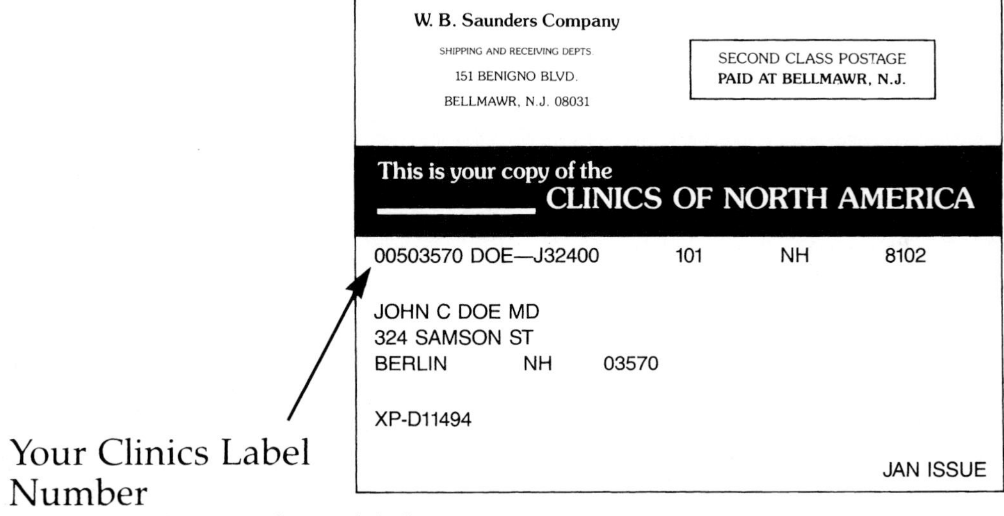


Your Clinics Label Number

Copy it exactly or send your label along with your address to:
**W.B. Saunders Company, Customer Service**
Orlando, FL 32887-4800
Call Toll Free 1-800-654-2452

Please allow four to six weeks for delivery of new subscriptions and for processing address changes.

**BUSINESS REPLY MAIL**

FIRST-CLASS MAIL PERMIT NO 7135 ORLANDO FL

POSTAGE WILL BE PAID BY ADDRESSEE

PERIODICALS ORDER FULFILLMENT DEPT
ELSEVIER
6277 SEA HARBOR DR
ORLANDO FL 32821-9816